INFECTION and PATIENT CARE

A Guide for Nurses

Dinah Gould
MPhil, BSc, SRN, DipN
Senior Lecturer in Nursing Studies,
Polytechnic of South Bank, London

HEINEMANN NURSING
LONDON

William Heinemann Medical Books
22 Bedford Square
London WC1B 3HH

ISBN 0–433–12450–4

© Dinah Gould, 1987

First published 1987

Typeset by Wilmaset, Birkenhead, Wirral
and printed in Great Britain by Anchor Brendon, Tiptree, Essex

Contents

	Introduction	iii
1	Microbiology and patient care	1
2	Infection: past and present trends	33
3	Nursing, research and infection	48
4	Providing a safe environment: the patient-centred approach	63
5	Providing a safe environment: policies and procedures	78
6	Isolation nursing	93
7	Response of the body to infection	104
8	Care of the patient with an indwelling urinary catheter	125
9	Wounds and infection	137
10	Using the infection control service effectively	161
11	Infection: education and counselling	185
	Appendix	199
	Index	203

Introduction

A great deal has been written about infection control in hospital over the years, but less attention has been given to the feelings of people who have developed infections in hospital or the community, or the effect of infection upon their lifestyle. The practice of immunisation and the mass production of antibiotics have caused premature death from tuberculosis and pneumonia to become things of the past. Cholera and typhoid are no longer scourges in the western world and the World Health Organisation has eradicated smallpox. Apparently, it is no longer necessary for nurses to learn about fevers, or to fear catching an infectious condition from their patients ... or is it?

In 1984 alone over 40 people died of acquired immune deficiency syndrome (AIDS), and the number of fatalities claimed by this 'new' disease has increased steadily ever since. Hospitals responded to the arrival of the disease in Britain by developing emergency guidelines, and the Royal College of Nursing set up a Working Party to explore all aspects of care required by these patients. Appropriate counselling, and the care of bereaved relatives, were tasks for which the average nurse was just not adequately prepared. The year 1985 was marked by numerous outbreaks of infectious illness, including a major epidemic of salmonella food poisoning and legionnaire's disease – both occurring in hospital. In the summer of 1986 there was a considerable increase in the number of cases of meningococcal meningitis (particularly in Gloucestershire). The number of cases notified had doubled over a period of three years.

It would appear, then, that nurses still need to develop skills necessary for the care of the infected patient, while at the same time it is the nurse's right to learn how to protect herself from infectious agents. The aim of this book is to discuss the many different problems associated with infection, from the perspective of both patient and nurse.

Entire books have been devoted to the topic of infection control in hospital. Others deal exclusively with communicable disease. This book is not meant to be exhaustive in its approach. Its purpose is to show how nurses may apply the principles of microbiology to the care of people who have already developed an infection, or who are at risk of developing infection by virtue of their condition or treatment.

Chapter 1 describes the characteristics common to all living organisms, with particular reference to microorganisms, pointing out how they can cause disease and why they do so with particular success in the hospital environment. Discussion of the growth requirements of microorganisms and the ways in which they are spread form the basis of underlying methods of control.

Chapter 2 deals with past epidemiological trends of infectious diseases in contrast to the situation today. The part played by immunisation, antibiotics and the generally improved health of the nation in the control of infectious illness is described.

Nurses today are urged to read research reports and to apply relevant findings to patient care. Chapter 3 outlines the main research methods used in nursing, with particular reference to infection control and care of the infected patient. The practical difficulties of conducting clinical nursing research are commented upon, together with the importance of infection control as part of quality assurance.

Chapter 4 assesses the risk of developing infection, both in hospital and in the community, using case studies to illustrate how this could evolve.

Chapter 5 describes the main ways of preventing infection in both hospital and home environments, building on the microbiological principles introduced in Chapter 1.

Isolation precautions receive detailed attention in Chapter 6, where case studies are used to illustrate the needs of individual patients.

The purpose of Chapter 7 is to describe the response of the individual to infection. Exposure to an infectious agent is a form of stress at both physiological and behavioural levels. Hence the psychological reactions of the patient need consideration, as well as the inflammatory and immunological changes that take place in the tissues.

Chapters 8 and 9 focus on nursing two groups of patients who are at particular risk of developing infection: those with an indwelling urinary catheter and those with a wound.

Chapter 10 draws attention to the effective use of the infection control service, both in hospital and in the community. All hospitals are required by statute to appoint an infection control officer; many also employ at least one infection control nurse, and have strict policies to help control and contain infection. The success of any policy depends as much upon the people who use it as upon the technical expertise of those responsible for devising it; all members of the health care team must be able to apply infection control policies critically, not follow them blindly.

Chapter 11 is concerned with counselling and teaching patients, relatives and other members of staff about infection.

Acknowledgements

I would like to thank Gower Medical Publishing Ltd for permission to reproduce adaptations of Figs 6, 7 and 11 from *Introducing Immunology* by N. Staines, J. Brostoff and K. James.

Chapter 1

Microbiology and Patient Care

INTRODUCTION

Infectious agents are responsible for approximately half of all known human diseases. As research continues, it is becoming apparent that they may also contribute to the development of neoplasms and to mysterious diseases of previously unknown aetiology. Bacteria, fungi and a few species of protozoa may complicate the course of illness and recovery among patients admitted to hospital for non-infectious conditions.

Infections that develop during hospital stay are called *nosocomial infections*, and these develop in about one patient in every ten who receives inpatient care. The cost of these infections per annum is difficult to calculate in the United Kingdom due to the absence of reliable data on a national scale. However, the infected patient usually stays in hospital for a longer period than patients with comparable illnesses who have escaped infection. The cost of the extra days is often used to measure the cost of infection according to the formula:

$$\frac{\text{Total patients}}{100} \times \frac{\text{\% nosocomial}}{\text{infection rate}} \times \frac{\text{extra}}{\text{days}} \times \frac{\text{cost of bed}}{\text{per day}}$$

In practice this equation represents a reduction in the number of beds available for elective patients on the waiting list for hospital admission rather than increased cost accrued by the hospital. Estimates of mean additional hospital stay due to nosocomial infection vary between 3 and 19 days, and the costs of stay also differ according to the particular hospital or unit. In addition to this, the infected patient drains the service by requiring antibiotic therapy, additional dressing materials, analgesia, more changes of bedclothes and more nursing time, especially if isolation precautions are required. A team of infection control experts (Ayliffe *et al.*, 1977) calculated from data they obtained from hospitals in the Midlands that approximately 4 million patients received acute hospital care between 1977 and 1978, and that a 5% infection rate causing an additional 3 day period of admission would cost £30 million for England alone. A 10% prevalence of infection would cost £60 000 000. These calculations took into consideration only the extra 'hotel' facilities required. Even though these findings are now out of date, the implications for cost-effectiveness within the health service cannot be disputed; cost to the patient, in terms of discomfort and prolonged hospital stay, cannot be quantified.

Despite technological advances which have made possible the mass production of antibiotics and vaccines, infection continues to be a major threat to people in western society, as well as to those in the third world – though manifesting itself in different ways. Knowledge of those factors likely to predispose the patient to infection is vital for nurses both in hospital and in the community. Acute infections such as meningitis usually have a rapid onset and afflict the young, especially children; they can be life-threatening, requiring intensive nursing care and support to the family. People who develop chronic or recurrent infections, or who have become asymptomatic carriers of infectious agents may need help to come to terms with their situation and to adapt to any necessary changes in their lifestyle.

Preventing the spread of infection both in hospital and in the community is a fundamental part of all nursing care and one of the most challenging, demanding as it does an understanding of the agents responsible for infection and a certain amount of self-discipline when theoretical knowledge is applied to the practical situation.

Within the last few years numerous nurse researchers have drawn attention to the nurse's apparent inability to apply theoretical knowledge, gained largely in the classroom, to the bedside. This observation was originally made in 1973 by Bendall, but has been supported by other authors who have examined the application of communication (Gott, 1984), general biological science (Wilson, 1975), and microbiology (Akinsanya, 1985) to everyday nursing care. Gould (1985) demonstrated that isolation techniques were poorly executed on the wards of a health district where infectious conditions were rife, although nurses at all levels of seniority had a very good knowledge of how these infections are spread.

The present system of nursing education in England and Wales is generally held responsible for these shortcomings. However, in the past many of the microbiology texts designed specifically for nurses have tended to concentrate upon the morphological characteristics of bacteria, rather than upon teaching infection control from first principles according to the physiological behaviour of microorganisms. Epidemiological trends and the impact of infection upon sick and healthy people living in the community have been ignored. In consequence, the information was often presented in the form of a catalogue. However, the shapes and sizes of bacteria constitute rather dry reading unless structure is related to physiology, as in the functioning of the bacterial cell. The physiology of microorganisms is of significance because it explains their ability to cause disease and their particular success in the hospital environment.

The characteristics common to all living organisms are described briefly below, to help illuminate the particular growth requirements of microorganisms, especially bacteria, which are discussed in detail.

THE CHARACTERISTICS OF LIVING ORGANISMS

These include metabolism, homeostasis, irritability, movement, absorption, excretion, respiration, growth and reproduction.

Metabolism

Thousands of chemical reactions take place simultaneously within all living cells. Collectively these are known as metabolism. New molecules are built up from raw building materials, a process called *anabolism*, in which energy derived from the respiration of food materials is required. Proteins are built from amino acids to make up both enzymes and the structural parts of the cell. Carbohydrates and fats in the main form the food reserves of living cells, carbohydrates being built from sugars, and fats from smaller molecules called fatty acids. *Catabolic reactions* are those that break down large, complicated molecules, releasing energy.

Homeostasis

Homeostasis is the ability of a living organism to maintain internal stability despite environmental fluctuations such as changes in temperature, humidity, oxygen levels and the availability of nutrients. This is made possible by the ability of the organism to detect, respond and compensate for external changes through the conservation of heat, moisture or the conversion of nutrients present in excess of immediate requirements to storage materials. These may be used when environmental availability becomes depleted.

The term homeostasis, originally coined by the physiologist Cannon in the 19th century, has generally been taken to imply characteristics of higher organisms. Man is regarded as the ultimate example of supreme environmental adaptation. However, microorganisms, especially bacteria, have evolved so that they are highly responsive to environmental change. *Escherichia coli*, a species inhabiting the human gut and commonly causing urinary tract infection, has, for example, the ability to metabolise a sugar called lactose, which is found in milk. When the bacteria are exposed to a substrate containing lactose they rapidly begin to synthesise the enzyme necessary to break it down. If lactose is removed from the medium, enzyme secretion promptly ceases. *E. coli* does not waste energy and raw materials to manufacture an enzyme that is no longer of immediate use.

Escherichia coli is widely used by research workers conducting experiments in biochemistry and molecular biology. Much more is known about the genetics and biochemical behaviour of this species of bacteria than of any human cell.

Irritability

Living organisms are characterised by their ability to respond to stimuli which occur through changes in the environment. Bacteria, like man, will actively move away from noxious stimuli, and be attracted to favourable environmental situations where moisture and nourishment are available. Response of living organisms in this way is an active process, unlike the passive movement of inanimate objects.

Movement

All living organisms have the ability to move, although this capacity is more developed in some than others. Vertebrates like man have evolved a musculoskeletal system to support the soft tissues and permit movement. Large muscles attached to the legs and arms permit sustained exercise; smaller, delicate muscles controlling the fingers, eyes and tongue allow fine, precisional movement. Similarly, many species of bacteria and most protozoa are highly mobile and have developed specialised structures such as cilia and flagella (see pp. 5 and 7) which help them move.

Absorption

All living cells have developed the ability to take up particles or molecules from the external environment, across the cell membrane, a property referred to as absorption. Cell membranes are semipermeable, so water is able to pass by *osmosis* from low concentrations of solutes outside the cell to the more highly concentrated solutions inside. Other molecules and ions may travel across the cell

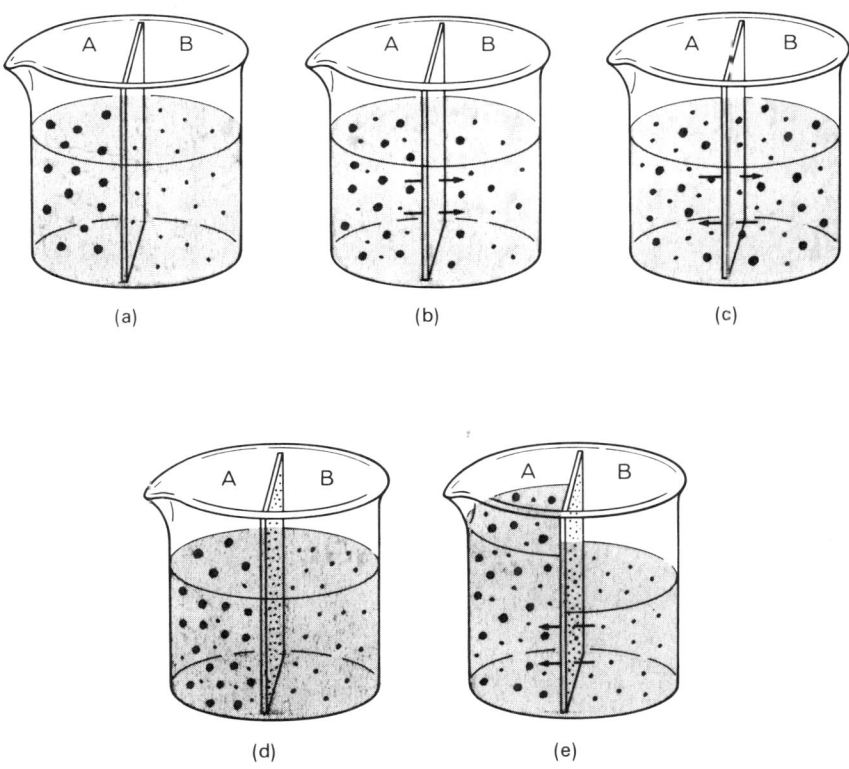

Fig. 1.1 *Diffusion* is the movement of the molecules of a liquid or gas randomly in all directions, until they achieve a uniform concentration throughout the space available to them. A semipermeable membrane in beaker (a) separates a salt solution (large molecules A) and water (small molecules B). In (b) the molecules can be seen moving through the pores of the membrane, until in (c) uniform distribution of both types of molecule has been achieved. *Osmosis* is the passage of solvent molecules (usually water) across a semipermeable membrane from low to high concentrations. In (d) small water molecules are separated by a semipermeable membrane from a strong salt solution. In (e) the water molecules are moving to the higher concentration.

membrane by *diffusion* from high environmental concentrations to lower concentrations within. Osmosis and diffusion are both passive physical processes which do not involve the expenditure of cellular energy (Fig. 1.1). Oxygen diffuses passively into living cells. Other substances may be absorbed against a concentration gradient, involving the expenditure of energy by the cell. In the human gut the molecules of various food materials, including glucose, are actively absorbed. The uptake of lactose by *E. coli* is also an active process.

Excretion

As well as absorbing materials, all living organisms must expel the waste products that result from metabolism, as they would otherwise accumulate rapidly, reaching toxic levels. In man the chief organs of elimination are the lungs, the kidneys and to a lesser extent, the skin. In the case of microorganisms, molecules escape from the entire surface of the cell.

Respiration

Respiration is a biological process which involves the oxidation of food substances. Water, carbon dioxide and the energy vital for metabolism are released. In the case of human beings, higher animals and plants, oxygen is always required for respiration, but some bacteria, including a few species of medical importance, can use materials other than oxygen to supply the cells with energy. *Clostridium welchii*, the bacillus responsible for gas gangrene, does not require oxygen for respiration, which is why it grows deep in the tissues. A further example is *Bacillus anthracis*, which causes anthrax, a serious disease of sheep and cattle that may occasionally be transmitted to humans.

Growth and Reproduction

All living organisms grow. Individual cells increase in size and divide. When bacterial cells reach a certain critical size they divide and the daughter cells separate, giving two independent but identical bacteria.

Genetic variation occurs among animals and plants. Exchange of genetic information is possible through sexual reproduction, which allows adaptation to the environment. Exchange of genetic information can sometimes occur in bacteria, and possibly among some fungi under laboratory conditions. This phenomenon is discussed below.

MICROORGANISMS RESPONSIBLE FOR INFECTION

Infection is caused by four main groups of microscopic organisms: bacteria, viruses, fungi, and protozoa.

Each of these groups is discussed in turn. Bacteria deserve primary mention because they are responsible for the majority of hospital-acquired infections; viruses are the cause of most common infectious conditions encountered in the community (colds, influenza, and childhood ailments such as measles and chickenpox).

Mycoplasmas are similar to bacteria but without thick cell walls. They also sometimes cause human diseases. Rickettsiae and chlamydiae are parasitic microorganisms, similar in some respects to viruses and in others to bacteria. Finally, parasitic worms may also be responsible for human infestation; they are multicellular, and many are clearly visible to the naked eye.

Classification of Bacteria

Bacteria are classified according to their shape (morphology) and general appearance. The main types are illustrated in Fig. 1.2.

Cocci

Round bacteria are called cocci (singular: coccus); in pairs they are known as *diplococci*. Examples of diplococci include *Streptococcus pneumoniae*, which can cause pneumonia, and *Neisseria gonorrhoeae*, which is responsible for gonorrhoea. Clusters of cocci are termed *staphylococci*, because of their supposed resemblance to bunches of grapes (from the Greek *staphylos*).

Staphylococcus aureus is widespread in hospitals where it causes many nosocomial wound infections. Streptococci consist of round bacteria attached to one another so that they form long chains. They cause boils, sore throats and a wide range of other

Microbiology and patient care

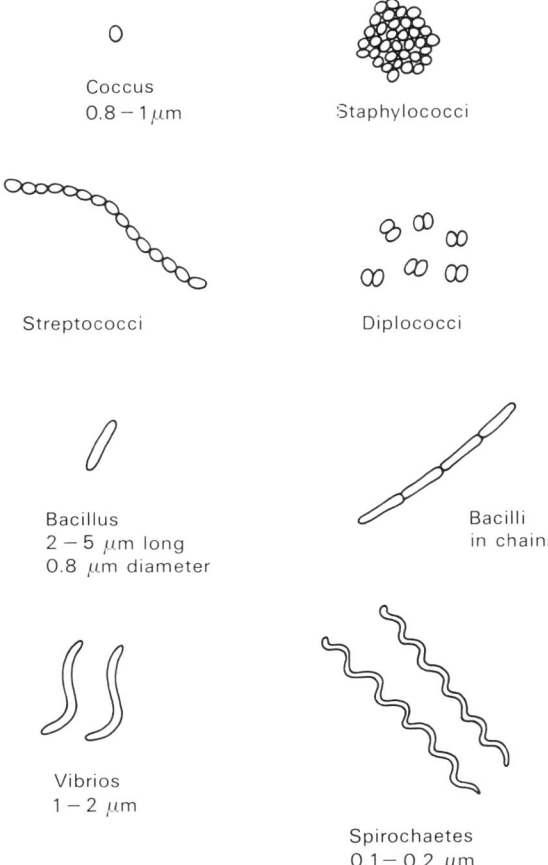

Fig. 1.2 Bacterial morphology.

infections commonly encountered both in hospital and in the community. An outbreak of streptococcal infection on a childrens' ward and the action taken by both nurse and microbiologist is discussed in Chapter 10.

Bacilli

Bacilli are rod-shaped bacteria, which can occur singly or in chains. They are notorious for their ability to cause infections in hospital, especially urinary tract infection. *Pseudomonas*, *Klebsiella*, *Proteus*, *E. coli* and *Salmonella*, the food-poisoning bacteria, are all bacilli. Many, such as *Proteus*, are highly motile.

Vibrios

Probably less familiar morphological types are the curved vibrios, like *Campylobacter*, which in recent years has been held responsible for outbreaks of food poisoning, especially those involving shellfish.

Spirochaetes

Spirochaetes are very small, flexible, spirally shaped bacteria. Examples of these are *Treponema pallidum*, which causes syphilis, and *Leptospira* which causes a disease in dogs, that when transmitted to man is called Weil's disease. *Leptospira* infects rats and is excreted in their urine; in man, infection can result in renal failure.

All bacteria are microscopic and therefore invisible to the naked eye. Approximate sizes are shown in Fig. 1.2.

Bacterial Physiology

In multicellular organisms like man cells are grouped together so that they make up different tissues, of which several types make up the various organ systems. These operate in conjunction with one another to promote the functioning of the individual as a whole, a system of organisation described as *division of labour*. Some cells are specialised to fulfil particular functions, but lose (or at least have a reduced) capacity to perform others. Nerve cells, for example, have become specialised to communicate information in the form of nervous impulses; but they lack motility and have lost the power of reproduction. The cells lining the respiratory tree have developed special structures (cilia) to sweep foreign particles out of the respiratory passages; they have retained the ability to make secretions to a much greater extent than have neurons, releasing mucus to trap the inhaled particles.

In contrast to the cells of higher organisms, all bacteria are unicellular; all the functions necessary to reproduce and to maintain life are performed by a single cell operating on its own. Even when bacterial cells grow together in clusters or chains they do not share a division of labour; every single one is capable of independent life and reproduction. This information is important for nurses as part of their responsibility in infection control (see Chapter 5).

Bacteria are visible under the high magnifying lens of the ordinary light microscope, providing they are appropriately 'fixed' (killed) and stained, but the electronmicroscope has made it possible to examine the fine detail or ultrastructure of all cells at much greater magnifications. Figure 1.3 shows a typical bacterial cell in electronmicroscopic detail. However, one of the major drawbacks of this instrument is that all living material to be examined must first be killed and stained. So the image which appears cannot, therefore, represent cells in their dynamic, *living* state.

The cells of multicellular organisms are distinguished by a nucleus containing the genetic material responsible for the unique characteristics of the species and of the individual organism. Cells of this type are referred to as *eukaryotic*. The nucleus is surrounded by a phospholipid membrane and the cytoplasm outside it contains a variety of complex organelles, which are also surrounded by phospholipid membranes.

Bacteria represent an earlier, more primitive form of life in evolutionary terms, and their cells are described as *prokaryotic*. The major distinguishing feature is lack of a clearly differentiated nucleus surrounded by a membrane. Instead, the DNA carrying the genetic information lies directly in the cytoplasm.

The bacterial cell is surrounded outside by a

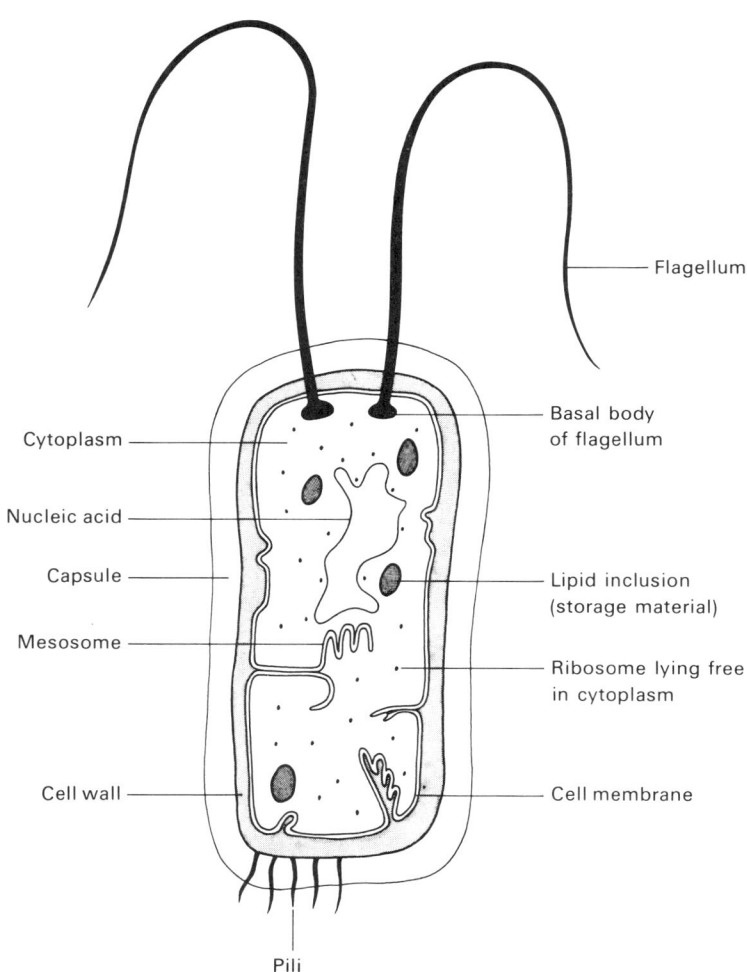

Fig. 1.3 Structure of a typical bacterial cell.

membrane made up of proteins and phospholipids. Exterior to the cell membrane there is a rigid cell wall which gives the organism its shape and a degree of mechanical protection.

In the laboratory, bacteria are classified according to their reaction when treated with a dye called *Gram's stain* (see Chapter 10). Response is determined by the properties of chemicals present in the cell wall. Bacteria which stain blue or purple with Gram's stain are said to be *Gram-positive*, while those which fail to take up the colour of Gram's stain and retain the red colour of the counterstain are said to be *Gram-negative*. Streptococci and Staphylococci are Gram-positive; *Pseudomonas, Proteus, Klebsiella, Salmonella* and *E. coli* are all Gram-negative bacilli. *Neisseria gonorrhoeae* is a Gram-negative diplococcus.

The classification of the main types of bacteria important as causative agents of human disease is given in the Appendix, which also indicates their Gram-staining properties.

Some bacteria secrete a mucilagenous capsule around the cell wall, which helps to prevent desiccation when the environment becomes dry (Fig. 1.4). As an example, *Streptococcus pneumoniae* is a diplococcus that can form capsules.

Under adverse environmental conditions some species of bacteria – such as *Clostridium* – survive by developing into spores. The vulnerable cytoplasm and cell wall of the cell are protected by a tough outer coat.

Molecules can be absorbed from the surrounding environment much more effectively by a unicellular organism than by a multicellular one, because the total surface area available for absorption is comparatively greater. It is for this reason that bacteria do not require complex transport systems like the circulatory system of higher animals, or mechanical respiratory apparatus such as lungs or gills.

The bacterial cell membrane dips down into the cytoplasm at various points, sometimes becoming invaginated to form a series of organelles called mesosomes. It is upon the increased surface areas afforded by the mesosomes that enzymes responsible for bacterial metabolism are anchored. Bacterial DNA is attached to the mesosomes. Protein synthesis takes place on small organelles called ribosomes, which, in bacteria, lie freely within the

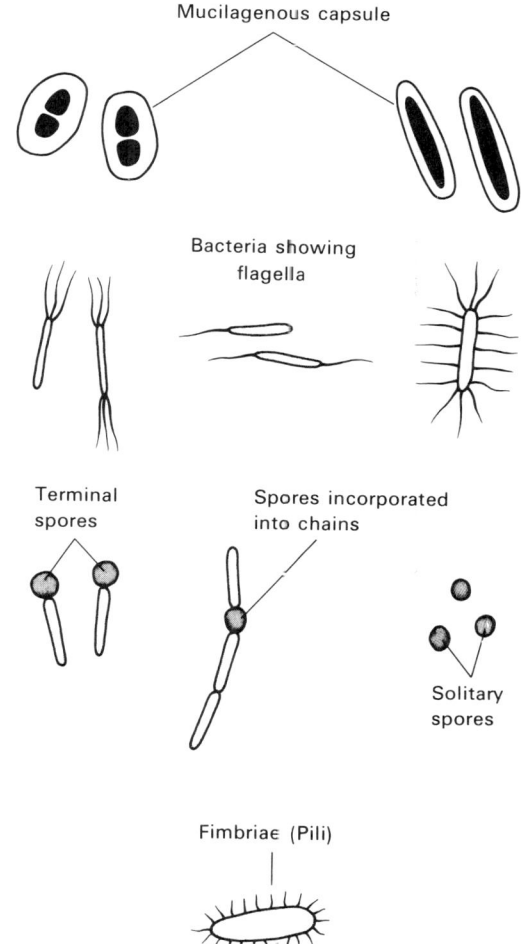

Fig. 1.4 Bacterial morphology.

cytoplasm. Lipids are stored in the cytoplasm as globules and inclusion bodies.

Some bacteria develop specialised organelles responsible for motility. The flagella typical of *Salmonella* and several other types of Gram-negative bacilli may be present singly or in large numbers, and are identical in structure to the flagellae of the spermatozoa of mammals and the cilia which line parts of the human body including the respiratory tree.

Other bacteria possess *fimbriae*. These are shorter, stouter structures (Fig. 1.4) which protrude out through the cell membrane and cell wall. They enhance the *virulence* (ability to cause disease) of the organism by helping it to attach itself to the membrane of the host cell. *Neisseria*, for example, uses fimbriae to attach itself to the mucous membranes of the host. Strains without fimbriae cannot cause disease. Virulence is discussed in greater detail in Chapter 8.

Bacteria vary greatly in their physiological requirements, some being a great deal more demanding than others. The relative simplicity of their needs compared to the demands of more sophisticated forms of life explain the success of bacteria and their ability to thrive in many diverse environments, some of which seem frankly inhospitable. However, like all living organisms they must have a supply of water, nourishment in a form that they can metabolise, and a substrate that can be oxidised during respiration. These requirements are discussed in greater depth below. It is vital for nurses to have an appreciation of bacterial growth requirements, so that infection control measures can be based on scientific principles, not ritual or mystique.

Bacterial Growth Requirements

Water

Biochemical reactions can take place only in solution. Water is an excellent solvent and is the chief constituent of all living cells. Molecules dissolved in water can move about freely and have the opportunity to collide with one another – collision is necessary before chemical reaction can occur.

A second advantage of water is that a considerable amount of heat is required to raise its temperature compared to other liquids. Living cells, with their high water content, can more easily regulate their temperature and maintain homeostasis.

In multicellular organisms, water continually bathes the surfaces of the tissues as extracellular fluid. Moisture must be present in the external environment if bacteria are to thrive and multiply. Gaseous exchange takes place only in solution.

Nourishment

Living cells derive their nourishment from three classes of chemical substances, all with large, complex molecules: carbohydrates, fats and proteins. Carbohydrates, the chief constituents of bread, white rice and potatoes, have molecules containing the elements hydrogen, carbon and oxygen, and they are classified according to the size of the molecule. The largest are polysaccharides such as starch and plant fibres made up of many individual sugar units strung together in chains.

Green plants synthesise sugars and starch from water and carbon dioxide, using the energy provided by sunlight. Some bacteria can derive their energy from sunlight in the same way. These are called *phototrophs*. However, the majority, including all those of medical significance, derive their energy from the oxidation of chemical compounds. These are called *chemotrophs*. The behaviour of a particular chemotroph will depend upon the source of food materials available and the ability of the bacteria to synthesise the enzymes necessary to digest these chemicals.

The growth requirements of medically important bacteria vary enormously. Gram-negative bacilli are robust bacteria well adapted to survival in the environment, and will flourish in solutions containing only glucose and a few inorganic ions. They will thrive everywhere in hospital, from fluid left to drain in the bottom of a washbowl, to intravenous fluids that have become contaminated. In contrast, the syphilis spirochaete is so exacting in its growth requirements that it has never been grown outside a living organism. In the laboratory, *Treponema pallidum* is grown inside the bodies of living animals, usually rabbits.

Attention has already been drawn to the ability of species like *E. coli* to switch on and off the enzyme systems required to digest a particular nutrient that happens to be available. *Treponema pallidum* is so delicate and so fastidious in its growth requirements that it will die rapidly once it has been removed from the protection of the living tissues of its host. Its mode of transmission is directly from one individual to another, either venereally or across the placenta from mother to fetus.

The growth requirements of different types of bacteria are extremely important in the laboratory, when a suitable growth medium must be selected. This is discussed further in Chapter 10, when the work of the diagnostic microbiology laboratory is described. Ability to ferment different food substrates is one of the tests used by laboratory staff to distinguish between different types of bacteria.

Respiration

Some bacteria, like higher animals and plants, demand oxygen in order to burn food materials to make energy. In the absence of oxygen they will not thrive or grow. These are called *obligate aerobes*. *Anaerobic* bacteria tend to be species which grow deep in the body, without oxygen; bacteria belonging to the genus *Clostridium*, responsible for gas gangrene, are anaerobic. Many bacteria, however, are *facultative anaerobes* – they use oxygen for respiration when it is available, but some other substance when it is not. *Staphylococci* and *Streptococci* are versatile bacteria able to grow in either the presence or absence of oxygen. Both are able to grow on the surface of the human skin, but both could cause a wound infection if inoculated deeply into the tissues during surgery or trauma.

In the laboratory, specimens obtained from patients are cultivated under both aerobic and anaerobic conditions (see Chapter 10).

pH

pH is the acidity or alkalinity of a chemical substance. The degree of acidity is a measure of the number of hydrogen ions available in a solution. The pH scale is a negative logarithmic scale, pH being the negative logarithm of the number of hydrogen ions available. This means that a very small change in pH has a dramatic effect on the number of hydrogen ions present. Solutions with a pH of less than 7 are acidic, and the lower the pH, the more powerfully acidic the medium; pH 7 is neutral, and above pH 7 solutions are alkaline. The most powerful alkalis have a pH of 14, the highest point on the scale.

Bacteria vary widely in the degree to which they will either tolerate or thrive at different pH values. Most bacteria of medical significance thrive best at a slightly alkaline pH. This is not an accident on the part of nature; the pH of blood and other bodily fluids are also slightly alkaline, with a pH of 7.45. There are exceptions, however. The vibrio which causes cholera (*Vibrio cholera*) is a waterborne infection, which causes particular problems in areas of the world where sanitation is poor. Vibrios enter the body via the mouth, and are unable to operate in the highly acid environment of the stomach. Activity is optimal at pH 8, and the bacteria begin to divide and set up inflammation in the small intestine, which provides an alkaline environment, since the bile and pancreatic secretions emptying into it contain large quantities of sodium bicarbonate. In the laboratory, the cholera vibrio is distinguished by its ability to grow in a culture medium rendered alkaline by the addition of bile.

Ecology

It is commonly accepted among the lay public that bacteria and other microorganisms do not necessarily cause disease. They are ubiquitous, having successfully exploited every ecological niche on the surface of the earth. Bacteria evolved millions of years before multicellular organisms and they continue to flourish, living freely in soil, water and air, as well as parasitising other living organisms.

Bacteria and fungi which live in the soil break down complex, organic molecules derived from dead animals and plants and recycle them. They are called *saprophytes*. Without their valuable work the earth would rapidly become cluttered with carcases that could not decay. Other microorganisms have become economically important in manufacturing processes: bacteria are now used to synthesise a variety of chemicals, including antibiotics; yeasts are important in breadmaking, and the fermentation of alcohol and cheeses.

In contrast, the parasitic bacteria which cause disease have become more specialised, and generally tend to be more exacting in their growth requirements (the extreme case of *Treponema pallidum* has already been mentioned).

Bacteria which cause disease are called *pathogens*; and those which are easily able to attack potential hosts are said to be *virulent*. Virulence is a complex phenomenon related to the physiology of the host as well as to that of the pathogen. The virulence of the species or strain of bacteria is thus directly relevant to infection control and planning individual patient care. This topic is discussed further in Chapter 4.

However, relatively few species of bacteria are pathogenic compared to the number that are free-living; a great many, especially those found in hospital, fall into the category classified as *opportunistic*. These have unexacting growth requirements and are free-living, but they are sufficiently virulent to successfully invade and cause clinical disease in the tissues of those who are already weak or debilitated. Several species of fungi, protozoa and viruses are now also known to be capable of opportunistic infection.

Opportunistic bacteria have become the scourge of hospitals, which provide ideal conditions for their growth and reproduction as well as large numbers of susceptible individuals as possible victims. Clearly some wards and units are more problematic than others from this point of view. An oncology ward where very sick people undergo radical surgery and intravenous therapy will almost certainly show greater evidence of hospital-acquired infection than a ward where patients are admitted only for observation and routine, minor surgery.

The Gram-negative bacilli are highly successful opportunists: *Pseudomonas*, *E. coli*, *Proteus* and *Klebsiella* all behave in this way. Other genera such as *Serratia* and *Acinetobacter* are less often implicated as the causative agents of opportunistic infection, but there is very good evidence to suggest that they can do so, and if the present trend continues, these Gram-negative bacilli will almost certainly feature more prominently in outbreaks of nosocomial infection.

An outbreak of hospital-acquired infection usually has serious consequences, irrespective of the organism responsible, although its nature and behaviour will influence the investigations undertaken and the steps recommended to halt further spread. The scientific journals contain numerous case reports of outbreaks that have actually occurred. Several case studies have been extracted as illustrative examples throughout this book, and to help clarify points discussed in the main text. Case study 1.1 below is a typical example of recurrent infection in hospital due to a Gram-negative opportunist.

Staphylococcus epidermidis lives harmlessly on the skin of healthy people and is described as forming part of the normal skin flora. In older textbooks it

---

Case study 1.1

Thirty-eight neonates developed infections after they had been admitted to a special care baby unit. There were 48 individual episodes of infection and one baby died. The remainder responded positively to antibiotic therapy. All the infections were due to *Staphylococcus epidermidis* (Davis, 1984).

---

may still sometimes be referred to as *Staphylococcus albus*, because it forms white colonies when grown on the surface of solid culture media in the laboratory. This distinguishes it from its close relation, *Staphylococcus aureus*, which produces yellow colonies. A second important distinguishing feature is the ability of *Staphylococcus aureus* alone to synthesise an enzyme called coagulase, which causes blood plasma to clot. Coagulase stimulates the tissues of the host to surround the focus of infection with fibrin. The clotting reaction initiated protects *Staphylococcus aureus* from being attacked and destroyed by the white blood cells of the host (see Chapter 7). *Staphylococcus epidermidis* is open to destruction by the host defences and, until a few years ago, it was considered to be strictly non-pathogenic. However, the evidence of case studies such as 1.1 above indicate that it can actively infect patients who are debilitated. Since technology is prolonging the survival of the very sick, the elderly and the prematurely born, opportunism is likely to pose an increasing threat to the future of hospital care. As case study 1.1 indicates, those at particular risk include patients who have undergone invasive techniques, such as mechanical ventilation or surgery, because these provide additional portals of entry into the tissues, against which the body has no active defences.

Exogenous and Endogenous Infection

Infections that have been acquired from the environment, or from another person, such as measles, whooping cough and influenza, are described as exogenous. However, many of the opportunistic infections rife in hospital originate from microorganisms that occupy the gut or live on the skin of normal, healthy people, and are transferred to another site on the same person, such as a wound, where they set up infection. These are called endogenous infections. Once a patient has developed an endogenous infection, the organisms can be spread to other patients, setting up a chain of infection. Bacteria that live harmlessly in one part of the body may behave destructively if transferred to a site where they are not normally found. Newsom (1979) reported the death of five patients in an intensive care unit after they had developed postoperative chest infections. Each patient was recovering from major surgery, had been given a tracheostomy and was undergoing mechanical ventilation. They all developed sore, dry mouths and had been given ice to suck. The ice had been contaminated with bacteria which normally live harmlessly on the skin, and these migrated into the respiratory passages of the vulnerable patients, setting up a series of fatal chest infections. The surgeons who worked on the unit added ice from the same machine to their lunch-time drinks, but did not even become ill.

Reproduction and Genetics

When the physiological requirements of bacteria have been met, they grow and divide. Under optimal environmental conditions each bacterial cell can split into two identical daughter cells about every 30 minutes in some species illustrating the rapidity with which bacteria can multiply in the warm, damp hospital environment (Fig. 1.5).

Genes determine the characteristics of living cells, from the structure of their membranes to the enzymes that they produce. In multicellular organisms, genes are organised into complex structures called chromosomes, but the bacterial chromosome is circular and less highly developed.

Bacteria reproduce by simple binary fission (see Fig. 1.5). First the chromosome divides into two, followed by the cytoplasm. A new cell membrane grows down between the two chromosomes, and a new cell wall develops like a partition on either side of it. The two bacteria then separate.

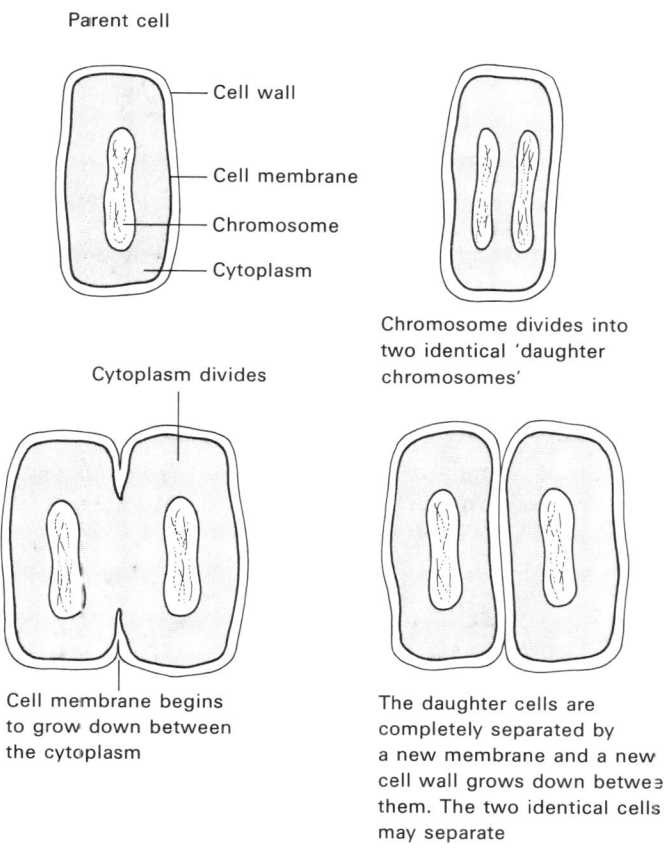

Fig. 1.5 Bacterial reproduction (binary fission).

Binary fission is asexual reproduction. Each new cell is identical to the parent cell from which it was derived and to its sister. Behaviour, as well as appearance, will be the same.

Asexual reproduction contrasts with the sexual reproduction of higher organisms, where there is exchange of genes between the two sexual partners, permitting genetic variation in the offspring. Some of the offspring may be less well adapted to their environment than the parents and may fail to thrive, dying before they in turn can reproduce. Most will be able to survive and grow with more or less the same advantages or disadvantages as their parents. Every so often, however, an individual will be subtly different from other members of its species in a way that will enhance its chances of survival. It thrives, and the beneficial characteristic favours the survival of any progeny inheriting it. The desirable trait tends to be passed on or, in genetic terms, to be 'selected' in favour of less desirable traits. Evolution has occurred.

Sexual reproduction has an obvious advantage in enabling the species to adapt to environmental change, because it provides greater scope for genetic variation than binary fission, where all the genes pass in identical combination to every generation.

Yet bacteria can respond swiftly to environmental fluctuations – that is why they are so successful at exploiting different conditions, including hospitals. It is also apparent that members of the same bacterial species do show some variation. For example, *Staphylococcus aureus* found in hospital is nearly always resistant to penicillin, but this is less often true of *Staph. aureus* isolated from people in the community. (This has not always been the case. When penicillin was first introduced into clinical practice, it was invariably able to kill all *Staphylococcus aureus* bacteria.)

The ability to survive in the presence of *antibiotics* is an obvious advantage to bacteria. There can scarcely be anyone alive in this country today who has not, at some stage in their life, received antibiotic treatment.

Antibiotics are produced commercially on a very large scale, and bacteria are used directly in the manufacturing process. Most bacterial DNA is present as a long, circular chromosome (see p. 6), but in many bacterial cells a very small amount of DNA (approximately 1%) lies freely in the cytoplasm. This extrachromosomal DNA is called a *plasmid* (Fig. 1.6). The extrachromosomal DNA carries genetic information in the same way as the circular DNA, and in a very few bacteria these genes may confer upon the individual bacterial cell the ability to resist destruction by antibiotics. Cells which happen to be resistant had no advantage over the normal 'wild' type, until antibiotic treatment became widespread. Under these circumstances, the resistant bacteria were able to survive where the wild type were not, and the population of resistant bacteria grew, especially in warm, damp wards and the tissues of debilitated patients, where division of the favoured cells could take place about once every 30 minutes. With the introduction of a manufacturing process in which bacteria were involved in the production of these drugs, the situation became worse. The microorganisms were exposed to antibiotics on a massive scale, and resistance developed virtually as soon as new antibiotics appeared on the market.

Plasmids probably played an important part. A bacterial cell without a plasmid is called an F^- or recipient cell; one that contains extrachromosomal DNA is an F^+ or donor cell. It is possible to regard F^- bacteria as 'female' and the F^+ donor cells as 'males'. A primitive type of sexual activity is possible between the two. The plasmid can be transferred from an F^+ cell to an F^- cell via structures called sexual pili. This process is called *conjugation*. If genes able to confer antibiotic resistance were carried on the plasmid then antibiotic resistance will be spread at the same time. There is evidence to suggest that this has happened both during drug manufacture, and in the clinical situation. Conjugation may have been responsible for some outbreaks of nosocomial infection.

Antibiotic resistance is a major problem in British hospitals, and the situation is not helped by the indiscriminate use of antibiotics, especially broad-spectrum antibiotics that can destroy a wide range of bacteria, rather than specific strains. Nurses are sometimes bewildered when a particular patient who has an obvious infection does not receive antibiotic therapy until a bacteriology report has been obtained from the laboratory several days later. This happens when the clinician is aware of the problem of antibiotic resistance, and

Microbiology and patient care 13

hopes to treat infection with an antibiotic that is specific to the bacteria responsible. Broad-spectrum antibiotics have to be used to treat serious, life-threatening infections even before the bacteriology results become available.

Many infection control committees (see Chapter 10) have now drawn up 'short lists' of the antibiotics which they advise doctors to prescribe routinely to treat uncomplicated infections and for those patients who require prophylactic antibiotic treatment before surgery. The population of bacteria in the hospital are therefore not exposed to the reserve antibiotics, and any bacteria which happen by chance to be resistant to them, having no special advantage, will not increase in large numbers. The reserve antibiotics are then available for problematic infections for which the usual range of antibiotics are not suitable.

Nurses have to contend with the problems of antibiotic-resistant bacteria in their work on the wards. Outbreaks of antibiotic-resistant bacteria have been reported, and a great deal of discipline is

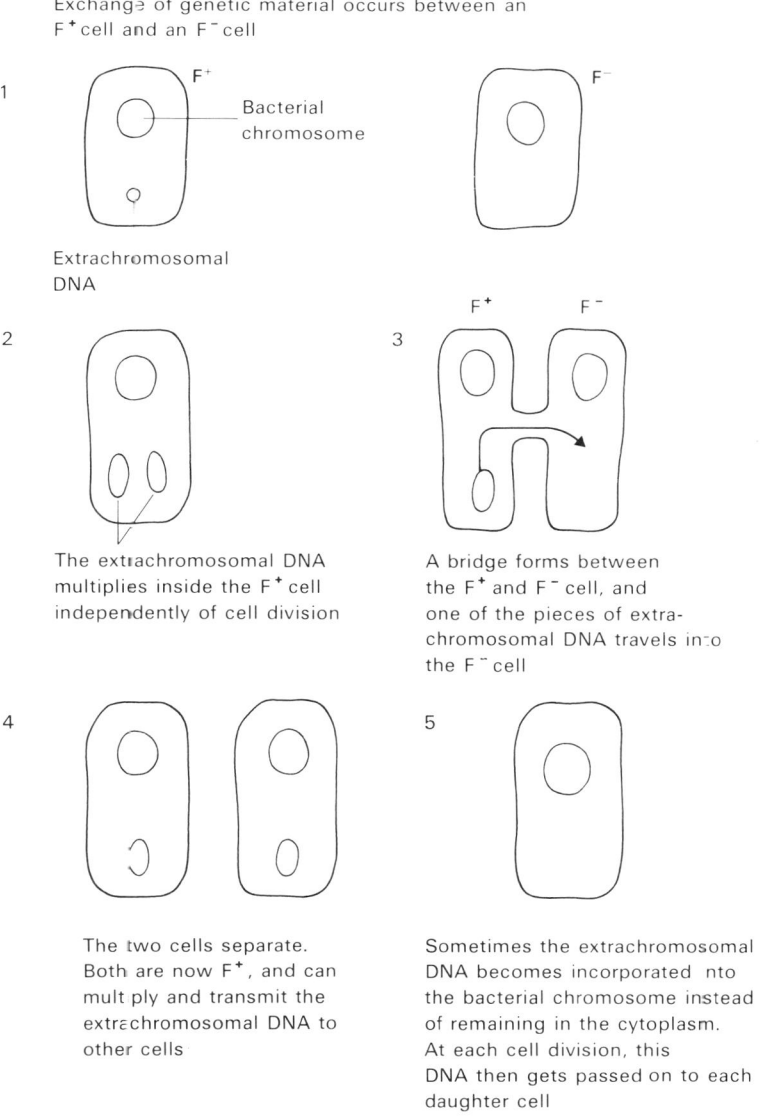

Fig. 1.6 Sexual reproduction in bacteria (conjugation).

required to control them. These outbreaks and the measures taken to contain spread are discussed further in Chapter 10. The consequences of infection that cannot be easily controlled can be tragic for the individual patient, as shown in case study 1.2.

Viruses

Viruses are minute particles responsible for a wide range of different infections in man, animals, plants and even in bacteria. Those which infect bacteria are called *bacteriophages* (*phages*). Sensivity to phages forms the basis of a valuable diagnostic laboratory test (see Chapter 10).

Structure and Life Cycle

Viruses vary between 20 and 200 nm in size and their structure has become apparent only with the high power of the electronmicroscope. Each virus particle consists of a protein capsule which surrounds a central core of nucleic acid (Fig. 1.7). Many viruses contain DNA, but a few, including the HIV virus responsible for AIDS, contain RNA. Viruses never contain both DNA and RNA, as do bacteria and all other living organisms. Structures attached to the surface of the capsule enable the virus to fasten itself to a host cell, and it then injects its nucleic acids into the cell, leaving the empty

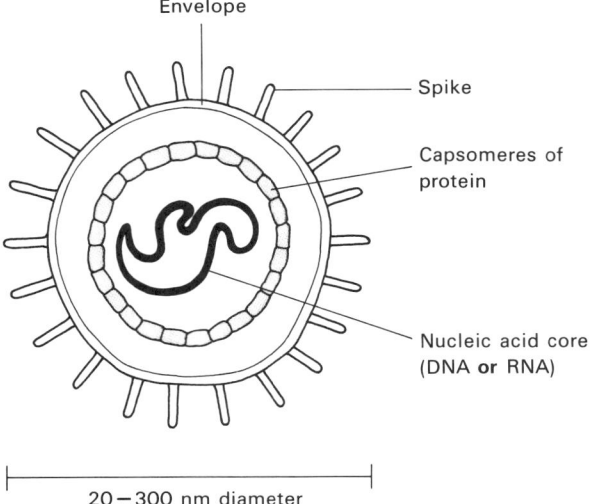

Fig. 1.7 Structure of a typical virus.

Case study 1.2

John took an extended holiday when he left university. He travelled across Europe with two friends of the same age and spent nearly a year abroad. During his travels he suffered from several episodes involving a cough and sore throat. He bought antibiotics from a pharmacy and treated the symptoms himself.

Towards the end of his holiday he was involved in a road traffic accident as a pedestrian, and was admitted to hospital with severe leg injuries. A decision was taken not to amputate his leg, but his recovery in hospital was fraught. He had an open fracture that had been heavily contaminated and the antibiotics he was given did not appear to combat the infection well.

John was frightened in hospital because he was in pain and because his understanding of the language, which was sufficient to communicate in shops and restaurants, was inadequate to obtain much information about the care he was receiving. He understood that he had nearly lost his leg, and because he had previously been an athletic young man, who had hoped to have a career as a sports master when he returned to England, this was important to him.

As soon as John's condition was stable, he was flown to a British hospital. There was evidence of severe infection in his injured leg, and an extensive area of tissue appeared black and necrotic. John was nursed in a single room, and when his family visited they, like the hospital staff, were requested to take isolation precautions. The nurses explained to them that John's leg was severely infected, and in view of the large quantities of antibiotics that he had received in a foreign country which appeared to be indiscriminate in the drugs used to treat even minor infections, there was a real danger that the bacteria in his wound might be difficult to control, and must be prevented, at all costs, from spreading to other people.

As soon as John arrived, wound swabs were sent to the bacteriology laboratory. When the results became available, they were telephoned to the ward. The bacteria were resistant to every antibiotic tested except for fucidin, a drug that can only be applied topically to wounds because it is severely toxic. The nurses were thankful that they had instituted isolation precautions. They now had to prepare John and his family for the possibility that the infection would possibly not be controlled by topical applications of fucidin. The doctors had hoped that following a course of intravenous antibiotics, skin grafts could be used to repair the wound.

Unfortunately, the infection could not be controlled, and John had to have a midthigh amputation.

protein capsule on the outside. Inside the host cell, the viral nucleic acids link up with the existing genes. Changes occur which prompt the host cell to stop synthesising its own characteristic proteins in favour of those of the virus. New virus particles are made instead. The life cycle of the virus is completed by liberation of the new virus particles, each ready to attack another cell (Fig. 1.8).

Viruses generally have a poor rate of survival outside living cells. Some, like the viruses responsible for respiratory diseases and childhood ailments, remain viable in droplets for some time, and they depend on airborne spread. Many others demand intimate contact between one host and the next potential victim before the successful passage of infection will occur. Reproduction outside living cells never occurs. Viruses are the ultimate, obligate parasites, and they are intentionally defined as

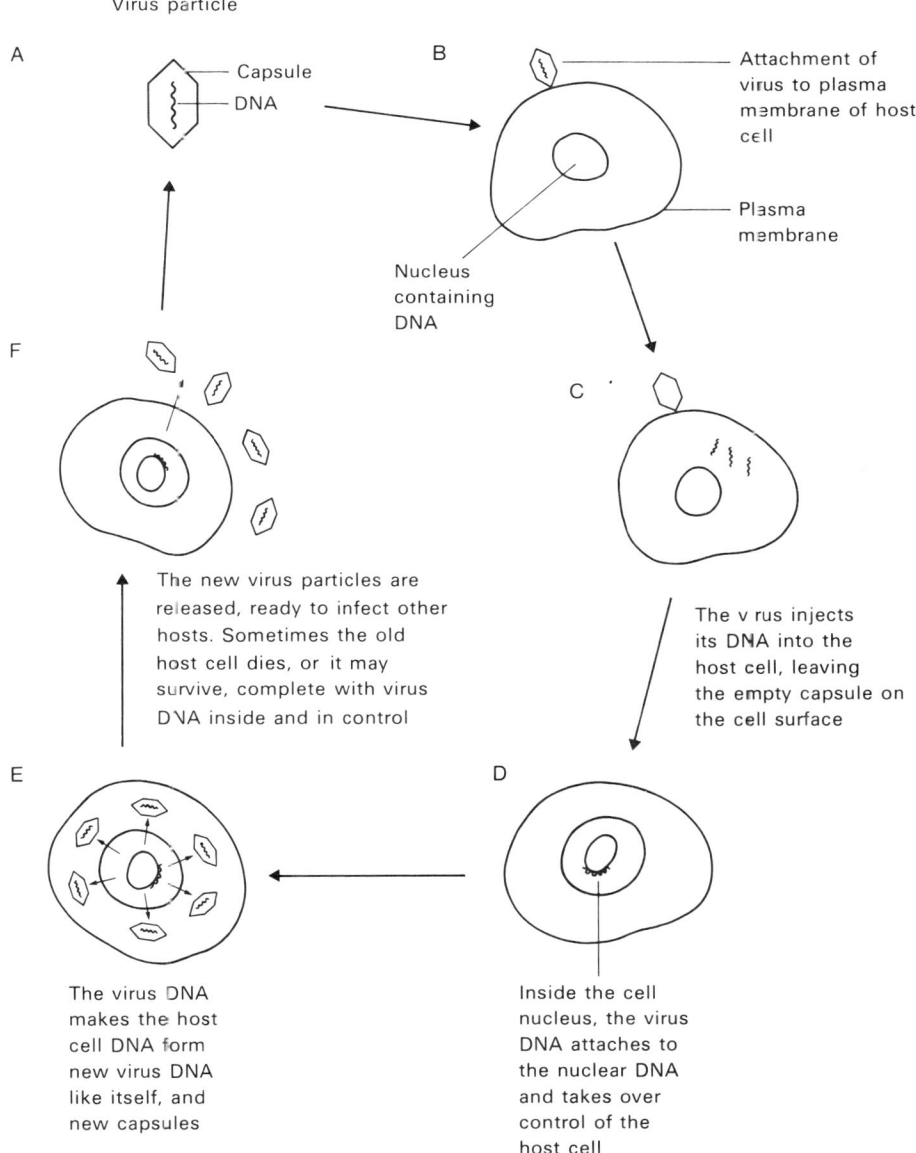

Fig. 1.8 Multiplication of a virus containing DNA.

'particles' rather than living organisms for they do not have a cellular structure and do not possess all the characteristics which apply to living organisms discussed previously in this chapter. Instead, viruses may be considered to occupy the grey zone which exists between the living and the non-living. This, in addition to their apparently primitive structure, has persuaded some people that viruses may have been the first 'living' creatures on earth. It has been speculated more recently that they may represent degeneration into a highly successful and quite sophisticated form of parasitism. Their existence as the earliest form of 'life' in the absence of potential victims is difficult to explain.

In the laboratory, viruses are grown in tissue cultures derived from the cells of animals. Before technology made tissue culture available, they were cultured by injecting infected extracts into eggs.

How Viruses Work

Viruses responsible for the common cold are inhaled as droplets via the upper respiratory tract. The particle attaches itself to the membrane of an epithelial cell lining the mucous membrane and invades. New virus particles are released and the host cell is destroyed.

Other types of virus may not necessarily destroy a host cell despite invasion and successful control of its genes. Instead, the parasitised host cell may survive and divide. The nucleic acid provided by the virus will divide too, and will be passed on to the two daughter cells and to their offspring when they in turn divide. A large number of cells builds up, each containing the foreign nucleic acids of the virus. The new, virally infected cells may look and behave rather differently from the cells of the original tissue from which they were derived. The virus may stimulate them to divide faster, forming a big mass of tissue, and it may make them synthesise proteins quite different from those normally manufactured by the host cells. This is a possible hypothesis for tumour formation (Fig. 1.9).

The Epstein-Barr (EB) Virus

The Epstein-Barr virus is attracted to human lymphocytes and is able to make them multiply rapidly. The same virus has been extracted from the cells which cause a tumour called Burkitt's lymphoma, and DNA from the virus is always found in malignant cells from patients who have developed Burkitt's lymphoma. This shows that the presence of the virus and tumour may be related, but it does not necessarily prove that one has caused the other.

The Herpes Simplex Virus

The Herpes simplex type 1 virus causes cold sores in a high proportion of the population. Its close relation, the Herpes simplex type 2 virus, is responsible for similar lesions in the genital region. People who have developed genital herpes develop antibodies to the virus which circulate in the bloodstream. Antibody titres to the virus are invariably higher among women who have developed carcinoma of the cervix. This indicates, although of course it does not prove, a relationship between the infection and later malignancy. The evidence is persuasive, however, since the incidence of cervical carcinoma is highest among women who have a history of promiscuous sexual behaviour, beginning early, with many partners. Sexual transmission is a probable, though perhaps not exclusive, method of spread.

Viruses and Cancer

It is important to keep this information in proportion. Malignant disease is of multiple aetiology, depending on the susceptibility of the host once it has been invaded by a possibly oncogenic virus. In view of this, it has not yet been possible to establish a definite link between human malignancy and viral infection. It is apparent that not every encounter, or even every invasion with a potentially tumour-inducing virus will result in malignancy. Research from the United States has indicated that about 80% of the population carries the Epstein-Barr virus in their lymphocytes, but it is latent. These people do not exhibit any signs of malignant disease. Burkitt's lymphoma is by no means a common tumour. Carcinoma of the cervix is, by contrast, an all too common form of malignancy. Attendances in 'special' clinics and histories taken from patients suggest that the number of women

Microbiology and patient care 17

who have frequent sexual encounters is high; yet many of them never develop carcinoma of the cervix.

The earliest relationship between viruses and cancers in animals was demonstrated in 1908. It was found that a type of leukaemia commonly found among chickens could be passed to healthy birds by treatment with filtrates of fluid from those that were infected. The filtrates did not contain living cells.

It has been known since 1938 that adenomas in mice can be induced by exposure to viruses. In humans the situation is more difficult to establish because malignancy, when it does occur, may not develop until long after the initial viral infection, and because human malignant illness does not appear to be contagious.

Fungi

Fungi are structurally more complicated than bacteria, and are higher organisms with true nuclei. Some branch in filamentous fashion (like mushrooms in the soil) and others, the yeasts, form buds. Both types are illustrated in Fig. 1.10. Fungi make spores with tough coats that can survive drying in an inhospitable environment. In the open air, fungal spores are dispersed in the wind; indoors, spread is in dust carried by draughts.

In Britain there are only a few species of fungi of

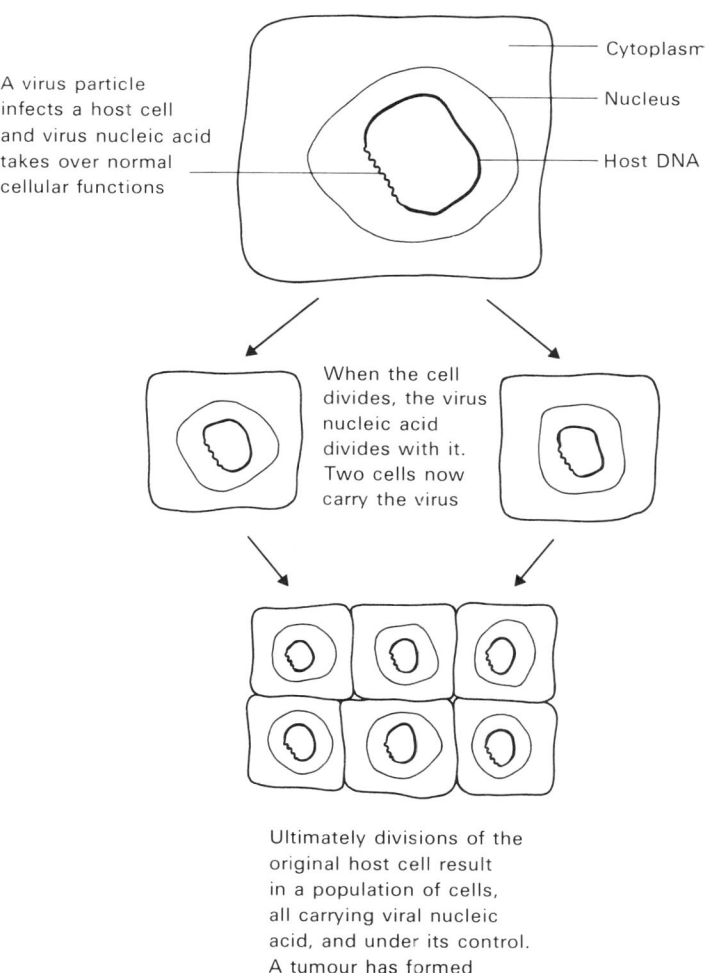

Fig. 1.9 Viruses and tumour formation – a possible mechanism.

medical importance. The most familiar is *Candida albicans*, the yeast responsible for vaginal thrush. *Candida* is a versatile opportunistic infection, fast becoming a scourge in hospitals, especially after patients have received antibiotics. These destroy the bacteria which normally live in the mouth, large bowel and vagina, so that *Candida* can take over. This fungus can invade the bladder to set up urinary tract infections, and is especially troublesome in special care baby and intensive care units.

The technical term for fungal disease is *mycosis*. Fungi may cause superficial or deep mycoses, depending on the ability of the organism to penetrate the deep tissues. *Candida* usually causes a superficial mycosis, with growth restricted to the surface tissues. Occasionally, in patients who have malignant illness or are taking immunosuppressive drugs, it can invade the deeper tissues. A few other fungi, such as *Cryptococcus* and *Aspergillus*, sometimes cause problems in the severely immunocompromised host such as the leukaemia patient. Tinea, the fungus responsible for athlete's foot, sets up a superficial mycosis, and often causes a painful, irritant rash in the skin folds of patients who have been inadequately washed and dried. Fungal disease, particularly deep mycoses, are not

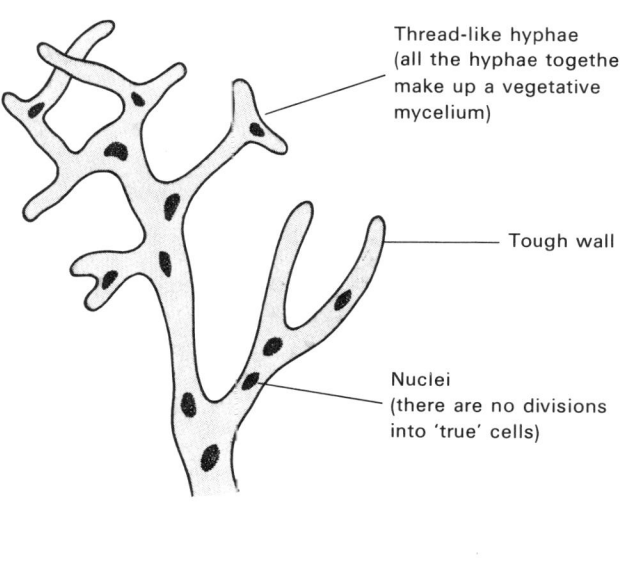

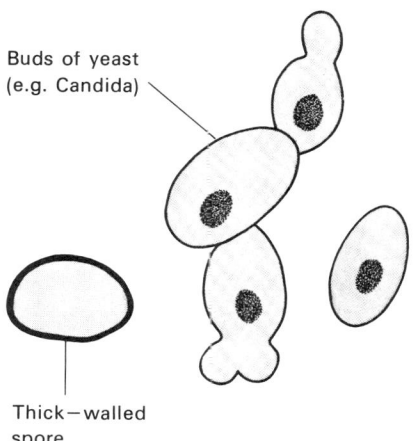

Fig. 1.10 Structure of fungi.

otherwise common in Britain, being generally more of a threat in hot climates. Treatment is with antifungal agents such as nystatin, clotrimazole and, for very severe infections, griseofulvin. When given systemically, most antifungal agents exhibit a variety of undesirable side-effects, e.g. vomiting, fever, renal damage, anaemia, rashes, thrombophlebitis of the injection site.

Protozoa

Protozoa are single-celled, microscopic animals, ranging in size from 5 to 50 µm (Fig. 1.11).

One of the most familiar protozoal infections is caused by *Trichomonas vaginalis*, which is sexually transmitted. Women develop a foul-smelling, irritating profuse vaginal discharge which has a characteristic yellow-green colour. Men generally remain asymptomatic. Treatment is with the drug metronidazole, often unpopular with patients, because they are advised to abstain from alcohol until the course is completed. Metronidazole taken with alcohol has been associated with fits.

Giardia lamblia is a protozoan which infests the large bowel, setting up bouts of mild diarrhoea, called giardiasis; this may persist for weeks or months and may be carried by some people asymptomatically.

Malaria is caused by a protozoan called *Plasmodium* (particularly *P. falciparum*), which has a complicated life cycle involving both man and the mosquito. Malaria is still endemic in many parts of the world, and rapid travel by air has resulted in people with the disease being admitted to British hospitals. Like trichomoniasis, malaria does not pose any risk of hospital cross-infection.

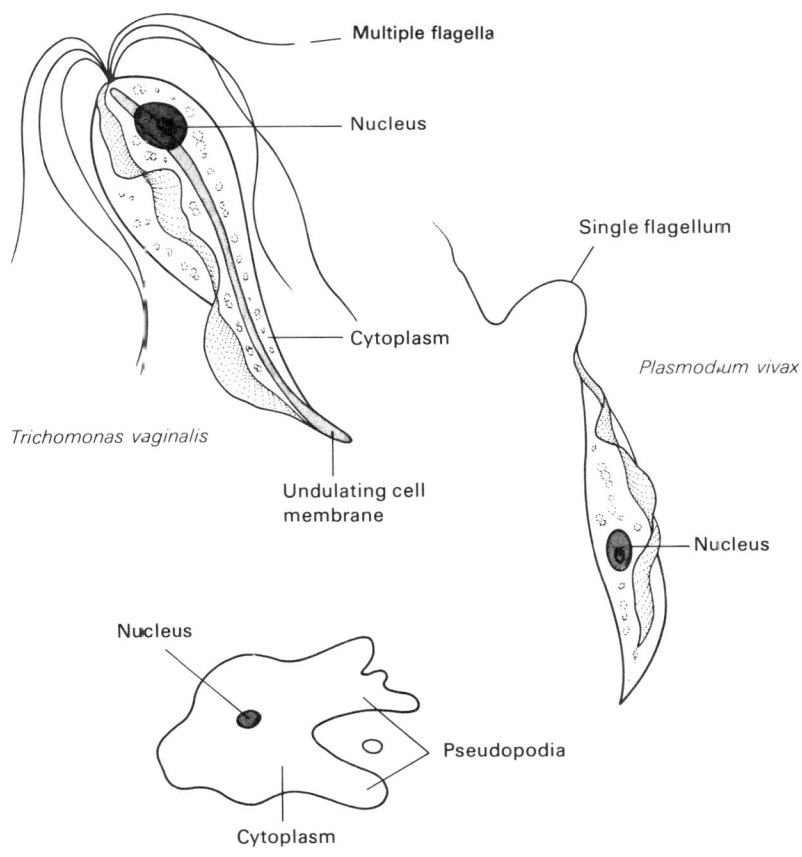

Fig. 1.11 Pathogenic protozoa.

Patients who have developed amoebic dysentry may also be admitted to British hospitals after travelling abroad. Here the causative agent is *Entamoeba histolytica*, which is present in the stools of infected patients. Both *Giardia* and *Entamoeba* could be transferred from one patient to another as a consequence of poor hand hygiene. *Pneumocystis carinii* is a protozoal infection responsible for pneumonia in severely immunocompromised patients, including those who have leukaemia or AIDS. The alveoli of the lungs become filled with frothy exudate, and untreated infections are usually fatal. Outbreaks of *Pneumocystis* infection have been reported from hospitals, implying that nosocomial spread is possible.

Another protozoan likely to cause problems among the debilitated is *Toxoplasma gondi*, a relation of the malaria parasite. It infects domestic cats, without causing apparent damage, but humans can become infected by contamination with cat faeces. Approximately 30% of the population carries antibodies for *Toxoplasma gondi*, indicating the existence of a significant incidence of subclinical, undiagnosed infections. Among the immunosuppressed, toxoplasmosis can be fatal.

Rickettsiae and Chlamydiae

The rickettsiae and chlamydiae are groups of microorganisms which both appear to bridge the gap between viruses and bacteria. They resemble viruses in their small size and their ability to reproduce exclusively within host cells. In their structure and other behavioural attributes they are reminiscent of bacteria.

Most rickettsiae are transmitted to humans by fleas or ticks. *Rickettsia prowazeki* carried by ticks will cause typhus in human beings.

Chlamydiae are transmitted from one victim to the next by airborne respiratory droplets. Psittacosis spread by cage birds is a chlamydial infection, and so is trachoma (caused by *Chlamydia trachomatis*), the most common disease resulting in human blindness, and widespread in the third world. Chlamydiae are also responsible for a number of sexually transmitted diseases; chlamydial species have been isolated from the genital tracts of men and women diagnosed with non-specific urethritis (NSU). There is evidence that this infection in women can lead to damaged fallopian tubes and infertility.

Mycoplasmas

Mycoplasmas are bacteria which lack cell walls. They change shape readily because they have no rigid outer supporting structure and are often filamentous. Most are very small. The most significant human mycoplasma is *Mycoplasma pneumoniae*, which can cause pneumonia.

Helminths (Worms)

Numerous species of worms cause human infection. They are multicellular animals, some quite large, and fall into two broad groups, roundworms and flatworms.

Ascaris worms and threadworms (*Enterobius vermicularis*) are both roundworms. Ascaris is a big white or pale pink worm which lives in the small intestine of humans and domestic animals, particularly pigs, and feeds mainly on semidigested food. Eggs, excreted in the faeces, can survive for long periods outside the body, until ingested by another host. Diagnosis is usually made when an adult worm is expelled in the faeces. Ascaris in Britain is found mainly among immigrants, affected before they arrive in this country. Prevention is by the provision of adequate sanitation.

Threadworms live in the large intestine, spending the entire life cycle in the human host. The female threadworm emerges from the anus, usually during the night, to lay eggs on the perianal skin. Irritation may cause the victim to scratch, setting up reinfection if eggs are transferred to the fingers and swallowed. Infestation occurs primarily among children because the eggs are able to withstand the slightly less acidic environment of a child's stomach better than that of an adult. Infection among members of the same family usually occurs through touching and from infected clothing. Diagnosis can be made by attaching a length of adhesive tape (such as Sellotape) to the perianal skin overnight. The following morning the tape can be stuck over a clean microscope slide trapping any eggs to its surface and the slide can then be examined by the laboratory staff.

Flatworms include flukes and tapeworms (Fig.

1.12). Both have complicated life cycles, involving animal hosts as well as man. In Britain, cases of liver fluke infection sometimes occur in humans when diseased animals are eaten or eggs swallowed. In Japan, lung flukes may cause respiratory illness when infested shellfish are eaten. Since Japanese people eat a good deal of their food uncooked, the incidence of this serious illness is high.

British people may ingest the cysts of tapeworms by eating infected, undercooked meat, especially pork, or by ingesting the eggs after handling infected domestic pets, particularly dogs.

From this discussion it should be apparent that infection with worms can be avoided by attention to hygiene, including food preparation, and adequate sanitation.

Throughout this description of the more commonly encountered groups of microorganisms, it has been emphasised at several points that infection depends on numerous factors involving both the host and parasite. Disease does not necessarily follow *every* encounter between a pathogen and potential host. The special circumstances necessary before invasion can occur is discussed below.

ESTABLISHING INFECTION: PREDISPOSING FACTORS

Before infection becomes possible a susceptible host must meet a virulent microorganism. This discussion will focus on bacterial pathogenesis, because our knowledge of bacterial virulence is

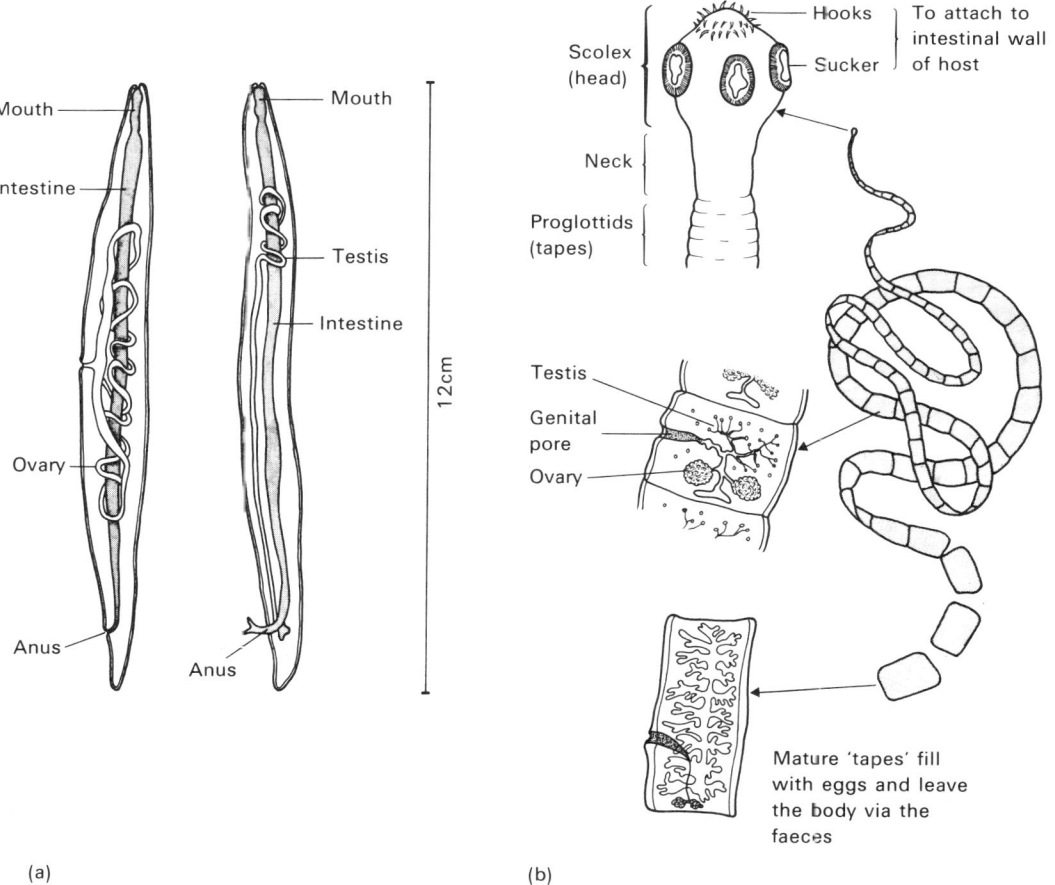

Fig. 1.12 (a) A pathogenic roundworm (*Ascaris lumbricoides*). (b) A pathogenic tapeworm (*Taenia*).

more complete than that of other kinds of micro-organisms. The pathogen must enter the tissues of the host and multiply successfully despite the defences mustered by the host. The life cycle of the pathogen is completed only by the exit of a new generation of bacteria and dissemination among other likely victims. Detailed knowledge of the life cycle of particular species of bacteria is of practical importance to nurses, since breaking the chain of infection at any point will help to control spread. Each of these stages will be discussed in turn, beginning with a description of those factors which contribute to virulence.

Virulence

Several factors contribute to the virulence of any pathogen:

(1) the size of the inoculating dose;
(2) ability to invade the tissues of the host while avoiding damage to the pathogen itself (invasiveness), and ability to damage the host tissues once established;
(3) damage to the host tissues, frequently achieved through the production of toxins.

Each of the above is described in turn.

Size of the Inoculating Dose

Perhaps the most obvious factor contributing to virulence is the number of pathogens available to establish infection. If only a few have access to the host, then it is unlikely that they will succeed in the battle against the host defences. Inoculation with a large number of bacteria is more likely to result in established disease.

Nurses often worry when a patient who has already spent some days in hospital is diagnosed with open pulmonary tuberculosis. Identification of the bacteria is usually difficult in these cases because the patient has difficulty in expectorating. Sometimes several specimens are sent to the laboratory before the acid-fast bacilli are seen. Under these circumstances it is rather unlikely that the patient is exhaling large numbers of bacteria in respiratory droplets. The size of the inoculating dose will therefore be small, and the risk of infection is probably slender.

Respiratory diseases of all kinds have a higher incidence in crowded communities, because people who live in close association are more likely to inhale a large inoculum. Meningococcal meningitis, for example, is a severe infection of the membranous layers enclosing the brain and spinal cord; the causative organism is *Neisseria meningitidis*. It may be carried harmlessly in the upper respiratory tract of healthy people, causing damage only when the bacteria gain access to the tissues of the central nervous system. The incidence rises dramatically among people who live and sleep together under crowded conditions, and that of clinical meningitis is then much increased. Reports from the First World War suggest that 20% of young men living in barracks became carriers, and that meningococcal meningitis was rampant among the troops; preventive measures included adequate spacing between beds. Today, fortunately, meningococcal meningitis is an uncommon disease in the western world, although epidemics have been reported in Africa and Brazil during recent years. There have also been recent disturbing reports of outbreaks around the town of Stroud in Gloucestershire, which remain unexplained.

Invasiveness

Invasiveness is the ability of bacteria to establish themselves within the host tissues, and to damage them structurally and physiologically through bacterial metabolism and multiplication. Some pathogens only colonise the bodily surface, others are able to penetrate deeply into the tissues. Several factors contribute to invasiveness. Ability to manufacture a tough capsule around the cell wall is a good example of this, as the capsule helps to prevent phagocytosis by the white blood cells of the host. *Streptococcus pneumoniae* and *Haemophilus influenzae* (which sometimes causes pneumonia or meningitis in children) both have capsules which contribute to their invasiveness. *Mycobacterium tuberculosis* has a particularly resistant, waxy wall, able to withstand prolonged attack by the host defences of the lungs. Pulmonary tuberculosis is therefore a disease of great chronicity.

Ability to synthesise particular enzymes may contribute to the invasiveness of some bacteria. Secretion of enzymes able to destroy host cells occurs onto the outer surface of the bacterial cell wall, where the enzyme may destroy cells of the host. *Staphylococci*, *Streptococci* and *Clostridium welchii* (which causes gas gangrene) all secrete enzymes known as haemolysins, which are able to destroy red blood cells. Coagulases are bacterial enzymes which make blood clot by their action on fibrinogen; the clot then protects the bacteria from phagocytosis, as well as isolating them from other defence mechanisms operating within the host. *Staphylococcus aureus*, for example, is a coagulase-positive bacteria, meaning it has the ability to 'wall off' boils; ability to secrete coagulase forms the basis of an important laboratory test. *Staphylococcus epidermidis*, on the other hand, is coagulase-negative, so its pathogenicity is correspondingly weaker than that of *Staph. aureus*.

In other species, pathogenic activity is related to the development of pili (hair-like processes) which bacteria use to attach themselves to the surface of the host cells before they invade; the diplococcus responsible for gonorrhoea depends upon pili. Mutant strains which lack pili also lose their pathogenicity.

Toxin Production

Toxins are poisons secreted by some, though not all virulent microorganisms. They may enter the bloodstream or lymphatic vessels, to be transported from the local site of bacterial activity to distant parts of the body. The resulting condition, toxaemia, can have serious, sometimes fatal consequences.

Toxins are classified according to the way in which bacteria synthesise them. *Endotoxins* are deposited into the bacterial cell wall and form part of its structure. *Exotoxins* are secreted outside the cell wall into the surrounding medium; they dissolve rapidly in the extracellular fluid, enter the systemic circulation and may be carried to all parts of the body. Under these circumstances it is usually the exotoxins which are responsible for the symptoms of disease rather than the bacteria themselves.

Exotoxins can destroy the cells of the host or inhibit specific metabolic functions, and they are among the most lethal chemical substances known. *Clostridium botulinum* (causing botulism) which occasionally survives in improperly canned food, secretes an exotoxin able to prevent the transmission of nervous impulses at the neuromuscular junction. The victim becomes paralysed, requiring mechanical ventilation when the effects reach the respiratory muscles. Botulism is a severe, often fatal condition.

Clostridium tetani manufactures tetanus toxin, which excites the neutrons of the central nervous system, causing muscular spasms and the deadly 'lockjaw'.

Several rather more mild infectious illnesses owe their symptoms to toxin production. Staphylococcal food poisoning is caused by a toxin that irritates the gastric mucosa, inducing vomiting.

Endotoxins are produced on the cell walls of numerous bacteria, including *Salmonella typhi* (typhoid), *Neisseria meningitidis* (meningitis) and some species of *Shigella* (dysentery). All endotoxins are responsible for the same symptoms of fever, and general malaise, regardless of the organism responsible.

Before bacteria can exert their influences on the tissues of a host, however, they must safely gain access. Their possible routes of entry into the body are outlined below.

Bacterial Invasion: The Portals of Entry

Bacteria can invade the body by the following routes: inhalation; ingestion; sexually transmitted infection; inoculation; congenital transmission. Each of these is dealt with in turn.

Inhalation

Pathogens may gain access to the respiratory tract by inhalation via the nose or mouth, a route taken by viruses causing influenza, measles and the common cold. Bacteria responsible for tuberculosis and diphtheria also enter by this route.

Ingestion

Many bacteria enter the gastrointestinal tract by ingestion with contaminated food or water. *Salmonella*, *Shigella* and the polio virus which causes poliomyelitis all gain access by this route.

Sexually Transmitted Infection

Sexually transmitted infections like syphilis, gonorrhoea and trichomoniasis (caused by *Trichomonas vaginalis*) are transferred from the genital tract of one partner to another during sexual intercourse. Gonorrhoea and syphilis are still both classified as venereal diseases, whereas trichomoniasis is regarded as sexually transmitted but non-venereal – the distinction is legal, of value in legal situations, but in medical terms of no real significance. Venereal infections are considered to be transferable (between adults) *only* by sexual intercourse, while sexually transmitted diseases may have additional means of spread. Gonorrhoea can be transferred to the eyes of the neonate during its passage down an infected birth canal, causing ophthalmia neonatorum.

Infection can also invade the bladder via the urethra, and may ascend to the ureters and kidneys. This portal of entry is of great significance to nurses, especially when patients are catheterised (see Chapter 8).

Inoculation

Inoculation via skin or mucous membranes can occur during surgical incisions, by accidental injury or by injection, either with a needle or through the mouthparts of an insect. This is how the mosquito spreads malaria, caused by the protozoan *Plasmodium*. Wound infections occur by inoculation in theatre and following accidental trauma; they are often caused by the skin flora of the patient himself or his attendants. The hepatitis type B virus can be inoculated through dirty needles. Infection can enter the body via the mucous membrane of the rectum – both syphilis and gonorrhoea have been isolated from female rectal swabs, where in some cases they may have been transferred in contaminated menstrual blood. The rising incidence of AIDS, and the high incidence of hepatitis B carriers in the homosexual population, have drawn more attention to the rectum as a possible portal of entry for infection into the body.

Congenital Transmission

Infections can be acquired congenitally across the placenta from the maternal to the fetal circulation. This is an uncommon mode of transmission which usually has a serious and tragic outcome. A familiar example is maternal rubella, especially if it occurs during the first trimester, when the baby's organ systems are developing. Blindness, deafness and mental retardation can result. Pregnant women who have developed rubella infections may receive counselling and therapeutic abortion if they desire it.

Treponema pallidum can cause congenital syphilis. Children born with this condition develop a particular facial appearance, said to be part of the stigmata of the congenital presentation of the disease. Today, all British women are routinely screened for syphilis, and fortunately the disease among children has become very rare because penicillin given to the mother will pass to the fetal circulation across the placenta.

Women who have developed AIDS may pass the disease onto their children. Whether this is truly congenital spread or the effect of close contact and breast feeding after birth has not yet been established. However, patients who have AIDS are a threat to the pregnant nurse because they so often carry cytomegalovirus, which can lead to mental retardation of the fetus.

Passive Defence Mechanisms Against Invading Pathogens

Living organisms actively defend themselves against pathogenic invasion (see Chapter 7). Additionally, the human body is designed anatomically and physiologically to provide passive barriers to microorganisms, which are now described. They involve the mechanical arrangements of the tissues and the secretion of fluids which help to wash infected particles from the body (Fig. 1.13). Discussion is in relation to the different systems of the body.

The Skin

The skin provides a mechanical barrier against infection provided that it remains intact. Secretions from the sebaceous glands are bactericidal.

Microbiology and patient care 25

The Gastrointestinal System

White blood cells present in the saliva destroy *some* of the bacteria present in contaminated food. Gastric secretions are highly acidic (pH 2) due to hydrochloric acid secreted by glands in the gastric mucosa. Consequently, bacteria are destroyed in large numbers in the stomach.

The walls of the small intestine contain small areas of lymphatic tissue (Peyer's patches) which destroy bacteria that have survived passage through the stomach. Bacteria can enter the bloodstream from the gut, but are carried to the liver via the hepatic portal vein, so they travel through the sinusoids of the liver before entering the systemic circulation.

In the sinusoids they are brought directly into contact with the cells of Kupffer, which are phagocytic, and can engulf foreign particles including bacteria.

The Respiratory System

The nostrils are lined with big, coarse hairs and cilia which trap large foreign particles. Inside the nose the turbinal bones are arranged so that smaller particles are trapped on them as the inspired air travels over their surfaces. Lymphoid tissue in the pharyngeal and nasopharyngeal tonsils is strategically arranged to trap inspired pathogens.

The entire respiratory tree, except for the alveoli, is lined with simple ciliated columnar epithelial cells. Goblet cells incorporated into this tissue secrete mucus in which particles from the inspired air become trapped. The cilia beat so that the mucus and particles are swept up the respira-

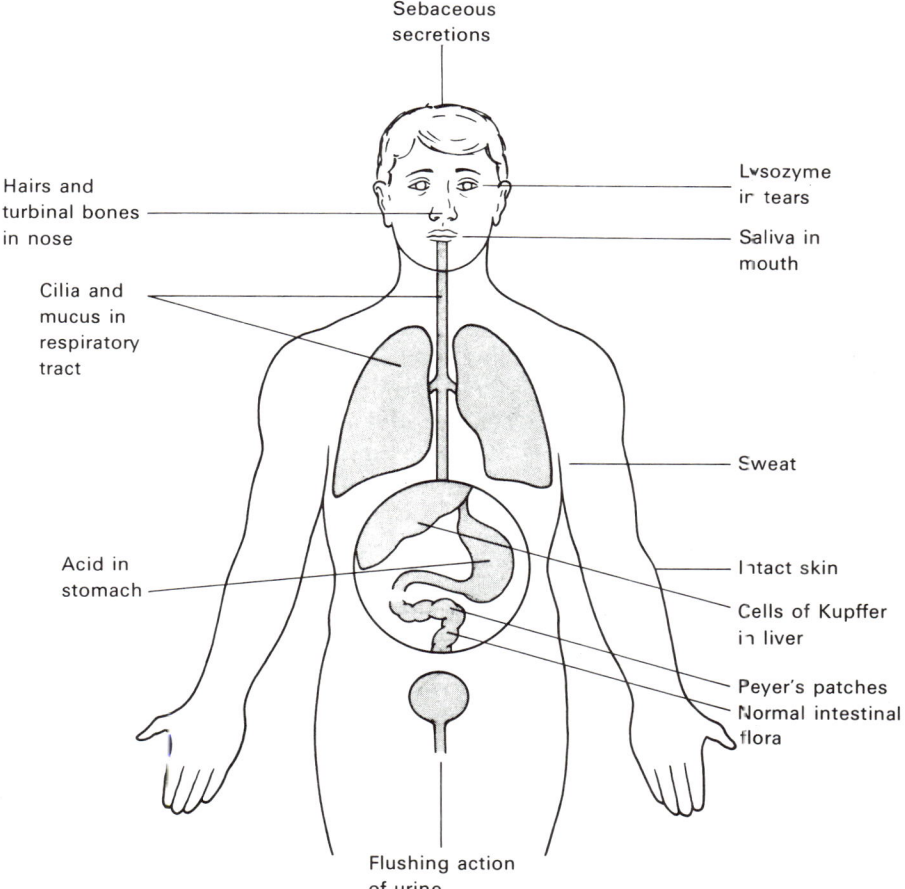

Fig. 1.13 Main physical barriers of the body against invading pathogens.

tory tree to the pharynx where they are swallowed. In a healthy person about 100 ml of mucus are secreted daily. The system is efficient and the alveoli are sterile, but excessive environmental pollution or cigarette smoking paralyse and eventually destroy the cilia. Excess mucus is secreted, sometimes as much as 1000 ml every day; this is coughed up, not swallowed. Excessive mucus production is one of the changes that accompany chronic bronchitis, a disease exacerbated by the damp British climate. Patients with chronic bronchitis are very prone to acute infections because of their impaired respiratory defence mechanisms.

Lung tissue is divided into segments by tough partitions of connective tissue which help to isolate foci of infection. This helps explain why local foci of infection set up by *Mycobacterium tuberculosis* tend to remain in the original segment of inoculation. White blood cells are present in the interstitial fluid which lies between the alveolar and capillary cells at the respiratory membrane.

The Genitourinary System

The vagina contains a resident population of bacteria which belong to the genus *Lactobacillus*, and metabolise the glycogen present in cervical secretions, forming lactic acid. The pH of the adult vagina is approximately 4.5, a level unfavourable for the growth of many other bacteria. In young girls and postmenopausal women, cervical secretions are scanty because the amount of oestrogen produced by the ovaries is a good deal less than during the reproductive years. The vaginal pH is correspondingly more alkaline, and vaginal infections are more common. Older women sometimes develop vaginal infections referred to as 'senile vaginitis'. Gonorrhoea, which attacks only the cervical cells in adult women, may infect the vaginal epithelium of girls who have not yet reached puberty.

The tip of the urethra contains the same types of bacteria usually present on the surface of the skin and mucous membranes, but in health the bladder is normally sterile. The length of the male urethra helps to prevent the migration of bacteria up into the bladder, but among women, who have a much shorter urethra, there is a very high incidence of urinary tract infection, for which all pregnant women are screened routinely.

In many respects the bladder appears to be defenceless against invading pathogens, a point that is explored in Chapter 8.

The Eyes

The enzyme lysozyme, secreted in tears, digests and destroys bacteria. Protection from large particles is offered by the eyelashes and blinking reflex.

Other Organ Systems

Other organs, protected deep within the body, contain cells which appear to be capable of phagocytic activity. The mesangial cells found between the nephrons in the kidney, and the microglia cells which help support and nourish the neurons of the central nervous system, can both engulf and digest foreign particles, and can apparently deal with pathogens too.

The White Blood Cells

White blood cells are manufactured in the lymph nodes and the bone marrow. They are present in the blood, lymph and the interstitial fluids which bathe the tissues, and they help to destroy any microorganisms which have successfully overcome the mechanical barriers that defend the body against invasion by foreign particles. Their contribution is discussed in much more detail in Chapter 7.

The Normal Body Flora

The external surfaces of the body, and many of its internal surfaces are colonised by a permanently resident population of bacteria, usually described as the normal flora. Far from being harmful, these bacteria help protect the body by offering resistance to any foreign microorganisms that might invade. Microorganisms that are beneficial to their host are said to be *commensal*. It is important to remember, however, that bacteria which behave as commensals in one anatomical location may cause damage if they gain access to another. The normal flora of the large bowel includes *E. coli*, which is of value to the host because it can synthesise vitamin B complex and vitamin K. But *E. coli* will generate urinary tract infection if it invades the bladder.

The normal skin flora varies from one location to another. Some bacteria live permanently on the skin, often deep in the sweat glands and are difficult to remove. These constitute the *resident* skin flora. Others, to a large extent contaminant bacteria, form the *transient* skin flora. The significance of permanent and resident bacteria to hand hygiene is discussed in Chapter 5.

Noble and Somerville (1974) have gathered evidence to show that no area of the skin surface is free of resident microorganisms except the nail plate. Density varies between different sites as well as between individuals. The arms and legs, which account for approximately half the total area of the skin surface, have only a low density of resident microorganisms (10^2–10^3/cm^2). On the forehead the distribution may reach 10^6/cm^2, and between the webs of the toes, 10^9/cm^2, especially if they are diseased.

The species of microorganisms carried on normal human skin varies according to the individual. Predominantly they are cocci, and include *Staphylococcus epidermidis*, *Micrococcus* and harmless members of the genus *Corynebacterium*, such as *C. diphtheriae* which causes diphtheria. All these bacteria are Gram-positive; the only Gram-negative bacillus often to be found as part of the normal skin flora is *Acinetobacter*.

Although these organisms present little or no threat during health, they may do so if the normal mechanical barriers of the body are breached by invasive techniques (surgery, intubation) performed in hospital on very sick people.

When the skin becomes diseased it may become colonised by other types of bacteria (Noble, 1979). For example, the hands of hemiplegic patients have been found to become heavily colonised with *Clostridium welchii*, perhaps in response to heavy perspiration (Chin and Davies, 1976). This has enormous implications for cross-infection when hemiplegic patients are admitted to hospital.

Asymptomatic Carriers

Apparently healthy people may be the unsuspecting carriers of bacteria that are potentially pathogenic. *Staphylococcus aureus* exists in the nasal mucosa of about 30% of the adult population, in the faeces of about 20%, and on the skin of 5–10%. Incidence tends to be higher both among people who work in hospital, and among men than women. Other common sites of carriage include the axillae, the toe webs and perineum. Carriers are not themselves damaged by the presence of the bacteria, but they may infect other people who are more susceptible and who respond by developing the clinical manifestations of disease. Different areas of the body disseminate these bacteria to different extents, and it tends to be greatest from the perineal area.

People who have had an infection may make an uneventful recovery, but continue to carry and to shed the bacteria responsible for weeks or months afterwards. As long as this situation persists they represent a potential threat to others.

Victims of food poisoning commonly become asymptomatic carriers, without signs of clinical illness. 'Typhoid Mary', a cook who worked in Boston earlier this century, has become legendary because of the large number of victims whom she infected during the course of her work. Asymptomatic carriers should not handle food intended for consumption by anyone other than themselves. Occupational health departments usually screen new employees before they are allowed to work in a catering department, and nobody known to have had *Salmonella* food poisoning may normally return to any type of work involving the handling of food until at least three consecutive stool cultures have been found negative. Finding out the precise nature of employment and persuading an individual to comply with infection control precautions may require a great deal of tact, as well as sufficient knowledge to ask pertinent questions. This is illustrated by case study 1.3 (p. 28).

Poultry is almost always infected with *Salmonella*, which may be present in raw chicken and turkey meat. Cooking at a high temperature for a sufficient length of time (until all the pink coloration of the flesh has disappeared) will destroy the bacteria and render the chicken safe. Thousands of people eat this relatively inexpensive source of protein every day and suffer no ill-effect. But failure to cook the meat sufficiently is a real hazard, and *Salmonella* food poisoning is a common occur-

Case study 1.3

Two young women who shared the same flat purchased a chicken pie from a takeaway restaurant, and ate half each. Both developed symptoms of food poisoning and went home to stay with their respective parents while they were unwell. Stool culture, arranged by their general practitioner, revealed that both had been infected with *Salmonella hadar*. After 2 weeks, stool cultures were again sent to the laboratory, and both girls were still found to be excreting bacteria, although clinically both were well. One of the girls was told by the doctor that she could return to work, but the other was told that she must remain at home until three negative stool specimens had been obtained in succession.

The first girl was employed in an office. In the course of her daily work it was never necessary for her to handle food for consumption by anyone other than herself. She always took sandwiches to eat at lunchtime. The second girl was a student nurse. At work she was expected to serve food to patients and if necessary to feed them, although she did not actually prepare their meals herself.

rence (see Chapter 10). To buy food, especially chicken, from a restaurant of dubious reputation is courting disaster, particularly if there is any possibility that it has been allowed to cool and then reheated. Bacteria are merely inactivated by the initial exposure to a low temperature, then multiply enormously unless the food is rapidly and thoroughly chilled. A second mild warming stimulates even more rapid cell division, and an even larger inoculum of bacteria will be ingested.

In case study 1.3 the general practitioner had taken the trouble to find out where the girls worked, and had given appropriate advice, but he had overlooked the fact that they shared the same home, and, presumably the same catering facilities in it. This was a serious omission, because the girls sometimes ate together – they might also collaborate in the preparation of meals, and run the risk of reinfecting one another.

Two cases of an infectious disease occurring in relation to one another in time constitute an outbreak, and this merits an investigation of the source. If the doctor had questioned the girls more thoroughly, he would have obtained a food history and arranged for the restaurant to be visited by the community health doctor (whose role is more fully discussed in Chapter 10).

MECHANISM OF SPREAD

Spread of infection from contaminated food is only one possible mechanism of transmission among microorganisms. They can also be passed from one victim to the next by both direct and indirect contact. Dissemination may be via the air, water, from insect vectors or by parenteral or venereal routes. Each of these mechanisms of dispersal is discussed below.

Direct Contact

Spread may be by direct contact between one person and another. This happens very frequently in hospital because patients are handled more often during a period of hospitalisation than at any other stage of the life cycle since infancy, and by a large number of different people. Those who are the most ill, and therefore most vulnerable, are inevitably handled most often. Crowding in old wards and shared facilities such as bathrooms exacerbate the problem.

Indirect Contact

There is a great potential for microorganisms to be spread to patients via inanimate objects (fomites). Bedclothes, pillows, soft toys, curtains, dressings and many other items can all act as fomites. However, nurses appear to exaggerate this threat, perhaps because they do not apply the principles of microbiology to their work on the wards. Bacteria, like all other living organisms, require warmth, moisture and a supply of nutrients before they will grow and multiply. Consequently they will flourish on warm bedclothes damp with perspiration, but will not survive for long on the cold, hard surface of equipment such as bedcradles or lockers. Provided that these are kept clean and dry, vegetative bacteria will die, and spores will remain inactive.

Airborne Spread

Droplets of infected material may be spread into the atmosphere by coughing, sneezing, or spluttered conversation, to be inhaled by another individual.

The extent to which different bacteria can remain viable in the air varies. This is related to the ability of the cell to resist desiccation by its thick cell walls, or the ability to form spores. Members of the genus *Clostridium* form spores, and so does the fungus *Candida*. Staphylococci and *Mycobacterium tuberculosis* cannot sporulate, but survive for long periods in the air because of their thickened cell walls.

Gaspar (1982) conducted an ingenious series of experiments using the non-pathogenic species *Micrococcus luteus* as a model to show how airborne bacteria may be disseminated. An airgun was used to spray the bacteria into a typical but unoccupied side room of a ward commonly used to isolate patients with infectious diseases spread by the airborne route. She showed that when conditions in the room remained still, the bacteria tended to drift around the room and outside into the ward corridor (the hospital was old, and the room was not fitted with an airlock). In a second experiment, where normal activity was simulated in the room after spraying, the bacteria settled more readily. However, climatic conditions may have influenced the result, since the weather had been clear and sunny throughout the first experiment, but had become hot and humid when the second experiment was conducted.

Other experiments have demonstrated that the number of airborne bacteria in a ward increase during periods of activity such as doctors' rounds and visiting time. Counts tend to be highest in the morning, often a time when dressings and invasive procedures such as catheterisation take place. The number of airborne bacteria is lowest at night. However, Ayliffe, Collins and Taylor (1980) present data to show that even when bedclothes are vigorously shaken they are unlikely to distribute microorganisms higher than the top of the bedside curtains drawn around a patient about to have a dressing changed.

Infection from Contaminated Food

Microorganisms or their toxins may be disseminated in contaminated food (see case study 1.3). A report by the British Association for the Advancement of Science (1977) pointed out that food poisoning may be the consequence of poor hygiene in shops, factories, restaurants, farms and in the home. At the conclusion of their report, the working party suggested that much could be done to eliminate food poisoning if the public could receive further education in matters of food hygiene – health visitors and district nurses could do much in this sphere. An example of food poisoning in conjunction with food manufacturing processes is given in Chapter 10.

Food poisoning may occur in any kitchen where large quantities are cooked under poor hygienic conditions. Unfortunately this sometimes happens in hospitals. Hospital kitchens have traditionally received crown immunity, which meant that they were not subject to periodic inspection by public health authorities and could not be sued for poor practices. However, following a recent severe outbreak of food poisoning in a large psychiatric hospital, which involved the death of 19 patients, it appears that the government may be persuaded to lift crown immunity. Hospitals, like restaurants, would then be forced to improve unhygienic conditions. Unlike restaurants, however, they make no profits to do so.

When a large quantity of food, perhaps stew or a joint, fails to reach an adequate cooking temperature, bacteria, especially spores deep inside, may escape unharmed. Slow cooking and storage in a warm place will allow them to multiply actively, contaminating the food. This is how *Clostridium welchii* causes food poisoning; since it is anaerobic, lack of oxygen in the middle of the food does not harm it.

Most people associate food poisoning mainly with meat and fish, particularly shellfish, but other food products are very often involved. *Salmonella*, for example, infects eggs as well as poultry. Cooked eggs are safe because the bacteria are destroyed, but custards, mousses, sauces like mayonnaise and other products which involve the use of raw eggs, or only very gentle heat to prevent the eggs curdling, can be dangerous.

Bacillus cereus is sometimes responsible for a mild form of food poisoning associated with Chinese restaurants. Spores of the bacteria are present in rice. These survive initial boiling and if ingested at this stage would cause no harm, being inactive, but if the rice is left in a warm room they will germinate and multiply. Gently frying previously boiled and stored rice will not destroy *B. cereus*.

Food poisoning described by the bacteria above is often mild, although *Salmonella* infections can be fatal among the elderly and infirm. However, some bacteria which cause food poisoning may represent a more serious threat. *Clostridium botulinum*, described earlier (p. 23), secretes a potent exotoxin able to block the release of acetylcholine from the synaptic ends of the nerve cells. Victims develop paralysis that may culminate in death from respiratory or cardiovascular failure.

Parenteral Spread

Some infections can be transmitted from one host to the next in infected blood and bodily fluids derived from blood – the viruses responsible for both hepatitis B and AIDS are transmissible in this way. Opportunities for spread by this route are greater in hospital than in the community. Hepatitis B and AIDS both have a higher rate of carriage in the homosexual population. Numerous explanations have been suggested for this phenomenon, but none has been entirely satisfactory.

The hepatitis B virus attacks the liver. Symptoms include general malaise, nausea, anorexia, headache, vomiting and diarrhoea. Upper abdominal pain is experienced as the liver enlarges and the victim becomes jaundiced due to the obstruction of the bile canaliculi. After the acute infection, patients can become asymptomatic carriers. The structure of the virus is complex, consisting of three antigens: surface, inner 'core', and 'e', which lies inside the core.

A shorthand notation is used to differentiate the three antigens. *HBsAg* denotes the surface antigen, identified in the plasma early during an acute attack of hepatitis B, and remaining in the plasma of all people who later develop into carriers. Not everyone who has become infected will become a carrier. To complicate matters further, some people experience only mild, or subclinical infections, becoming carriers with no recollection of ever having the disease. *HBeAg*, the e antigen inside the core, is present when the virus is actively replicating, and is a sign of active hepatitis and of high infectivity.

The core antigen, *HBcAg*, may appear transiently in the serum, and coincide with the appearance of antibodies. Presumably the antibodies are destroying the virus, so that its particles disintegrate, exposing the core. The core antigen is usually present in patients who are winning the battle against the infection, lending support to this hypothesis.

HBsAg patients are a good deal less infectious than those who carry the e antigen. Nevertheless, health care workers today would be advised to regard all blood as potentially contaminated, and to avoid direct contact with it.

Since 1971 the British Blood Transfusion Service has tested the blood of all donors for hepatitis B antigens, and people found to be positive are no longer able to donate. However, nurses and doctors have tended to overreact to threats of hepatitis B carriers, perhaps because the mortality rate originally associated with the disease was estimated to be much higher than has subsequently proved to be the case. Prevention of parenteral infections is fully discussed in Chapter 4, with particular reference to hepatitis B. AIDS is discussed in more detail in Chapter 2.

Sexual Transmission

The number of people who develop sexually transmitted infections is increasing on a worldwide scale, probably due to a more liberal approach towards sexual behaviour and attitudes. Contraception has become more effective, removing the fear of pregnancy. Condoms provide a barrier to infection, but oral contraceptives and intrauterine devices do not. Loneliness among people travelling or living away from home may promote sexual experimentation. Other factors to consider are the increased number of cases revealed by effective contact tracing, that may previously have gone unrecorded and untreated, and the increasing resistance of *Neisseria gonorrhoeae* to penicillin.

Throughout 1980 500 000 patients in the United Kingdom attended an STD clinic. The majority had a negative diagnosis, and many wanted reassurance following sexual contact with someone other than their usual partner, or because they had had multiple sexual contacts. Others attend with psychosexual problems.

Gonorrhoea is highly infectious, affecting approximately 60 000 patients every year. But in women many infections may remain undiagnosed so the exact number of cases is difficult to estimate.

The annual incidence of patients presenting with early syphilis is about 1300 males, mainly homosexuals, and 200 females. Antenatal screening programmes have been successful, and congenital syphilis is now rarely seen in Britain.

Genital herpes affects 2% of those who attend STD clinics. The incidence is said to be increasing, but again this is difficult to prove since publicity may have encouraged more patients, especially those with mild symptoms, to seek treatment.

Waterborne Infection

Infections disseminated in water are a good deal less problematic in Britain than in parts of the world where sanitation is poor. Cholera is endemic throughout Asia, but there are only occasional outbreaks in western countries, generally associated with lapses in sanitation. The eradication of cholera in London in the 1800s is discussed in Chapter 2, to illustrate how the threat imposed by infection has changed emphasis over the years due to improved health of the nation.

Spread by Vectors

Vectors are animals, usually insects, that carry infection from one host to another. Vector transmission may be either mechanical or biological.

In the case of *mechanical transmission*, pathogens are carried either on the feet of the insect or on some other surface part of its body. If the insect comes into contact with food, the pathogens may be transferred on to it and ingested. In this way, houseflies may be vectors for *Shigella*. In hospital, cockroaches and Pharaoh's ants may spread infection. Both insects are extremely difficult to eradicate.

In *biological transmission*, the insect bites an infected host, ingesting some of its blood which will contain pathogens. These reproduce inside the body of the vector, increasing in number so that more are available for contact with possible future hosts. Often reproduction takes place inside the gut of the vector, and new pathogens leave via the faeces. If the insect defaecates when it feeds, the pathogen can enter the wound. Malaria (described on p. 19), typhus and bubonic plague all have biological transmission via vectors. Typhus, spread by rickettsiae, and bubonic plague, caused by *Yersinia pestis*, both have the rat flea as their vector.

Many of the vector-borne infections, occurring to a large extent in tropical areas of the world, are life-threatening. However, for some of these man may be infected only occasionally, and accidentally. The virus causing Lassa fever, for example, normally infects a small rodent called the multimammate mouse, which lives in scrubland in Nigeria. Sometimes the mouse invades dwelling places and humans become infected, probably by contact with its urine. Lassa fever carries a heavy mortality rate, at least among Caucasian people.

CONCLUSIONS

In this chapter the characteristics common to all living organisms have been described, but with particular reference to microorganisms, especially bacteria. Factors contributing to virulence have been discussed, with a description of the normal flora of the human body and the way in which microorganisms are disseminated. In the next chapter, epidemiological trends are examined, to illustrate how the impact of infectious disease in Britain and the western world has gradually changed over the years.

References

Akinsanya, J. (1985). Learning about life. *Senior Nurse*, 2: 24–75.

Ayliffe, G. A. J., Collins, B. J., Taylor, L. J. (1982). *Hospital-acquired Infections. Principles and Prevention*, p. 50. Wright PSG, Bristol.

Ayliffe, G. A. J., Brightwell, K. M., Collins, B. J., Goontilake, P. C. L., Etheridge, R. A. (1977). Survey of hospital infection in the Birmingham Region. 1. Effect of age, sex, length of stay and antibiotic use on nasal carriage of tetracycline-resistant *Staphylococcus aureus* and on post-operative wound infection. *Journal of Hygiene*, 79: 299–314.

Bendall, E. (1973). *So You Passed Nurse?* Royal College of Nursing, London.

British Association for the Advancement of Science (1977). Salmonella, the food poisoner; a review.

Chin, P., Davies, D. G. (1976). Skin flora of paraplegic patients. *Journal of Hygiene*, 77: 93–96.

Davies, A. J. (1984). Is coagulase-negative staphylococcal bacteraemia in neonates a consequence of mechanical ventilation? *Journal of Hospital Infection*, 5: 260–269.

Gaspar, S. (1982). Is barrier nursing effective? In: *Proceedings of the Royal College of Nursing Research Society Thirteenth Annual Conference, 1982*, pp. 181–195. University of Durham, Macmillan Press.

Gott, M. (1984). *Learning Nursing*. Royal College of Nursing, London.

Gould, D. J. (1985). Isolation procedures in one health district. *Nursing Times Occasional Paper*, 81(7): 47–50.

Newsom, S. W. B. (1979). Review of the problems of cross infection. In: *Problems in the Control of Hospital Infection*. International Symposium Series No. 3. The Royal Society of Medicine, London.

Noble, S. W. B., Somerville, D. A. (1974). *Microbiology of the Human Skin*. Saunders, London.

Wilson, K. J. W. (1975). *The Biological Sciences in Nursing Education*. Churchill Livingstone, Edinburgh and London.

Further Reading

Postgate, J. (1972). *Microbes and Man*. Revised edition. Penguin, Harmondsworth.

Chapter 2

Infection: Past and Present Trends

INTRODUCTION

This chapter describes the major threat to life presented by infection in the past, and contrasts it with the present situation, showing that despite the advent of immunisation and antibiotics, infection continues to afflict western society in the 20th century.

Epidemiology can be defined as the study of the distribution and causes of disease in a human population. Historically, epidemiology developed from the study of contagious disease, although today its scope has expanded to include all diseases, whether they are infectious or not.

EPIDEMICS, PANDEMICS AND ENDEMIC DISEASE

An *epidemic*, or outbreak of an infectious disease, refers to two or more cases which appear to be related in space or time. Epidemics of infectious illnesses like typhoid, cholera, typhus and meningococcal meningitis remain an important threat in many tropical countries, but in western society their place as major killers has largely been taken by other diseases. Some of these are caused by infectious agents, and they are described later in this chapter. Several modern epidemics may be attributed to lax health habits and are open to improvement through health education – dental caries, which has been blamed on a diet high in sugars and poor dental hygiene, is a good example of this.

A *pandemic* is the simultaneous occurrence of a large number of infections from the same source. The Black Death which swept across Europe, reaching England in the 13th century, is a classic example of a pandemic.

In contrast to epidemic diseases, an *endemic* disease is one that is always present in the population to a greater or lesser extent. Malaria, for example, remains endemic throughout many parts of Africa.

It is possible to draw a graph to illustrate the typical epidemic curve (Fig. 2.1). To the left-hand side of the curve, the numbers of infected people rise gradually, reaching a peak at its midpoint. On the right-hand side, recovery proceeds faster than the appearance of new infections and the epidemic dies away. The courses of epidemics have been studied in isolated parts of the world such as Spitzbergen, Tristan da Cunha and the Faroe Islands.

Spitzbergen is an island on the edge of the Arctic Circle, which as recently as the 1930s was isolated from the rest of the world over the 6 month winter period. Toward the end of the winter, upper respiratory tract infections were absent from the community. The first colds and coughs appeared with the arrival of the first trade ship in spring, carried by members of the crew. As more of the islanders caught colds from one another, the

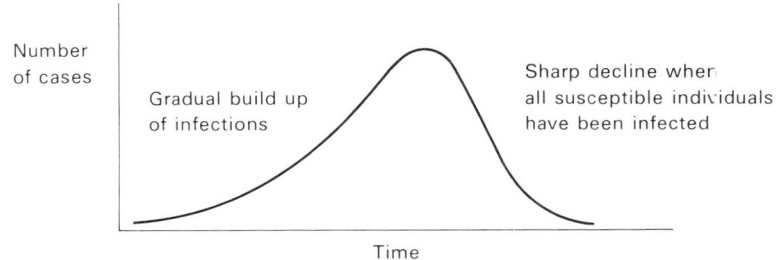

Fig. 2.1 The classic epidemiological curve.

epidemic curve rose, to reach its peak. As the year progressed, increasing numbers of people would catch colds and recover, having developed immunity to the virus. The epidemic curve would begin to decline again as the number of people recovering began to exceed the number infected. After the departure of the last trade ship, the community plunged back into Arctic winter, but it was free from upper respiratory tract infections.

Not all infections follow the classic model described above. If a number of people eat rice infected with *Bacillus cereus*, for instance, the epidemiological curve rises much more sharply, because the period of incubation is short, and all the infections develop together (Fig. 2.2). Recovery is also swifter and simultaneous, so the number of infected cases fall sharply again. When infections have a long incubation period and there is the possibility of secondary spread, the epidemiological curve will resemble the one shown in Fig. 2.3, which illustrates the response of a community to a wave of hepatitis infections. However, many epidemic illnesses occur in cycles every few years, measles and whooping cough, for example (Fig. 2.4). When an outbreak of measles occurs, every child not immune through previous exposure to the disease, and who has not received artificial immunisation (see Chapter 4), will develop the infection. The epidemic curve will rise, then fall when every child has caught measles. New cases will occur only sporadically until the next cohort of unimmunised children succumb 4 or 5 years later.

The way in which infectious illnesses spread throughout the community and the nature and behaviour of microorganisms remained shrouded in mystery until comparatively recent times. Many

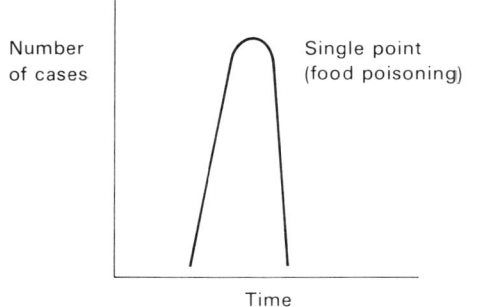

Fig. 2.2 Epidemiological curve to illustrate food poisoning (single point).

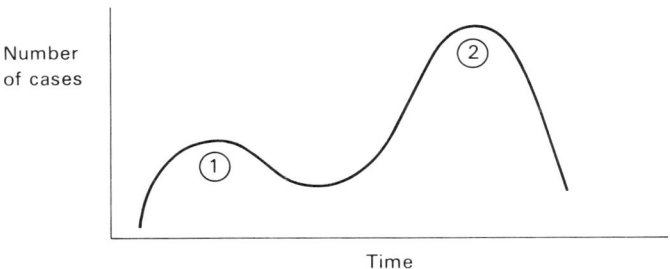

Fig. 2.3 Epidemiological curve to illustrate secondary spread.

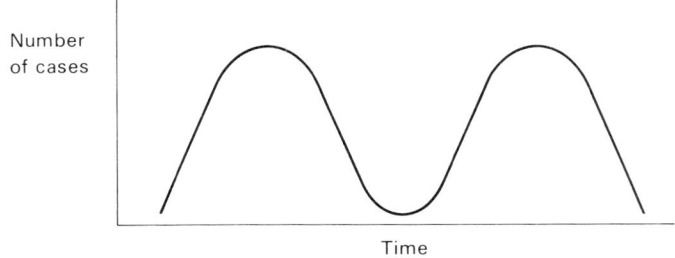

Fig. 2.4 Epidemiological curve to illustrate periodic outbreaks.

lay people today, and sometimes nurses, still have misconceptions about bacteria. Perhaps living organisms that are too small to see with the naked eye, but which continue to influence the health and welfare of people in the community and to alter the course of disease, seem to have mysterious qualities. Microbial behaviour has had an impact on the health and lives of ordinary people for centuries, and misunderstandings continue to influence current nursing practice. The history of microbiology and current research findings are therefore highly relevant to nurses working in every specialty (see Chapter 3).

HISTORICAL ASPECTS OF INFECTION

Since biblical times attempts have been made to limit the spread of infection. Lepers were forced to live apart from the rest of society and to warn other people of their presence. Ironically it is now known that leprosy, caused by *Mycobacterium leprae*, results in an indolent, chronic illness that does not appear to be highly contagious.

Infection has always generated fear, however, and sometimes this has been unreasonable; public response to AIDS is perhaps the best modern example. Today it is often difficult to staff hospital wards where infectious patients are nursed, and the problem is not new. In 1867 when an act of Parliament required fever hospitals to be built, nurses could seldom be found to work in them. They could not attract charitable funds (virtually the only source of revenue open to them at the time) and nobody wanted one built near their land. Nor would the voluntary hospitals available to the sick poor admit people with contagious illness.

The Work of Early Researchers

Francastro

As early as 1546, Francastro, observing that infection spreading between one person and another always manifested itself with the same typical symptoms, proposed that infection consisted of minute particles which could be transferred between one person and another. This idea was vastly ahead of its time.

Keddi

Throughout the course of history there has been a tendency to associate illness with punishment through divine intervention. When the inhabitants of an entire village became stricken with infection, the outbreak would frequently be blamed on 'foul vapours' or 'miasmas'. The relationship of disease to uncleanliness was generally recognised, but it was often attributed to the odour spread from swamps or areas where sewage had been allowed to drain.

Among other misconceptions was the belief, once widespread, that living organisms could develop spontaneously from non-living materials. It is not difficult to appreciate how this idea evolved. The eggs of flies deposited on meat are small and inconspicuous, but the maggots that emerge from them move and can be noticed as soon as they begin to grow. However, the theory of *spontaneous generation*, as it came to be known, was dispelled by an Italian called Francesco Keddi in 1668. He filled jars with meat and sealed them tightly. Control jars, also filled with meat, were left uncovered; maggots only appeared in the uncovered controls. Despite Keddi's work, many people remained unconvinced until Louis Pasteur's experiments in 1861.

Pasteur

Pasteur filled laboratory flasks with beef broth and boiled the contents, some left open to the air and allowed to cool; control flasks were sealed. Several days later, broth in the open flasks had obviously become contaminated, but not the controls. From his results, Pasteur hypothesised that spoilage in the open flasks had been caused by microorganisms present in the air, but that air itself could not generate microorganisms. In a second set of experiments Pasteur used flasks with long necks (Fig. 2.5), which could be bent into S-shaped curves after they had been heated. The contents of the flasks were boiled and cooled, but the openings were not sealed. Air could enter, but the shape of the neck would trap airborne particles. The broth within the flasks did not decay. Even today Pasteur's original flasks, on display in the Pasteur Institute in Paris, show no signs of contamination.

Pasteur's work demonstrated the presence of microorganisms within non-living substances, showing that they could be destroyed by heat. This led to a suggestion that heat could be used to prevent decomposition. These discoveries are of great significance to nurses because they have provided the basic principles of asepsis.

In later experiments Pasteur demonstrated the fermentation of sugar to alcohol by yeasts in the absence of air, showing once again that the change was dependent upon air. Aerobic bacteria spoil alcohol by converting it to acetic acid, so that it tastes sour; wine that has been uncorked for several days will develop a 'vinegary' taste. Pasteur

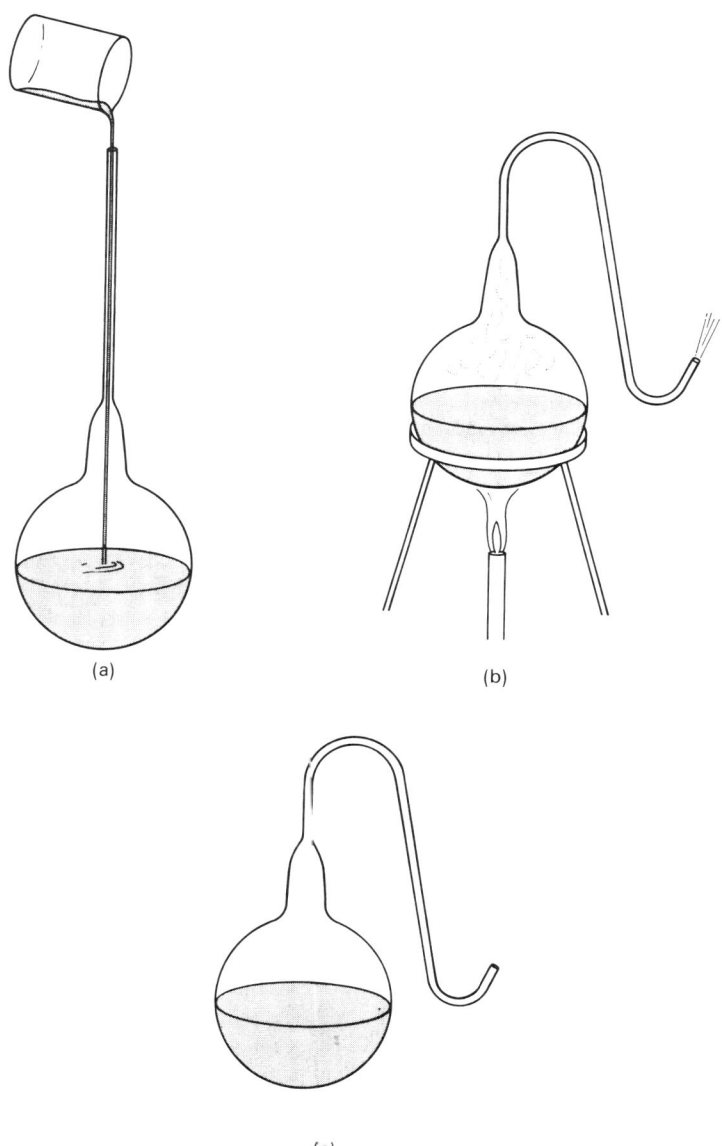

Fig. 2.5 Pasteur's experiment disproving the theory of spontaneous generation. (a) Nutrient broth poured into long-necked flask. (b) Flask contents heated, and the neck drawn into an S-shaped curve. (c) Cooled broth. No microorganisms grew because they had been destroyed by the heat. No spores or microorganisms could enter through the S-shaped neck of the flask.

developed a technique of heating alcohol to a temperature high enough to destroy most of the bacteria in it, yet without altering its taste. Today, milk as well as alcohol is pasteurised routinely. The same principle can be used to render safe crockery used by infectious patients in hospital, so that they do not have to eat from disposable plates.

Van Leeuwenhoek

Microorganisms were first drawn and described by Anton van Leeuwenhoek, a Dutch merchant with a keen interest in amateur science. He used ground glass to develop a magnifying lens, which enabled him to examine a variety of materials as diverse as rain water and the scrapings from his own teeth. From his original drawings, dating around 1673, it is possible to identify several common species of bacteria and protozoa.

The evident importance of yeast during fermentation suggested that microbial activity might be connected to physical and chemical changes in other substances, such as food spoilage. Gradually people began to realise that microorganisms might share the properties common to all living organisms, and also be responsible for disease. However, the relationship was demonstrated not among human victims of infection, but among silkworms used in the French textile industry at a time when its prosperity was threatened by an outbreak of protozoa. Pasteur devised a method of identifying the ailing silkworms, so that they could be separated from healthy ones, blocking the route of transmission.

Koch

Unequivocal proof that bacteria are responsible for the transmission of infection was provided in 1876 by Robert Koch in Germany. He identified bacteria in the blood of cattle destroyed by anthrax and grew them on an artificial culture medium (see Chapter 10) outside the tissues. He was later able to isolate the typical Gram-positive rod-shaped bacilli from the culture, inject them into healthy animals and reproduce the same symptoms of disease; the bacilli appeared in the bloodstreams of the inoculated cows. This sequence of experimental steps, affording the first really direct evidence of the relationship between specific microorganisms and a given disease, has become known as *Koch's postulates*, and they remain a vital tool in diagnostic medical microbiology. However, Koch's findings were puzzling to a number of other researchers.

Klebs and Loeffler

In 1881 Klebs and Loeffler isolated *Corynebacterium diphtheriae*, the bacillus which causes diphtheria. Fluid taken from the laboratory cultures reproduced the disease, even when all the bacteria had been filtered from it. This happened because the symptoms of diphtheria are due not to the bacteria themselves, but to their exotoxins. As a consequence of this work bacterial toxins were eventually discovered.

Semmelweiss

However, methods designed to prevent the transmission of microorganisms continued to be haphazard because they were imperfectly understood. Advances came slowly during the 18th and 19th centuries and, at first, the proponents of the theories were greeted with disbelief. In 1847 the Viennese obstetrician Semmelweiss noticed an association between the delivery by doctors and the high puerperal mortality of women. The rate of sepsis among women who had been delivered by midwives was much lower by comparison. Semmelweiss concluded that the puerperal fever which killed them had been transferred on the hands of the doctors, because they did not wash their hands between attendance in the post-mortem and delivery rooms. Semmelweiss tried to introduce a strict regime of handwashing, but he was ridiculed by his colleagues and died without ever knowing how important his work would become.

Snow

A few years later (1854), Dr John Snow demonstrated in London a geographical relationship between the occurrence of cholera and the number of people who used the Broad Street pump to obtain their household water supplies. He halted the epidemic by removing the handle of the pump. This was the first real evidence to suggest that infection can be waterborne. Snow had enacted the basic principles of epidemiology: he had identified the source of the infection, determined the population most likely to be at risk, and removed the source, although the bacteria were not identified at that time.

Snow's work prompted an improvement in sanitation in towns, and led to the introduction of an arterial system of drainage. Today, cases of cholera occur only sporadically in Britain, mainly introduced by overseas travellers.

Infection and the General Public

The dampness of the British climate unfortunately favours the survival of bacteria carried by the droplet route, since the droplets are prevented from rapidly drying out; most infectious diseases in the community are caused by respiratory pathogens spread via the air. In hospitals, infection is spread mainly by direct contact, usually on the hands of staff. Extensive research undertaken by infection control experts during the 1950s has influenced the development of nursing procedures and precautions taken to limit spread.

Any historical discussion about the transmission of infection is bound to include figures who have been remembered for their scientific discoveries. However, no discussion about trends of infection in the past can ignore their impact on ordinary people. The threat of infection cast a shadow over the population for centuries, and its influence was far stronger than it is today.

The problem of infection does not exist in a vacuum. The natural history of communicable disease is inseparable from social, political, economic and climatic influences. Battles have been won or lost because one army proved more or less susceptible to an infectious agent than the enemy. An example is the story of the early American pioneers, who carried smallpox to the Red Indian populations. The pioneers, who had been exposed to smallpox in childhood were immune, but the Red Indians had no immunity, and the infection had a devastating effect on their numbers. According to legend, the pioneers sold their smallpox-infected blankets to the Red Indians, knowing that they had no natural immunity.

Epidemics and Endemic Diseases

History is riddled with accounts of epidemics. Sometimes these are vague, others give a remarkably clear description not only of the disease, but of its likely method of spread and the havoc that followed. It is known, for example, that Athens was devastated by bubonic plague in 419 BC. Greek physicians at this time did not understand the cause of infectious disease, but they noticed a clear link between hygiene and health and took steps to improve their standards of civic sanitation. Doctors were appointed to administer all matters related to health in the towns; they were expected to check the cleanliness of drinking water, to ensure that marshes were drained, and make provision for burials. Some of the ideas current at this time have a surprisingly modern flavour: the Greeks developed the idea of holistic health; physical and mental well-being were considered to be equally important, and education was extended to encompass physical training.

Accounts of epidemics are widespread in historical writing. In contrast, endemic diseases have attracted less attention, because rather than creating a sensation they form part of everyday life.

Early man was undoubtedly plagued by parasitic disease, but epidemics probably did not develop to the extent possible in large communities because the spread of infection is dependent upon a continuous supply of new victims. Early man lived in small groups that moved between one locality and the next. Contagious disease became more of a problem when increase in the population resulted in settled townships and people crowded together, especially when the standard of living was poor. When towns and villages grow up haphazardly without civic planning, the chief problems, as the Greeks had discovered, lie in achieving an adequate method of sanitation and obtaining clean water supplies. It is for this reason that periods of economic and social change, resulting in urbanisation, are generally accompanied by outbreaks of infection. Many accounts have been described from the 14th century, since this period was marked throughout Europe by a population growth and a series of extremely poor harvests. The net result was an insufficient supply of food, and faced with prospects of starvation large numbers of peasants moved to the towns.

The Middle Ages

Throughout the Middle Ages there were epidemics of leprosy, syphilis and smallpox, but the greatest scourge was bubonic plague caused by a Gram-negative bacillus called *Yersinia pestis*. These bacteria are carried by rat fleas, and one of the ways in which accounts of plague can be recognised from old documents is through descriptions of the characteristic red and yellow discolorations of the victims' skin. In Browning's narrative poem 'The Pied Piper', the eponymous 'hero' is symbolically dressed half in red and half in yellow, representing the plague that followed the rats; the 'door in hillside' where the piper lured the town's children is a communal grave.

Bubonic plague is a particularly virulent infection because the bacilli can grow and divide in the white blood cells instead of being destroyed by them (see Chapter 7). Even today plague has not been totally eradicated from the world. It is still carried by rodents in some hot climates, and the rate of mortality among human victims is about 75% unless treatment is prompt. Death usually occurs less than a week after infection.

The Black Death in 1348 was caused by the spread of bubonic plague to England by rat-infested ships arriving from the East. No reliable mortality rates are available, but estimates suggest that in Europe, and possibly in England, at least one-third of the population died. The spread of infection was increased because frightened people already incubating plague fled from one locality to another in search of safety.

The Industrial Revolution

The Industrial Revolution, another era of population change, is associated with an upsurge in the number of infectious illnesses. British prosperity was increasing through growth of economy and increasing foreign trade. Until this time, England had been an agricultural nation; people who worked on the land or in cottage industries lived in small, isolated communities. But from the 17th century onwards, the nation became increasingly dependent on the sale of manufactured goods abroad to purchase essential food materials for the home market. Acceleration in capital investment brought a change in emphasis from farming to industry. By the turn of the 17th century, new advances in technology permitted manufacturing processes on a large scale; some people accrued wealth, and a greater gulf separated the rich from the poor. But in spite of the overall development of prosperity in Britain, poverty was widespread. People flocked from the land to work in the towns, and as these increased in size, citizens were herded together on a previously unprecedented scale. There was no civic planning and very insanitary conditions developed rapidly, further enhancing the risk of infection. Life expectancy was short and the neonatal and childhood mortality rates were extremely high. It was against this background that John Snow halted the cholera epidemic in London, and Dickens wrote his novels, nearly every one containing a description of the death of a child or young adult from tuberculosis, another typical contagious disease of the times.

The 19th Century

Although the 18th and 19th centuries described in these terms seem grim, there were glimmers of light. The age of philanthropy was dawning, and many notable people were inspired to do 'good works'. Florence Nightingale laid the foundations for a systematic and improved nurse training. Although she is remembered chiefly for her work during the Crimean War, and subsequently for founding the training school at St Thomas's Hospital in London, she was responsible for a good many more projects, including setting up a health visiting service to advise mothers about hygiene. Nightingale scorned the idea of 'germs', but she was a great proponent of hygiene. She noticed that some soldiers who occupied particular beds in wards at Scutari would succumb very quickly, and she realised that this was because they were inhaling air direct from the sewers. Her famous statement 'The hospital should do the sick no harm' has been used most aptly for at least one modern series of nursing articles on the prevention of infection in hospital.

In Florence Nightingale's time wealthy people avoided hospitals at all costs. Admission was the road to fatality. Hospitals were the havens of the very poor, and although contagious cases were not admitted, overcrowding, malnourishment and the general lack of hygiene all contributed to an exceptionally high rate of infection. Nurses, prior to the system introduced by Nightingale, slept on or near the wards, and were remunerated partly in rations of gin.

The incident of the Broad Street pump, and the threat of cholera outbreaks led to an appreciation of the need for civic planning. At this time Edwin Chadwick developed an arterial system of water supply. It is important to remember the Victorian attitudes on poverty and ill health, which were generally taken to be the direct fault of the very people who had to endure them. Chadwick, however, was more charitable. He visited the slums himself and in 1842 published a report called *Sanitary Conditions of the Labouring Population of Great Britain*. Chadwick believed that good health was dependent upon good civic engineering. So he advocated a continuous system of drainage, with separate arrangements for the supply of drinking water and the disposal of sewage; these were placed under the control of local authorities. Chadwick's report brought 19th-century Britain on a par with the standards attained centuries before by the ancient Greeks.

Advances in medicine and microbiology during the 19th century were sufficient to make an impact on public understanding and attitudes towards infection. Until the beginning of this century, the only public health machinery in Britain were quarantine regulations instituted in 1743, the regulations for health within the naval service and a newly created vaccine board. As the century unfolded attention was gradually drawn to the vital need for radical new health policies. In 1804 yellow fever was carried from overseas by ships from the West Indies to the Mediterranean; the increase in trade brought with it a greater risk of importing infection. Over a third of the population in Gibraltar died, fear spread to England, and the College of Physicians advocated the establishment of a Central Board of Health, a world-wide epidemiological centre, rigid separation of the sick and healthy, hospitals for treating infectious patients, which were to be maintained at public expense, and strict rules for fumigation and decomination. Towns where 'fevers' had been reported were advised to set up local boards, and rules for isolation were to be enforced by justices of the peace.

The Central Board of Health was established in 1804, but was disbanded soon afterwards because of its high administrative costs, and because of a false sense of security – yellow fever never actually reached British shores. In fact, throughout history Britain has managed to escape some of the worst epidemics experienced in Europe because of its geographical isolation and cool climate, unsuitable for insect vectors. This is still an important protective factor today, for example, helping to keep rabies out of the country with the aid of strict animal quarantine rules. Our major threat now is air travel, because of the speed at which foreign travellers, possibly incubating tropical fevers, can enter the country.

However, instead of an epidemic of yellow fever, Britain was plagued with cholera in the 1820s, the result of a pandemic sweeping across Asia. Despite rigorous regulations to enforce the identification and segregation of victims, and 'fumigation', the epidemic proceeded slowly but relentlessly. Cases were not easy to diagnose in the early stages, and this was possibly a major contributory factor; 5000 people had died by 1832, when the Cholera Act replaced the Central Board with local ones. Enthusiasm for these also waned with the epidemic; however, memory of the devastation perhaps contributed to acknowledgement of the work of Chadwick and Snow.

By the end of the 19th century attitudes towards hospitals were changing too. Improvements in medicine and nursing meant that for the first time treatments could be given more reliably outside the home. In fact, with the development of new diagnostic tools like X-rays, and successes in surgery made possible by Lister's discovery of the antiseptic properties of 'carbonated lime', some procedures were now impossible outside hospital. For the first time, wealthy people were admitted, and doctors became increasingly able to gather together 'interesting' cases for study under one roof. In a sense, the age of care had ended, to be replaced by the era of 'cure' so familiar today.

Health Today

For many years, the improvement in health that

took place at the end of the 19th and the beginning of the 20th century was attributed to medical advances. It was generally accepted by social historians that the increase in the size of the population was caused by a decline in the death rate made possible through advances in medicine. This traditional view has been questioned by Thomas McKeown in a series of scholarly articles, culminating in the publishing of his book *The Role of Medicine* (1979). The hypothesis put forward by McKeown, and the evidence which he uses in support of it, are of great relevance to the provision of nursing care today. Before discussing them, however, it is necessary to describe the advances in immunisation and the development of sulphonamides and antibiotics that are still important for keeping infectious illnesses at bay.

MEDICAL ADVANCES

The 18th Century

Country people have known for years that immunity to the lethal disease smallpox could be achieved by scratching the surface of the skin and introducing serum from cows which had the related but much milder cowpox infection. During the 17th century, the practice of inoculation was introduced from Turkey to the more genteel classes. It found favour among the nobility, but a good deal of confusion arose because it was not always successful. On some occasions, the process of 'variolation' led to severe and sometimes fatal infection. Jenner showed the concept of immunisation to be feasible as a preventive measure at the end of the 18th century. The secret of success lay in ensuring that the cow serum was injected deeply into the dermis of the recipient; failure often occurred because the serum was scratched ineffectively on to the epidermis.

Throughout the 18th century there is evidence that large numbers of people were immunised against smallpox (Razzell, 1977), and multiple screening programmes were organised in villages and towns. The impact of these programmes on the morbidity and mortality attached to the disease are difficult to estimate, because parish records, the only documents kept at the time, are so often incomplete. However, records from the United States suggest that the number of people who developed smallpox, as well as the number who actually died from it, declined rapidly during the 18th century.

The 19th Century

During the late 19th century, Pasteur, among several other contemporary scientists, showed that the serum of immune animals contained substances that would neutralise the toxins of the microorganism originally responsible for the infection. Pasteur developed vaccines against anthrax and rabies. Artificial immunity is now possible against a wide range of bacterial and viral diseases. To illustrate the value of immunisation the conquest of diphtheria is described below.

Diphtheria

Microscopic studies as long ago as 1882 revealed characteristic bacilli in the grey 'false membrane' which forms over the tonsils of diphtheria victims. The pathological changes were soon found to be due not to the bacteria themselves, but to a filterable toxin that they produced; a solution of the toxin could reproduce the characteristic symptoms of the disease in experimental animals. Soon it was established that animals could be immunised to make an antitoxin able to neutralise the damaging effects of the toxin. Experiments showed that this was possible in humans using the serum from immunised horses. Before this work could benefit the public, however, it was necessary to examine the natural history of diphtheria bacilli within the community, to find out the proportion of asymptomatic carriers (if any) and to determine to what extent children of different ages were able to develop natural immunity. This is the type of information still needed today in the event of a diphtheria outbreak. Carriers were identified by swabbing and culturing secretions from the back of the throat. When diphtheria was prevalent in a community in the days before immunisation, it was common to find by this method that up to 5% of apparently healthy children were carriers of the bacillus. Since individuals were generally found to carry the bacteria for only a few weeks, it was felt that children must have been reinfected on numerous occasions throughout childhood. However, even before immunisation was introduced, it was extremely rare to find that more than 10% of the children in a community were suffering from clinical diphtheria at any one time. Thus, asymptomatic carriage was for most of the time harmless.

The *Schick test* was devised to determine the presence of diphtheria antitoxin in the blood. It involves injecting a very weak solution of toxin into a child's skin; if there is sufficient concentration of antitoxin in the blood, the result is negative, because the toxin is neutralised. In the absence of antitoxin, injected toxin produces a positive result: inflammation occurs.

Epidemiological studies in New York before the introduction of diphtheria immunisation showed, as a result of Schick testing, that neonates were usually immune; they received the antitoxin from their mothers and retained it until they were about 6 months old. The lowest proportion of negative reactions occurred for children around the age of one year, but soon afterwards the process of active immunisation began to occur through casual, generally asymptomatic infection. This nearly always happened before adolescence. The epidemiological curve is shown in Fig. 2.6. In retrospect it seems that children only developed clinical manifestations of the disease if they received a particularly large infective dose, or encountered an especially virulent strain of bacteria before developing adequate immunity through harmless asymptomatic infections. Schick-negative children rarely develop diphtheria.

Clinical research has shown why there is this difference in susceptibility. If a large infective dose of diphtheria bacilli lodge on the tonsils of a child who has not yet developed immunity, they multiply on the surface of the tissues and rapidly gain access into the lining of the throat. They release toxin which destroys adjacent cells, including white blood cells. Necrosis results, providing an ideal medium for the bacilli to continue growth and toxin production. As tissue destruction accelerates, the typical 'grey' membrane forms because the bacteria and dead cells spread over the palate. Toxins leak into the blood, and the general symptoms of the disease manifest themselves.

In a child who has already managed to develop immunity, diphtheria bacilli may establish themselves temporarily in the throat, but cause only trivial damage. Antitoxin in the blood protects the superficial tissues of the tonsils from damage. Dead tissue cannot accumulate and in its absence the bacteria have only limited opportunity to multiply and are soon destroyed by phagocytosis (see Chapter 7).

In the light of this evidence it follows that in order to prevent diphtheria it is essential to ensure that every child within the community develops antitoxin *before* encountering a large infective dose

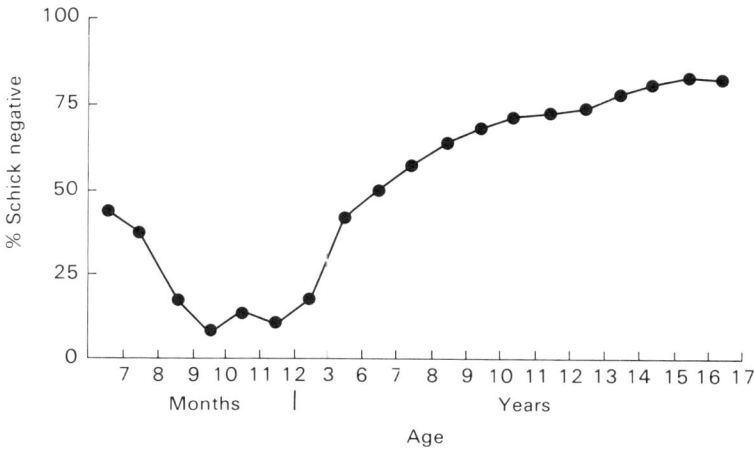

Fig. 2.6 Percentage of children developing immunity to diphtheria by age (shown by results of Schick test). If a child is immune to diphtheria, the Schick test will be negative. In the first few months of life passive immunity was conferred by maternal antibodies, but gradually lost again. Subsequent immunity was acquired from infections which were mainly subclinical.

of bacilli. This has been made possible by inoculation with formalin-treated toxin. Formalin does not destroy the ability to stimulate antitoxin production, but it destroys the harmful properties of the toxin itself.

Immunisation against diphtheria was introduced in the early 1920s. The trend of mortality for the disease in England and Wales from 1910 to 1960 is shown in Fig. 2.7.

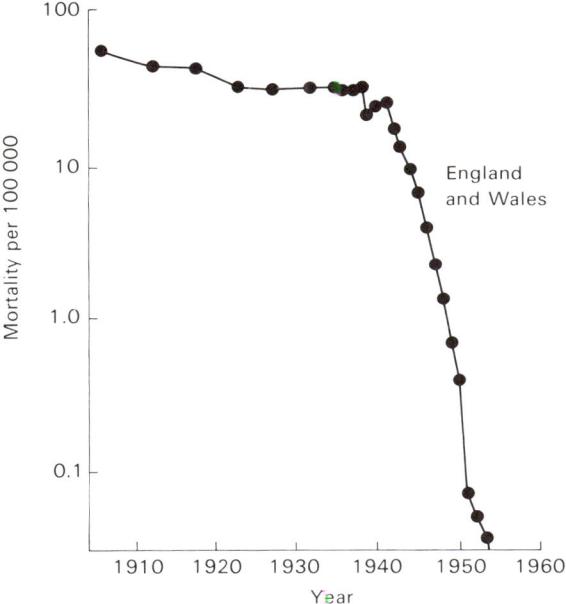

Fig. 2.7 Mortality per 100 000 from diphtheria between 1900 and 1950 (England and Wales).

Immunisation in the 20th Century

Unfortunately, the number of diseases for which immunisation is possible remain limited, mainly for technical reasons involving production. However, there are several infections for which immunisation is both feasible and desirable, yet the public is slow to seek protection from them.

Whooping Cough (Pertussis)

In 1941 there was a big epidemic of whooping cough, probably exacerbated by the evacuation of young children from cities during the early years of the war. This provided impetus for the development of a vaccine, followed by introduction on a national scale in Britain in 1957.

The incidence of whooping cough began to fall and by 1974 eight out of every ten children had been given the triple vaccination which incorporates immunisation against whooping cough (see page 91). Extensive clinical trials had suggested that the vaccine was safe, but the results of studies in the 1960s indicated that the protection was not as great as had been anticipated, so its composition was altered to increase its strength.

Side-effects have been reported following vaccination, but they are nearly always mild and do not generally last long. Concern was expressed following reports of sporadic, but serious, permanent brain damage after administration of whooping cough vaccine; 36 cases were reported by Great Ormond Street Hospital in 1974, occurring over a period of 11 years. This culminated in the formation of the Association of Parents for Vaccine Damaged Children, which demanded an enquiry into the use of the vaccine. These anxieties received serious consideration, but it was pointed out that one child in every hundred may experience an episode of convulsions during the first part of its life, and this may happen purely *by chance* shortly after the whooping cough vaccine has been given. In order to prove immunisation is the unequivocal cause of brain damage, it would be necessary to show that children who have recently been immunised have a higher incidence of neurological problems compared to a second group of children identical in every respect, apart from *not* receiving the vaccine. This was the task of a major epidemiological study entitled the National Childhood Encephalopathy Study (Alderslade *et al.*, 1981).

The details of this study can be found in Chapter 3. The research team concluded that whooping cough vaccine is only very occasionally associated with serious neurological problems and that permanent damage is very rare indeed. Parents can be reassured by health visitors that they are not placing their children at risk if they decide to have them vaccinated.

Although this research was undertaken in the 1970s, and its results have been made available to health care professionals, in recent years many parents have been reluctant to have their children vaccinated. Coverage by the media has not helped. Initially large numbers of babies received the triple vaccine, so that many health visitors, as well as young parents, have never encountered a case of whooping cough and remain ignorant of the serious and alarming nature of this infection. Antibiotics make little impression on the causative organism, *Bordetella pertussis*, so that babies become ill rapidly and may still die, especially if the family circumstances are poor and the home damp. The risks of *not* being vaccinated far outweigh the very small danger attached to the vaccine.

Measles

The situation is much the same with the measles vaccine, one of the leading public health developments of the 1960s. This disease has long been considered one of the standard episodes of childhood; lifelong immunity follows an attack of the virus. A swing of opinion took place with the growing realisation that brain damage may sometimes develop after measles. Roughly one child in every thousand will develop the severe effects of measles encephalitis, but mild brain damage seems to occur quite frequently and can alter the normal pattern of EEG waves. Uptake of measles vaccine is still disappointing; health visitors and school nurses have a leading role to play in developing awareness among young parents.

Antibacterial Drug Therapy

Immunisation is a preventive measure; antibacterial drugs can also be used in this way, but they are more often used to treat established infection.

The belief that specific substances exist to cure diseases is well established in folklore. Cookery books dating from the 17th and 18th centuries contain as many recipes to cure disease as of gastronomic interest. Little logic existed for these remedies until the end of the 19th century and the acceptance of the germ theory. Concurrent advances in organic chemistry then set the stage for effective chemical treatment of disease.

Ehrlich's Work

The father of modern chemotherapy is Paul Ehrlich, whose work in Germany showed that a drug called Salvarsan would cure syphilis. Prior to this discovery, patients were given poisonous mercury compounds. Sometimes these killed the spirochaetes, sometimes the patient!

Ehrlich observed that the dyes used in diagnostic microbiology (see Chapter 10) worked because they were taken up very strongly by bacteria. It occurred to him that if microscope dyes could be made poisonous, they might be used to destroy bacteria in living patients. He developed a yellow-coloured dye called acriflavin which is still sometimes used as a disinfectant for superficial wounds. To his disappointment it proved too toxic for internal use.

Dormagk's Work

A spectacular advance in this field was made by Dormagk in 1935. He synthesised protonsil, the first chemotherapeutic agent to be strongly effective against bacteria. Protonsil was effective because it was broken down in the liver to sulphonamide. The impact of these sulphonamide drugs was enormous. Their introduction in the 1930s made pneumonia a curable disease for the first time. The chemical structure of sulphonamides is very similar to that of para-amino benzoic acid (PABA), a growth substance essential to bacteria which the bacteria are unable to manufacture themselves. When sulphonamides are present, bacteria try to use them instead, and fail to grow.

Fleming and Penicillin

Therapeutically, sulphonamides were rapidly superseded by antibiotics. Alexander Fleming, working at St Mary's Hospital in London, also dreamed of a drug that would inactivate bacteria yet leave the patient unharmed. His laboratory was situated on the corner of the building, overlooking a busy street. Dust swirled in through the windows. Spores of the mould *Penicillium notatum* carried by the air currents settled on to a culture plate of *Staphylococcus aureus* and inhibited its growth. However, Fleming was unable to isolate the antibiotic in 1928; this was left to Ernest Chain and Howard Florey working at Oxford, and the first penicillin was purified in 1939. During the Second World War development of the drug continued in the United States. Penicillin became universally available after the war, and many other synthetic antibiotics are now available.

McKeown's Ideas

McKeown (1979) argues that the development of medicine, with the advances made in immunisation and antibiotics, are insufficient to explain the increase in birth rate and decline in death rate that occurred towards the end of the 19th century. He believes that these advances occurred at the wrong times: smallpox was conquered *before* the population changed, and antibacterial drugs were discovered *after* the event. Instead, according to McKeown, population changes occurred secondary to industrial and economic developments. Gradual improvements in nutrition, hygiene, and education (which became compulsory just before the turn of the century), increased survival rate in infancy and prolonged old age. Environmental modification also helped to control the spread of infectious diseases. This is still important in the third world, where the World Health Organisation is striving to quantify the number of infections that occur, raise public awareness, identify efficient and economic methods of prevention, and implement control measures.

MODERN PROBLEMS OF INFECTION

In Britain today, most people die of degenerative diseases, malignancies and other conditions brought on with advancing age. The aetiology of many of these conditions remains obscure. In many cases environmental influences of a lifetime interact with genetically determined factors to result in not one, but a variety of related disorders. But closer examination indicates that contemporary Britain has not yet escaped from the perils of infection. Infectious agents may contribute to diseases that for years were thought to be degenerative. Moreover, the control of infectious diseases remains very much a product of the way they are spread. Transmission of waterborne infection can be interrupted quite easily by controlling public water supply. But foodborne diseases are more difficult to prevent because strict personal hygiene is necessary. Airborne infections are often impossible to control. Upper respiratory tract infections still account for the majority of days absent from work in this country.

Two recent examples are used below to illustrate the continuing problems of infection. These have been chosen because of their notoriety, but many more exist, although they have received less media coverage.

Acquired Immune Deficiency Syndrome (AIDS)

AIDS is caused by a virus, the human immunodeficiency virus (HIV), the close relatives of which cause leukaemia. HIV attacks the T helper cells of the immune system (see Chapter 7), so that it can no longer operate. Patients become extremely susceptible to certain types of microorganisms, mainly those responsible for opportunistic infections. They do not die from AIDS itself, but from infections generally harmless to healthy people which overwhelm their immune system.

The history of AIDS in the west is brief, although it has been the subject of an enormous number of scientific articles. In 1981, clinicians and epidemiologists noticed that an unusual type of pneumonia, caused by the protozoan *Pneumocystis carinii*, was developing with surprising frequency among young, previously healthy homosexuals. It was often seen in combination with Kaposi's sarcoma, a rare tumour generally reported among the elderly. News of the disease spread to England, where the first reports of AIDS were from homosexuals who had had sexual contact with people from the United States. By 1983 a definite disease syndrome had been identified and towards the end of the year HIV had been identified as the causative agent. An antibody test was developed in 1984, the only laboratory investigation currently available. It is not a test for AIDS itself, but for the antibodies produced in response to the virus. Hence a positive result indicates merely that an individual has been exposed to HIV and responded to it. It does *not* automatically mean that this person has AIDS.

From the data available at the present time, it appears that for every hundred people in whom antibody has been detected, 75% will remain well; 15% will probably develop generalised lymphadenopathy, and the remaining 10% will develop

AIDS itself, which will probably be fatal; patients who develop its characteristic infections generally die within approximately 2 years. However, the history of AIDS is so short and data so limited that predictions are difficult. Information available from California since 1981 suggests that people who have developed lymphadenopathy do not necessarily progress to the full disease. A prospective study is still in progress; cases are being examined and data collected as the patients are diagnosed. Despite the mass hysteria that has accompanied AIDS, and gloomy predictions of exponential spread, numbers involved in the study are too small for generalisations to be made. It is not clear whether patients with lymphadenopathy are infectious, but it is assumed that they are. The condition is mild: lymph glands in the neck, groins and axillae swell; the patient may feel vaguely unwell.

AIDS has been defined by experts in communicable disease as 'The presence of a reliably diagnosed disease at least moderately indicative of a cellular immune deficiency'. The typical opportunistic infections are shown in Table 2.1. No single patient will develop them all, nor will they develop the same health problems. In Britain AIDS most commonly presents with respiratory or gastrointestinal infections. Treatment and nursing care vary with every patient. The infections may be treated with specific drugs, but no cure has yet been found for the underlying immune deficiency. The types of people most commonly affected are shown in Table 2.2.

HIV is destroyed at 80 °C and by disinfectants containing hypochlorite (Spire *et al.*, 1984). Infection control is not a problem. In hospital, precautions that are customarily taken against hepatitis B are sufficient (see Chapter 5). In the home a dilution of one-part domestic bleach (such as Domestos) to ten parts of water will destroy the virus.

Since AIDS first hit the headlines, there has been much speculation about its likely mode of spread. It is known to be disseminated in blood and blood products, and by semen during sexual activity. Spread from infected mother to baby is possible, though whether this is via the placenta or in breast milk remains to be established. HIV has also been detected in saliva and other bodily fluids, but it is not certain whether these can act as vehicles of transmission.

Similarly, there has been much preoccupation with the source of the disease. Most authorities agree that the virus has always been present somewhere in the world, recently causing havoc because it has inadvertently entered the homosexual population, becoming able to exploit the sexual mode of spread. A high incidence of opportunistic infections, coupled with Kaposi's sarcoma, has been reported among certain African tribes in

Table 2.2 Groups at Particular Risk of Developing AIDS

Homosexual/bisexual men
Haemophiliacs/recipients of blood transfusions/blood products
Intravenous drug abusers
Sexual partners of people who have AIDS
Travellers abroad, e.g. Africa

Table 2.1 Opportunistic Infections that Have Been Reported Among Patients with AIDS

Microorganism	Classification	Nature of infection
Cryptosporidium	Protozoan	Gastrointestinal infection
Pneumocystis	Protozoan	Pneumonia
Toxoplasma	Protozoan	Pneumonia CNS infection
Strongyloides	Helminth (worm)	Pneumonia, CNS or disseminated infection
Aspergillus	Fungus	CNS or disseminated infection
Candida	Fungus	Oesophagitis
Cryptosporidium	Fungus	Pulmonary, CNS or disseminated infection
Mycobacterium	Bacteria	Atypical tuberculosis
Cytomegalovirus	Virus	Pulmonary, gastrointestinal or CNS infection
Herpes simplex	Virus	Mucous membrane, pulmonary or gastrointestinal tract infections

which young women are traditionally available only to elder members; consequently, young men resort to homosexuality.

Food Poisoning

Salmonella food poisoning has been mentioned in Chapter 1, and is discussed again in Chapter 10. In the summer of 1985 19 people died in a hospital for the mentally ill in the north of England. Salmonellae in uncooked chicken were transferred to cold roast beef, either on the hands, or on the blade of a slicing machine in the kitchen. The patients died through failure of staff to observe the commonsense rules of kitchen hygiene, a result of poor supervision on the part of the catering managers. The outbreak began over a bank holiday weekend, soon after the contaminated meat was eaten. The report describing the outbreak stated that it was 'frightening' in its scale and rapidity of onset. By 7 am the following morning the first patient was ill and 2 hours later 36 patients in eight wards were affected. By the end of the first day, 94 patients had become ill and one had died. Altogether, over 400 patients and staff were affected, and 19 patients died.

The nurses who worked on the wards were placed under tremendous pressure, but very little cross-infection occurred, and their efforts were commended in the inquiry which followed the outbreak. Senior nurse managers were heavily criticised, however, and the outbreak sparked a national inquiry into the role of public health doctors and the control of communicable disease.

CONCLUSIONS

Clearly the prevention of infection and education of the public are major nursing tasks in both hospital and in the community. To understand the principles of prevention, nurses must have a knowledge of clinical infection and epidemiology. Information about both these subjects has been provided by research studies. Some of these have been good, some less good, because the method used to obtain the information has been flawed, interfering with the interpretation of results. In order to judge whether or not research findings are sound, and fit to be introduced into clinical practice, it is necessary to be aware of the shortcomings of the studies. Chapter 3 deals with research appreciation, so that information in later chapters can be held in proper perspective.

References

Alderslade, R., Bellman, M. H., Rawson, N., Ross, S. B., Miller, E. M. (1981). The National Childhood Encephalopathy Study. In: *Whooping Cough. Reports from the Committee on Safety of Medicines and the Joint Committee on Vaccination and Immunisation.* HMSO, London.

Burnet, M., White, D. O. (1972). *Natural History of Infectious Disease*, 4th edn. Cambridge University Press, Cambridge.

Chadwick, E. (1842 reprinted 1965). *The Sanitary Conditions of the Labouring Population of Great Britain.* Longmans, London.

McKeown, T. (1979). *The Role of Medicine*. Blackwell, Oxford.

Razzell, P. (1977). *The Conquest of Smallpox*. Caliban Books, Firle, Sussex.

Spire, B. *et al.* (1984). Inactivation of lymphadenopathy-associated virus by chemical disinfectants. *Lancet*, 2: 899–900.

Further Reading

Burnet, M., White, D. (1972). *Natural History of Infectious Disease*. Cambridge University Press, Cambridge.

Khatib, H. (1986). Acute gastroenteritis in infants. *Nursing Times*, 82 (23): 31–32.

McNeil, W. (1979). *Plagues and Peoples*. Penguin, Harmondsworth.

Miller, D., Webber, J., Green, J. (eds) (1984). *The Management of Aids Patients*. Macmillan, Basingstoke.

Morgan-Capner, P., Griffiths, G. (1984). Foetal and neonatal infection. *Nursing Times*, 80 (45): 28–32.

Pancham, J. (1986). Complications of measles. *Nursing Times*, 82 (23): 42–47.

Peckam, C. (1986). Immunisation. *Nursing Times*, 82 (34): 29–34.

Chapter 3

Nursing, Research and Infection

INTRODUCTION: WHERE DOES INFORMATION COME FROM?

How do we obtain our knowledge? Generally people notice things from personal experience and direct observation. Nurses who work with a particular patient or client group may become aware of similarities between the people they care for, so that certain broad generalisations can be made. A nurse who has had experience with the terminally ill may notice that a high proportion develop pain that they describe in a particular way. Eventually, by trying out different approaches, she may find some measure that seems particularly helpful in relieving this type of pain. Some of her ideas may be obtained from colleagues or from information in nursing books and magazines. In time, she will contribute her ideas to other nurses, and if they seem particularly interesting or unusual, she might feel encouraged to publish them.

Few people would deny the value of personal experience gleaned over time, especially that of people who work in a specialist field. This has always been true of nursing, which has been described as an art as well as a science (Crow, 1981). However, too great a reliance upon anecdote and casual observation can be dangerous, as it may lead to ritualistic behaviour practised without question. This, again, happens a lot in nursing. One example will be sufficient (case study 3.1).

The article published as a result of this success is a typical case study featuring the care of just one patient, with sweeping generalisations made on behalf of the new and novel treatment it describes. Published case studies and reports provide a good deal of information about the individual patient described, but they are concerned with only one incident or one individual, and have obvious limitations. No real scientific evidence could be suggested to explain why stericula treatment had been effective, and other factors that might have

---

Case study 3.1

A nurse was delegated responsibility for the care of an extremely sick patient who had an extensive pressure sore, positioned so that dressings were difficult to apply. She felt that as the patient was terminally ill, his wound would probably not heal well, and that her main task should focus on measures designed to promote comfort. She had previously had experience of dressing stoma wounds, which may sometimes become badly excoriated, and had found that this could be relieved with stericula powder (Wallace and Hayter, 1984). She applied this powder to the pressure sore, and was surprised that over a few days the wound showed signs of marked improvement.

Similar results were obtained when stericula was used as a topical preparation for the pressure sores of other patients on the same unit. An article was published describing its efficiency, and stericula gained an enthusiastic following for pressure sore treatment throughout the hospital.

---

enhanced healing were not taken into account. Improved nutritional status or the increased availability of nursing aids to relieve pressure might have been important, or possibly all three factors operating in combination. Perhaps, after the initial unexplained success, nurses on the unit began to take greater interest in patients with pressure sores, so that a better standard of care was received overall, as often happens when new methods of treatment are introduced (David, 1982).

There is always the danger that interest in a new treatment may wane once its use has become commonplace, accompanied by a decline in the level of attention received by the patient and recurrence of pressure sores that seem intractable. Judging by the number of 'wonder treatments' reported for established pressure sores, this may be a common occurrence.

Wallace and Hayter (1984) did not conduct any trials to determine the effectiveness of stericula as a topical treatment for pressure sores before advocating that it should be used for this purpose, despite the fact that it is not in fact manufactured for treating this type of lesion. Not surprisingly, many other nurses attempting to use stoma care products to heal established pressure sores have been disappointed with their results. A ritual for treating this type of lesion has developed, and its actual value has not yet been conclusively demonstrated.

Observations can be beneficial if they spark off a line of enquiry that results in controlled testing of a new product or new procedure, planned so that its value can be explored. Some of the practical problems encountered during trials to examine the effectiveness of topical wound care agents and disinfectants are discussed later in this chapter.

THE NEED FOR NURSING RESEARCH

It is evident that patient care should be based on methods that are, wherever possible, of demonstrable value, and this is one of the functions of research undertaken in the field of nursing practice. Clearly, if stericula, for example, is not really helping wounds to heal, then an expensive product is being used wastefully. Since the effect of stericula on the tissues of an established pressure sore has never been properly investigated, it is also possible that this preparation might have a deleterious effect. Indiscriminate use of equipment in this way is thus unprofessional and potentially dangerous.

McLeod-Clark and Hockey (1979) provide one of the most satisfactory definitions of research, which they describe as a 'planned, systematic activity' with the aim of increasing our 'available body of knowledge'.

The key words of their definition are 'planned' and 'systematic'. The term research implies a highly organised, tightly controlled process, irrespective of the subject of enquiry or the method of investigation. In reality this description is often distorted. Visiting a library to obtain a few selected articles about a topic or asking a small number of conveniently available people for their opinions do *not* constitute research.

According to McLeod-Clark and Hockey, research is necessary to extend knowledge in some chosen sphere. More specifically, in clinical nursing, research is required to ensure that the patient receives care of demonstrable value. In direct contrast to this situation, however, a great many nursing practices and procedures depend heavily upon rituals and traditions like the one described above, and they continue to be conducted in a prescribed manner because they were once found to be beneficial for just a few individual patients.

Button (1986), attempting to review the literature to describe the theory and rationale underlying the aseptic dressing procedure, found a dearth of research reports. Hunt (1974) had conducted a study in three schools of nursing which conclusively demonstrated that learners employed a different technique on the ward from the one they had been taught in schools of nursing. The procedure was different in each of the three hospitals visited. The only other references relating to the conduct of the procedure dated from the very early 1960s and the Second World War (one paper in each instance). Although Hunt cited both of these as evidence in support of the aseptic dressing technique, they cannot really be regarded in this light, since both were published prior to the introduction of central sterilising services department (CSSD), and the earlier report describes a situation in which dressings were conducted by a doctor, with the aid of two nurses – one handling clean dressings, the other contaminated ones.

A decrease in the number of wound infections was reported in the earlier study after the introduction of aseptic technique, but several other changes were instigated at the same time, so that it is impossible to determine the real reason for improvement. In view of the flimsy evidence available to support the value of the dressing technique as it is currently practised, it is difficult to envisage how the complicated procedures involving clean and dirty forceps and other refinements could have evolved. The value of the aseptic dressing technique is further discussed in Chapter 9.

The degree to which patients actually benefit from many other nursing practices and procedures is unclear. For example, a team of nurses led by David *et al.* (1983) indicated that nurses working in different hospitals throughout the country used a total of 98 different products to treat established pressure sores. Many of these were restricted to one particular ward or unit.

A nurse and consultant exploring the care of catheterised patients found procedures to be unstandardised and without rationale (Kennedy and Brocklehurst, 1982).

The length of time that patients are starved prior to surgery and diagnostic investigations also appears to be haphazard (Hamilton Smith, 1972). When they were questioned, student nurses seemed largely unaware of the reason for starvation prior to anaesthesia, or the minimum length of time necessary for fasting. Jones (1975) found the nutrition of patients in medical wards to be neglected, and there is evidence that this is still the case (see Chapter 4).

A great many misconceptions have developed over the years, and become incorporated ritualistically into patient care. The results of a study published in 1975 (Wilson, 1975) suggested that nurses' overall knowledge of the biological sciences was poor and significantly less complete than that anticipated by their medical colleagues. Since biology helps to lay the foundations of good bedside nursing care it is likely that patients may have suffered through this omission. It appears that this situation is perpetuated: Akinsanya (1985) found that student nurses had a poor understanding of biological principles, one of the greatest deficiencies being in microbiology. Understanding the nature of infection and its prevention may well be hindered under these circumstances. In Akinsanya's study one of the main problems seemed to be that nurse teachers felt they had been insufficiently prepared to teach physiology, microbiology and pharmacology. All these subjects have direct relevance to the care of patients who are susceptible to infection or who have an established infection.

Good nursing care depends not merely on the ability to understand the pathophysiology of a given disease and applying this knowledge, but on the ability to understand the needs and feelings of the person who receives care. Communication is the essence of nursing. It is crucial to the care of a patient who has an infection because he will need to understand the reasons for the restrictions imposed upon him and, if at all possible, be encouraged to participate in his own care. Unfortunately, there is some suggestion that nurses do not transfer the information relating to communication that is provided in the classroom to the practical care of patients in the wards (Gott, 1984).

The need for nursing research has been much publicised among members of the profession, and nurses at every level today are encouraged to become 'research-minded'. In the light of the studies described above, this does not appear to be an unreasonable request. However, when interpreting the results of any study, much will depend upon the way in which the findings have been presented, and the ability of the reader to interpret them in a meaningful way. Much also depends on the method used to collect the data, for this may bias the results. Not all nurses need or wish to conduct their own research studies, but all need to understand how research findings are obtained and analysed, so that they can interpret findings intelligently and determine their applicability to the particular situations in which they work.

The main research methods employed in nursing are outlined briefly below. They are explained in other textbooks in greater detail than is possible here; a selection is provided in the further reading list at the end of the chapter.

RESEARCH METHODS IN NURSING

Most of the research methods used in nursing investigations have their origins in social science. Epidemiological studies and those which demand laboratory techniques have been conducted less often, chiefly because most nurses in a position to undertake research have had more education in the sphere of social rather than biological science, endorsing the findings of Akinsanya (1985).

Different authors have categorised research studies in a variety of ways. Perhaps one of the most helpful is to distinguish between the following approaches:

- exploratory (descriptive) research,
- experimental or intervention studies,
- evaluative research.

Each is discussed briefly in turn, wherever possible drawing upon studies that have been concerned with problems relating to infection.

Exploratory Research

Research that is of an exploratory nature seeks to document an existing situation without manipulating it or introducing change. Presly (1984) refers to this rather aptly as 'look and see' research. Examples include the study by David *et al.* (1983) previously described, in which the authors documented the care of established pressure sores in England and Wales (see Chapter 9) and Gould's investigation (1985) of nurses' ability to undertake isolation nursing precautions (see Chapter 6).

Studies like these are valuable because they highlight problems and lay the foundations for further work of an experimental nature. For example, there are plans to investigate in greater detail the effect of different topical agents on pressure sore healing.

The methods most commonly used when carrying out this type of research are shown in Table 3.1. They are frequently used in conjunction with one another, to help corroborate findings. A researcher wanting to find out how often ward sisters throughout one health district viewed the services offered by the infection control team might lack the time to visit each ward. Instead questionnaires might be used to gather opinions, but a percentage of the sisters might be interviewed in depth. Possibly some interviews might also have been conducted in a preliminary pilot study to find out the type of information likely to be collected. This would help with the design of the questionnaire used for the main study. Ward records might also be examined, to determine how often the infection control nurse and microbiologist had visited each ward.

Table 3.1 Research Methods

Questionnaires
Surveys
Participant and non-participant observation
Content analysis of existing documents

Exploratory studies are a typical feature of newly developing academic disciplines, because they help to map out territory for future experimental work. It is not, therefore, surprising that more nursing research studies fall into this category than into any other. Several researchers have approached infection control in this way.

A small-scale study undertaken by a clinical teacher to enquire into the hand hygiene of hospital patients found that facilities for handwashing were seldom provided for bedfast patients after they had used a bedpan. When the same patients became ambulant their hand hygiene was observed to be satisfactory and all said that they would wash their hands after using the toilet at home. They thought that the nurses were 'too busy' to bring bowls of water every time a bedpan was used, a view shared by the ward nurses (Lawrence, 1983). Jackson (1983) used a questionnaire and laboratory methods involving microscopy, culture and antibiotic sensivity testing (see Chapter 10) to compare the effects of cleaning sheepskins on the ward and in the hospital laundry. Practices on 33 wards were examined: seven wards did not use sheepskins as a nursing aid; on nine wards sheepskins were always processed in the hospital laundry, where acceptable levels of disinfection could be achieved; on the remaining 17 wards, sheepskins were generally cleaned in a bathroom or sluice, then dried on radiators. Use of the laundry was avoided because the nurses did not understand the supply system for obtaining nursing aids within their hospital. Some attempted to disinfect as well as to wash sheepskins, but the disinfectants employed were either inappropriate or diluted beyond effectiveness (see Chapter 5).

Bacterial contamination of sheepskins is inevitable in view of the patients (often immobile and incontinent) who need them most. Jackson found that sheepskins in use were contaminated with both *Staphylococcus aureus* and Gram-negative bacilli. More disturbingly, three of the 23 newly cleaned sheepskins that she subjected to bacteriological testing were also contaminated, indicating that this procedure was inadequate when conducted on a ward.

The study took place throughout the summer months. In winter, when more patients may require sheepskins, levels of contamination may be higher.

Contaminated sheepskins may also act as reservoirs of infection (Meers and Stronge, 1980). They represent a hazard to patients by acting as fomites (see Chapter 1). The serious nature of this situation was reflected in Jackson's findings, since a high proportion of the bacteria isolated from the sheepskins were resistant to many of the clinically important antibiotics.

In another study, conducted by an infection control specialist (Greaves, 1985), questionnaires, methods of observation and laboratory studies were used to examine the risks of infection presented by bedbathing. By unobtrusively marking a washbowl it was possible to determine the purposes for which it was used on several consecutive days. Many were unaesthetic: for example, using the same bowl to soak the underwear of a patient who had been incontinent, then to wash patients. Observation showed that flannels were seldom rinsed, and disposable paper clothes proved to be less of an infection control hazard, as well as being acceptable to patients. The water was rarely changed during the bedbath, and at the end of the procedure sampling revealed heavy contamination by Gram-negative bacilli.

The findings of exploratory research are frequently distressing to nurses because they have so often drawn attention to practices that are poor, not always taking into consideration the resources available. Authors have sometimes made rather idealistic suggestions for future practice. All the studies discussed above had negative findings. Those conducted by Lawrence and Jackson speak for themselves. David's team found that nurses employed 98 different preparations to treat established pressure sores. There was little rationale behind their choice. Gould showed that isolation precautions were poorly understood, although the hospitals in which she conducted interviews were situated in an inner city area where the prevalence of infectious disease was high. Kennedy and Brocklehurst could point out many instances of thoughtless catheter care.

Despite an increasing body of research reports to highlight indifferent nursing care, little exists to provide clear evidence of practices that are sound. There is, for example, no lack of information about possible methods for the treatment of established pressure sores in the nursing and medical journals (see David, 1982), but it is often contradictory and confusing. Despite more than 20 years of enquiry, commencing with the pioneering work of Norton *et al.* (1962) information exists mainly about what should *not* be done to pressure sores, rather than emphasising local treatments that may reduce infection rates and promote healing.

There is a dearth of clinical nursing research in comparison with the amount that is concerned with nursing education and management, possibly because most nurses in a position to undertake research have been prepared in the social rather than the natural sciences and draw heavily upon sociological and psychological research methods. The work of infection control nurses is exceptional in this respect.

Questionnaires

The earliest research studies to enter the nursing literature in Britain explored the reasons behind the high wastage rate in nurse training. They were conducted not by nurses themselves, but by sociologists. Questionnaires were generally used, as these have the advantage of being relatively cheap (postage rates are not costly compared to the length of time required for interviews and the inevitable travelling) and convenient for the researcher conducting the study.

The disadvantage of questionnaires is that the rate of response may be low. If only 60% of the subjects contacted return questionnaires, then the views of the remaining 40% will never be known. The very reason for failing to respond to the questionnaire may set non-responders as different from the responders. If, for example, a questionnaire was designed to find out the average income of a given sample of people, those who were low wage earners might feel inclined not to respond about this sensitive area. In this case, if a 60% rate of response was obtained, it might cause the researcher to suppose that the subjects in his sample were more affluent on average than was in fact the case. Alternatively, those with modest incomes might not be alone in their failure to return questionnaires. Subjects with very high incomes might prefer not to do so in the fear that they would be traced by the Inland Revenue.

The information provided by responders may well be incomplete or an approximation of the truth, or the subject may fail to understand the questions. The opportunity to probe and rephrase questions possible in an interview will inevitably be lost.

Questionnaires remain an extremely popular method of data collection among nurse researchers; most of the studies mentioned so far in this chapter involve the use of a questionnaire as part of the research design. The frequency with which questionnaires are employed tends to overlook the skilled and time-consuming nature of their construction and the fact that the responders – often patients or other nurses – are expected to spend considerable time completing them.

The results of any questionnaire or interview study depend very much upon the way in which questions are asked. Different types of questions are illustrated in Table 3.2, which show how subjects may provide different information when faced with an open-ended question that leaves them free to choose their own words, or when confronted with a closed question forcing their choice of response.

The responses of closed questions are obviously very much easier to analyse. For open questions, which have not been formulated in a skilful manner, analysis will be complicated to the point where findings are no longer very meaningful. Examples of poor question wording are shown in Table 3.3.

Interviews

Interviews involve direct communication between the researcher and the research subjects. The researcher will write down (or tape record) verbal information provided by the subject. The rapport achieved between the two is very important. A researcher who seems brusque or uninterested is not likely to obtain good cooperation. Skill is needed when framing questions, even if they have been prepared in advance, and the conversation must be guided carefully back to the topic if the subject is inclined to provide a great deal of extraneous information. When the interview is planned, embarrassing or thought-provoking questions are best left towards the end, so rapport has been established and the subject is talking freely. However, the final questions should be of a bland, general nature, since the subject could be left feeling angry or unsatisfied if controversial points were raised at this late stage.

Data collected by interviews are generally more

Table 3.2 Closed and Open Questions

Closed question:
   Have you been given much information about the infection?:
   Please tick
      Yes
      No
      Not sure

Open question:
   Have you been given much information about the infection?

Some possible responses to this question:
(1) Yes, the doctor said that the wound would hurt for several days and to go on taking the antibiotics.
(2) Yes, but I don't remember much. The doctor mentioned something about tablets.
(3) No, I really wanted to ask, but the doctor is always so busy.
(4) No, only about taking the tablets.
(5) I can't remember.
(6) I can't remember, really. They told me the wound would hurt, and that I would need antibiotics for about a week, but that was all.

Table 3.3 Question Construction: Some Common Errors

(1) Have you been given any information about the infection and the wound?
    This is a double-barrelled question. Later the researcher will have no way of knowing whether the information recorded was specifically in relation to the infection, the wound, or both.
(2) You *have* been given information about the infection?
    This is a leading question. A timid person might not feel able to contradict, even if the information provided had not been sufficient. Even a question that has been carefully constructed can be leading if some of the words are heavily emphasised during an interview.

Poorly worded questions may also be ambiguous, particularly if double negatives are used.

rich than from questionnaires but there will always be some topics that certain people will not feel happy to discuss, and they *may* be more likely to provide information on an anonymous questionnaire. In a big study conducted by professional interviewers this is not a problem, because subjects will always be assured of confidentiality. However, when the researcher happens to be a nurse in the same hospital, her colleagues may be wary of saying too much. It is worth noting at this point that several of the small studies previously described in this chapter were undertaken by nurses working in precisely this situation. Another important point to be taken into consideration when asking *any* question is the place where the encounter occurs. Patients and nurses may feel rushed when interviews take place on a busy ward, or inhibited if it is likely that the conversation will be overheard.

Sometimes, when large-scale studies are conducted, it will be necessary to employ more than one interviewer. Problems can arise because of differences in interview technique. One interviewer may be extremely sympathetic in manner, encouraging subjects to talk more and enlarge upon their experiences. The additional encouragement may not be verbal. The way that the interviewer sits, or her facial expression, may suggest greater empathy to the subject. Some interviewers may write faster than others and manage to record more information when questions are open.

These difficulties are referred to collectively as *interviewer bias*. They are eliminated as far as possible by training interviewers, and emphasising that *everything* the subject says in response to an open question must be recorded. The attitude of the interviewer is very important. In the study by David *et al.* (1982) the research team believed that the nurses they interviewed felt able to discuss the treatment of pressure sores, often regarded as a symptom of indifferent nursing care, because of the non-judgemental attitude of the interviewers.

Observation

Observation is a major research method in social science that has not been used to any extent in nursing. In participant observation, the researcher works alongside the subject, looking out for the points of interest at the same time. In non-participant observation, like the study of wound dressings conducted by Hunt (1974), the researcher watches the subjects and records her findings at the same time, introducing less bias because she does not depend on memory. A checklist of points to watch must be devised. The researcher will otherwise be extremely selective in her recordings.

In nursing, non-participant observation is particularly hard to do, since most nurses would feel uncomfortable if they noticed that a patient was in discomfort or placed at risk and were obliged by the requirements of their study not to intervene.

Research Instruments

Questionnaires, interview schedules and checklists are research instruments. Psychological tests of personality, IQ, anxiety, depression, etc. are further examples of research instruments originally developed by social scientists that have been used in nursing studies. A well-designed research instrument must be valid, reliable and sensitive. These terms are explained and examples given in Table 3.4. With all these points to bear in mind it is clear that a research report cannot be read and 'absorbed' like a novel: the way in which the study was conducted is of central importance to the way in which the results are interpreted. If Lawrence (1983), for example, had asked nurses how often they offered patients the opportunity to wash hands instead of observing what they actually did, the findings of her study might have been different.

Table 3.4 Research Terms: Validity, Reliability and Sensitivity

Validity: A valid research instrument is one that actually measures what it sets out to measure. There are, for example, two reasons for anxiety. An individual may feel anxious when faced with a threatening situation (state anxiety) or feel anxious most of the time, because this is an inherent part of his personality (trait anxiety). A questionnaire designed to measure state anxiety administered during the hospital admission procedure would not give very meaningful information about trait anxiety since hospital admission is highly stressful. It would not, therefore, be valid.

Reliability: The reliability of a research instrument is its repeatability, under the same conditions, with comparable subjects over time. For example, a questionnaire that showed that a particular group of hospital patients were knowledgeable about their illness one day, but lacking knowledge the next day, would not be reliable.

Sensitivity: The scale of the measuring instrument should be sufficiently fine to detect differences in the amount of the variable that it is measuring. An instrument designed to measure boredom among patients nursed in isolation would not be sufficiently sensitive if it showed that mildly and heavily affected people both had the same degree of boredom.

Sample Size

Sample size is another important issue, and is often a problem in nursing research, where samples have sometimes been so small that the results cannot be generalised to other situations. In the study by Gould (1985), for example, only 60 nurses were interviewed about isolation nursing techniques, and the number of sisters included in the study was very small. This was thought to constitute a major problem, since it is generally the sister who decides how procedures will be conducted on her ward. Gould visited wards in the afternoon, when they were less busy and interviewed any nurses that were available. Her sample was therefore one of convenience, and this could have introduced bias into her findings; nurses who preferred not to be interviewed could have made themselves too busy.

Random Samples

To avoid this type of bias, a random sample should be used wherever possible. A random sample is one in which every subject in the entire population that could be examined is given an equal chance of inclusion. If Gould had had sufficient time to do this, she would have taken the name of every nurse in the hospital and interviewed the first 60 to be pulled out of a hat, making sure that the slips of paper on which they were written had been thoroughly jumbled up. A more sophisticated approach would be to assign every nurse a number and use a published list of random numbers to select 60 subjects. A series of numbers written down out of the researcher's head would be no substitute for a published list compiled by computer, because people have preference for particular numbers (for example, three and seven) and this could introduce a subtle bias.

A second problem that affects the generalisability of Gould's findings was the health district in which the study took place. It was situated in an inner city area where the prevalence of many communicable diseases was unusually high and isolation was often arranged on a special ward. Many hospitals do not have a separate isolation ward (see Chapter 10). The results cannot, therefore, be extrapolated to the situation in other health districts, and care was taken to point this out in the original report. The study by David et al. (1983) was able to surmount this problem. A large number of pressure sores were examined, and many nurses interviewed in a sample drawn from hospitals throughout England and Wales.

This study was funded externally by the DHSS, and the work was conducted by a team of experienced interviewers. All too often in nursing, small-scale studies are undertaken as a matter of necessity, frequently by people with limited resources and little experience. This is potentially a dangerous situation when the shortcomings inherent in the study are not taken into account. Another related difficulty is the lack of replication of nursing research studies. Many are conducted by nurses required to undertake a special project as part of a course requirement or higher degree, and they are never repeated.

Intervention Studies

In contrast to exploratory studies, the results of intervention studies are often more interesting and encouraging to clinical nurses. In this type of study the researcher sets out to test a hypothesis: 'If x is done to patients in this sample, then y will follow'. From this, it would be possible to conclude that the intervention x caused y to follow. A control group would be used, identical to the experimental subjects, except that they would not experience the intervention y.

The main difference between exploratory and intervention studies is that causal relations become much more clear, since the researcher introduces control into the situation as well as asking questions or making observations. For example, a researcher might set out to test the hypothesis: 'If a new disinfectant D is introduced to treat wounds that have become infected, then the infections will clear up in n number of days'. An experiment would be set up where the researcher deliberately manipulated one major factor (called the independent variable), the application of the new disinfectant, in order to assess its effect on a second factor (the dependent variable) which is the number of days required for infection to resolve.

Before embarking on the full study, the researcher would probably wish to carry out a smaller scale pilot study on a few subjects, to ensure that the design of the experiment was feasible. This could help to answer a number of important practical questions.

The nurses using the disinfectant must all apply it in the same way, as laid down by the experimental design, and they must be trained so that they all recognise the point when inflammation and other symptoms of infection disappear. If questions are to be asked, for example to patients, to find out whether they find application of the disinfectant painful, it must be ensured that they can understand the questions and are willing to answer them honestly.

Some kind of assessment and measurement will be necessary in a study of this kind. This may be qualitative. The research subjects may be categorised only as behaving or not behaving in a particular way – for example, being infected or not being infected after the specified number of applications of the disinfectant. In other cases, quantitative measurements may be required. Bacteria cover the entire surface of the human skin, including a wound, but whether they are actively damaging the tissues and setting up infection is a different matter. In the laboratory, the number of bacteria present, and the white blood cell count obtained from a wound swab, are used to determine the presence of clinical infection. These are quantitative measurements. It follows that the measuring device must be reliable, valid and sensitive (see Table 3.4).

After the data have been collected, they will be analysed and presented in a final report, which may be published. The stages of the research process, which are common to both exploratory and intervention studies, are shown in Table 3.5.

Table 3.5 Stages of the Research Process

(1) Asking the research question
(2) Literature search
(3) Choosing data collection methods; planning the research design
(4) Data collection
(5) Analysis
(6) Presentation of results – written report and publication

Boore's Study

An important intervention study in the British nursing literature is Boore's (1978) investigation of the effect of information-giving on stress during postoperative recovery. Physiological stress decreases the immunological defence mechanisms and delays healing (see Chapter 7) and the recovery of postoperative patients. Boore hypothesised that providing preoperative patients with specific information about what to expect on the day of the operation and during the postoperative period would decrease the amount of stress experienced and promote recovery. Information was given to an experimental group of patients, undergoing either cholecystectomy, or hernia repair (herniorrhaphy). To rule out any advantages the experimental patients might gain simply because someone was taking special interest in them, a control group of cholecystectomy and hernia patients spent the same time chatting to a researcher, but did not receive information.

The effects of psychological stress were assessed by asking patients how they felt and reports from ward staff who did not know the group to which the patients had been assigned. Indicators of physiological stress were obtained by collecting 3 hourly urine samples to measure the levels of steroid hormones (which increase with additional stress), temperature, the number of doses of analgesia, and the incidence of complications.

The day-to-day work was conducted by two research assistants: one assigned the patients randomly to either the experimental or control group and was responsible for the intervention; the other collected the data without knowing the group to which the patient had been assigned.

In the experimental group only two patients developed wound infections compared to eight in the control group. Two of the experimental patients developed respiratory infections, but five respiratory infections developed among control patients. Taking the other measures into consideration, the control patients appeared to make less good recovery and to experience more stress, since their urinary output of steroids was overall higher than that of the experimental subjects. When the herniorrhaphy patients were considered separately, there were few differences between experimental subjects and controls. However, two cholecystectomy patients in the experimental group had wound infections compared to seven control patients while only one experimental subject had a respiratory infection compared to four controls.

Structuring the Study

The same careful attention must be paid to intervention studies as to exploratory ones. Questions must be framed as unambiguously as possible; measuring instruments must be valid, sensitive and reliable; wherever possible samples should be obtained randomly and subjects allocated to control and experimental groups in a random fashion.

In addition to the problems shared with exploratory research, intervention studies present a number of difficulties of their own, particularly in relation to ethics. In a study of the kind undertaken by Boore, how can a researcher justify giving some treatment which is considered to be beneficial to one group of patients while withholding it from another? It is of course possible to argue that the control patients in Boore's study were not actually denied anything that they would normally have received; the information provided to experimental subjects by the research team was *additional* to the information routinely supplied by the medical and nursing staff, so this was not withheld during the study. Another point is that no intervention can definitely be regarded as beneficial until the findings of the study in question have been analysed. Numerous research findings have indicated the provision of information to surgical patients to have been beneficial (see Dumas, 1963; Lindeman and van Aernan, 1971; Hayward, 1975). Others, probably less often mentioned in the literature, tend not to support these findings (Ozbolt-Goodwin, 1979; Webb and Wilson-Barnett, 1983).

Perhaps a more difficult question is the amount of information that should be provided to people who are asked to take part in a research study. The decision of whether or not to participate is entirely theirs, and they must be assured that findings will be confidential. People who take part in an exploratory study can be told about the aims of the research without jeopardising findings. The same might not be true if subjects were told that the purpose of the study was to find out the influence of a particular variable considered to be beneficial, and then realised that they either were or were not to receive that treatment.

Practical Problems

Intervention studies can present grave practical difficulties. The lack of scientific evidence in support of the use of topical wound disinfectants and other agents has already been commented upon. The situation with chronic wounds is particularly difficult to investigate, because the incidence of sepsis and the rate of healing will to a large extent reflect the patient's underlying condition, and may be a reflection of the original cause of the lesion (see Chapter 9). To determine the effectiveness of a given preparation x on the healing of a pressure sore it would be necessary to allocate patients to an experimental control group in numbers large enough to ensure that meaningful statistical analysis could take place. The underlying aetiology of wound-formation would have to be the same for subjects in both groups; the progress of a varicose ulcer cannot be compared to that of a pressure sore. The sores would have to be in the same anatomical position. Vasculation, degree of movement of the affected part and the likelihood of contamination (considerable for a sacral sore) may all influence ability to heal. In Chapter 4, the influential effects of dehydration and nutrition on the incidence of sepsis and their relationship to healing are discussed. Only patients of similar nutritional status with equivalent fluid balance can therefore be compared to one another.

The technique demanded by this type of investigation is that of matching pairs; for every patient receiving preparation x who has a sacral pressure sore, who is female, aged 75, obese and who has adult onset diabetes mellitus, a similar patient must be placed in the control group, and not receive preparation x. Comparison to a male patient, or someone of different body build, who lacks the same metabolic disorder will not do, for valid comparisons cannot be made between like and unlike. The sores must be of comparable size and depth, and the patients must be treated in the same way. If pressure-relieving aids are employed for one patient, but not another, then any differences in the rate of healing could be attributed to this, and not to the topical application. Although pressure sores continue to develop more frequently than nurses would like, it is not difficult to see why few experimental trials of this nature have taken place.

Many trials of new preparations and equipment reported in the literature have not been controlled properly. Some have not been controlled at all, although the authors have made claims for the success of the treatment they are testing. The effect attributed to the treatment might have been associated with some other uncontrolled variable such as nursing management which the researcher did not measure.

In other studies, the healing of dissimilar wounds has been compared and many samples are small. Inevitably samples of convenience have been used on the majority of occasions.

Nurses need to be aware of these pitfalls, because the choice of topical wound treatments, like many other clinical commodities, is now vast. Advertising campaigns are cut-throat. References are often made to published research studies allegedly showing the product to be of proven value, but it is up to the nurse practitioner, responsible for planning patient care, to read the literature and assess the value of the product to the patient. If nurses are to be accountable for the care they give, they must know the rationale behind it.

Yet another difficulty encountered with clinical research trials is the problem of measurement (see above). The number of bacteria and white blood cells in a wound can be counted, but how deep is the wound? Are its edges at the point where broken skin ends and inflammation begins, or should the inflamed lips of the wound be included in its surface area? At what stage is a wound truly healed?

Where different researchers are working together on a project and do not employ the same criteria, bias will creep in. Computer techniques for assessing the contours of a wound are described by Anthony (1985).

Good planning and the acceptance of common definitions by all members of the research team are clearly vital. Despite the drawbacks of intervention studies their results seem to hold more promise for the future than exploratory studies which criticise, but offer little in the way of solutions.

Evaluative Research

The term evaluation has become familiar to nurses because it has been given to the final stage of the nursing process. Evaluation is a judgement of worth, or an attempt to determine whether previously defined objectives have been met. The care given to an individual patient can be evaluated, or the effectiveness provided by a particular medical or nursing service to a large number of people – for example, the effectiveness of an immunisation programme. Implicit in this approach lies the importance of determining objectives when planning either the care of an individual or the provision of a service.

According to Waters and Cliff (1983), evaluation of health care services is part of a continuous cycle (Fig. 3.1); as a service is planned, objectives should be set, so that once the service has been implemented for an agreed length of time, evaluation and recommendations for future practice can be made. In this way, evaluation becomes an instrument for planning. Where a service has been in operation prior to the days of formal planning and objective-setting, an initial, exploratory evaluation will be justified.

With the introduction of performance indicators

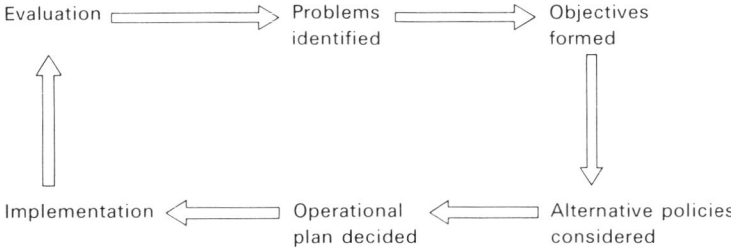

Fig. 3.1 Evaluation of health services – the planning cycle.

and quality control into the NHS in the mid-1980s, evaluative studies at all levels are likely to become more important. If nurses working in the wards are to have the service which they provide assessed, or are to be involved in collecting information periodically or routinely for assessment, then it is important that they understand the framework of evaluation of the service as a whole, as well as evaluation of the individual patient. Although the implementation of the Griffiths Enquiry threatens to erode the nursing voice at district level, it is still important that nurses who advise health service managers about provision of the services should recognise the importance of evaluation and the need to introduce new studies sensitively so that the people responsible for providing the service should not feel unduly threatened or negative about suggestions for change.

The importance of handling other people's feelings, sometimes in the light of unpalatable findings, has been recognised for years by nurses working in the field of infection control. They have been carrying out evaluation for a long time – for example, the collection of clean wound and urinary tract infection rates among inpatients (see Chapter 10). If present trends within the health service continue, it is likely that greater attention will be paid to these statistics in the future.

At the present time, however, evaluation remains more the tool of epidemiologists than of the individual researcher. This is in many ways inevitable. To give meaningful results, epidemiological studies must be planned on a large scale, demand several different methods of data collection, and have a team approach. Good statistical advice at ever stage, including analysis, is vital. Little can be achieved without adequate financial support. Nurses may be important members of the team, especially during data collection, so their understanding of the study and their ability to obtain cooperation from other people will be of major importance. Hamilton (1986), a professor of community medicine working from a London teaching hospital, argues that in future nurses should be given greater opportunity to learn about epidemiological methods because in their day-to-work with patients and clients they have the opportunity to observe patterns of ill health. This enables them to help identify trends.

Epidemiological Studies

Nurses who work in the community have recognised the importance of collecting accurate statistical data for years, reflected in the theme of their very successful Primary Health Care Conference organised by the Royal College of Nursing in London in 1985. In view of this, the main types of epidemiological studies will be outlined below. They include: descriptive surveys, analytical studies, and experimental studies.

Descriptive Surveys

Descriptive surveys document the amount and distribution of disease in a sample of the population. Three main characteristics are described:

- *Who* is affected,
- *Where* the disease occurs,
- *When* the disease occurs.

The last point is particularly important in the case of infectious diseases, which may appear in the community at fairly regular intervals (see Chapter 2).

The methods used in descriptive surveys depend on the disease investigated. Often questionnaires are used or basic clinical measurements, such as bacteriological screening. In a study to document the occurrence of urinary tract infection in a sample of young women within a general practitioner's caseload, women making up the sample would have a specimen of midstream urine sent for bacteriological examination. They might also be questioned about symptoms like dysuria and frequency. These tests are typical of epidemiological studies; they are reasonably cheap and can be applied quickly to a large number of people. Perhaps one of the best examples to illustrate a descriptive survey of this kind is the National Survey of Infection in Hospitals, conducted by Meers *et al.* (1981).

This study was designed to determine the prevalence of infection among hospital patients in England and Wales. Funding was necessary from an external body, and following a pilot study, visits were made to 43 district general hospitals; 18 186 patients in acute wards were included.

The method used to obtain the sample could be criticised, for it was not random. Infection control officers (see Chapter 10) were contacted by the research team and asked if they would like to take part. Bias was almost certainly introduced since these infection control officers may have been particularly concerned about nosocomial infection and more likely to participate. Since the members of the research team were visitors in the hospitals and depended upon the cooperation of the hospital staff, it is difficult to see how this problem could have been avoided.

In each hospital the survey was conducted by a member of the research team, the infection control officer, a nurse (usually the infection control nurse) and a second member of the nursing staff drawn from the particular ward visited. An average of 423 patients were surveyed in each hospital and they were placed in categories according to medical specialty.

The decision to classify each patient as infected or not infected was made in the ward, often at the bedside, based on information from nursing and medical notes, laboratory reports and clinical examination. Clear definitions of infection were formulated before the study commenced and they were tested in the pilot study. They seemed to be adequate since people in different hospitals had little difficulty in applying them, and the rates of infection recorded in all hospitals were very much the same. Each infection was further identified according to whether it had developed in hospital or in the community before admission. Respiratory infections were more difficult to categorise in this way than urinary tract and wound infections. The causative organism (if identified) and details of antimicrobial therapy were also recorded.

Although the amount of work generated by the study was considerable, data collection was accomplished swiftly to avoid seasonal variations. As with so many exploratory investigations, the results are sobering, and they are of importance to all nurses who plan and deliver care.

The overall rate of infection was 19.1%, half of which were estimated to originate in hospital. Respiratory infections were the most frequently recorded, but the majority had developed before admission. Urinary tract infections were the most common hospital-acquired infections, accounting for 22% of the infections recorded overall, and for 30.2% of all those which developed *after* admission.

Nearly all those who had urinary tract infections were catheterised.

Wound infections were the second most common category of hospital-acquired infection – overall, 5% were judged to be clinically infected. Surgical wounds are categorised according to whether they are clean or contaminated (see Chapter 9). According to the National Prevalence Study (Meers *et al.*, 1981), infection was recorded frequently in wounds that, according to their site, should have been free of sepsis.

A prevalence study documents the number of cases of disease in a population at one particular point in time. The National Prevalence Study provides information only about the number of cases of infection in hospital *on the day that each hospital was visited*. It cannot be stated categorically that the same rates of infection occur at this moment in time. Descriptive surveys conducted at one point in time are sometimes called cross-sectional studies.

If the study could be repeated on the same patients several times throughout their hospital stay, this would constitute a longitudinal study. Another type of descriptive survey is the incidence study. The difference between prevalence and incidence studies is explained in Chapter 9.

It is important, however, to emphasise that a descriptive survey, like any exploratory study, cannot establish a cause-and-effect relationship. The fact that urinary tract infections occurred mainly among catheterised patients strongly *suggests* that some relationship may exist between the two, but does not *prove* it.

Analytical Studies

Analytical studies set out to test a hypothesis about the cause of disease. In a case-control analytical study, people who have a given disease (cases) are compared with controls who do not. Differences that might explain why the cases became ill are then sought. The cases are matched with controls in terms of age and other variables as far as possible.

This was the approach taken by the National Childhood Encephalopathy Study (Alderslade *et al.*, 1981) which set out to find whether or not serious brain damage occurred more often after whooping cough immunisation than would occur by chance.

In general, reactions to the killed, purified bacteria which constitute the vaccine can take two forms. Approximately 5% of children can be flushed and irritable for a few hours after vaccination, and a few have short episodes that could be described as a very mild form of febrile convulsion. More worrying have been the very occasional reports of children developing severe, permanent brain damage after receiving the vaccine. Over a period of 11 years Great Ormond Street Hospital in London heard of 36 cases of this kind, although they were reported from several different countries. The research team had to bear in mind the various other forms of brain illness that may lead to damage in the first year of life. Sometimes severe convulsions can occur for no apparent reason, resulting in lasting damage. If, by chance, the baby had received the vaccine shortly before the convulsions, vaccination could be held responsible, even though it was *not* in fact to blame. To demonstrate that vaccination is the true cause of brain damage it would be necessary to show that vaccinated children (cases) develop neurological problems more often than control children matched to the cases in every respect other than *not* receiving the vaccine.

Every consultant of paediatrics, neurosurgery and infectious diseases in the United Kingdom was invited to tell the research team about each child with neurological symptoms or febrile convulsions seen over a 3 year period commencing in 1976. In view of the nature of the investigation, cooperation was excellent.

Analysis of the first thousand children suggested that the cases could be divided into two groups, almost equal in size: those whose neurological problems had resolved after 15 days, and those whose problems had not.

Children whose problems were longer term were visited at home and examined in detail by a paediatrician. Two visits were made: one as soon as possible after notification, the other one year later. Children who seemed well after 15 days received follow up visits at home by health visitors, because they are trained in the observation of normal child development.

For every child notified to the researchers, two control children were matched on the basis of the data collected by the paediatricians and health visitors, and they were also visited at regular intervals. Immunisation histories were obtained by writing to their general practitioners.

Of the 1000 cases of serious neurological disorders made known to the researchers, and analysed in detail, the peak age of onset for those children who did not recover fully tended to be lower than for those who did. Of these children, 35 had received the vaccine within 7 days of the onset of acute illness, while the remaining 965 had not. Statistical tests revealed that there was no characteristic illness associated with the vaccine that did not frequently occur in non-vaccinated children.

Of the 35 cases found to be associated in time with vaccination, three could have been regarded as neurologically abnormal *before* its administration. Out of the 32 remaining previously normal children, 21 had recovered completely within 15 days. Only nine children could be identified for whom no explanation other than vaccination could be found for their neurological damage. Three had minor defects, six major defects; this number was not statistically significant – that is, it could have occurred by chance.

On the evidence of this study, health visitors can advise parents that the whooping cough vaccine is safe.

Experimental Studies

These are generally concerned with the treatment or prevention of disease. The randomised controlled trial undertaken to test the effectiveness of new drugs is the best example of this kind.

Clearly, epidemiological studies bear similarities to those previously discussed. To differentiate strictly between different research methods is artificial; studies that take an experimental approach will involve many of the same data gathering instruments as, for example, exploratory or evaluative studies.

CONCLUSIONS

The purpose of this chapter has been to illustrate the importance of reading and understanding research methods, because of the way that this influences the results obtained. In other chapters, research studies are discussed, sometimes in depth, and shortcomings in the research design are indicated where necessary.

References

Akinsanya, J. (1985). Learning about life. *Senior Nurse*, 2: 24–25.

Alderslade, R. et al. (1981). The National Childhood Encephalopathy Study. In: *Whooping Cough: Reports from the Committee on Safety of Medicines and the Joint Committee on Vaccination and Immunisation.* HMSO, London.

Anthony, D. (1985). Measuring pressure sores. *Nursing Times*, 81 (24): 57–61.

Boore, J. (1978). *Prescription for Recovery.* Royal College of Nursing, London.

Button, D. (1986). Paper presented at the Royal College of Nursing Annual Research Society Conference, Reading University.

Crow, R. (1981). Scientific nursing research: art and science. In: *Nursing Practice*, Smith, J. P. (ed.), pp. 29–31. Butterworths, London.

David, J. (1982). Pressure sore treatment: a literature review. *International Journal of Nursing Studies*, 19: 183–191.

David, J. et al. (1983). An investigation of the care of patients with established pressure sores. Report of the Northwick Park Nursing Practice Research Unit.

Dumas, R. R., Leonard, C. (1963). The effect of nursing on the incidence of post-operative vomiting. *Nursing Research*, 1: 12–15.

Gott, M. (1984). *Learning Nursing.* Royal College of Nursing, London.

Gould, D. J. (1985). Isolation procedures in one health district. *Nursing Times Occasional Paper*, 81 (7): 47–50.

Greaves, A. (1985). We'll just freshen you up, dear. *Nursing Times Journal of Infection Control Nursing*, 81 (36): 1–4.

Hamilton, P. (1986). Identifying trends. *Nursing Times*, 82 (8): 31–32.

Hamilton Smith, S. (1972). *Nil by Mouth.* Royal College of Nursing, London.

Hayward, J. (1975). *Information – A Prescription Against Pain.* Royal College of Nursing, London.

Hunt, J. (1974). *A Study of Surgical Dressings in Three Hospitals.* Royal College of Nursing, London.

Jackson, J. (1983). Sheepskins – a potential hazard? *Nursing Times Journal of Infection Control Nursing*, 79 (18): 2–6.

Jones, D. (1975). *Food for Thought.* Royal College of Nursing, London.

Kennedy, A., Brocklehurst, J. C. (1982). The nursing management of patients with long term indwelling catheters. *Journal of Advanced Nursing*, 7: 411–417.

Lawrence, M. (1983). Patient hand hygiene – a clinical enquiry. *Nursing Times*, 79 (22): 24–25.

Lindeman, C. A., van Aernan, B. (1971). Effects of structured and unstructured pre-operative teaching. *Nursing Research*, 20: 319–332.

McLeod-Clark, J., Hockey, L. (1979). *Research for Nursing. A Guide for the Enquiring Nurse.* HM and M Publishers, Beaconsfield, Bucks.

Meers, P. D., Stronge, J. L. (1980). Hospitals should do the sick no harm – 3. Where does infection come from? *Nursing Times*, 76 (19): 12–13.

Meers, P. D. et al. (1981). Report of the National Survey of Infection in Hospitals. *Journal of Hospital Infection*, 2: 23–28.

Norton, D. et al. (1962). *An Investigation of Geriatric Nursing Problems in Hospital. National Corporation for the Care of Old People.* Reprinted 1975. Churchill Livingstone, Edinburgh and London.

Ozbolt-Goodwin, J. (1979). Programmed instruction for self-care following pulmonary surgery. *International Journal of Nursing Studies*, 16: 29–40.

Presly, A. (1984). Common terms and concepts in nursing research. In: *The Research Process in Nursing*, Cormack, F. S. (ed.), pp. 30–36. Blackwell Scientific Publications, Oxford.

Wallace, G., Hayter, J. (1974). Karaya for chronic skin ulcers. *American Journal of Nursing*, 74: 1094–1098.

Waters, W. E., Cliff, K. S. (1983). *Community Medicine. A Textbook for Nurses and Health Visitors.* Croom Helm, London and Canberra.

Webb, C., Wilson-Barnett, J. (1983). Hysterectomy. A study in coping with recovery. *Journal of Advanced Nursing*, 8: 311–319.

Wilson, K. J. W. (1975). *A Study of Biological Sciences in Relation to Nursing.* Churchill Livingstone, Edinburgh and London.

Further Reading

Bynner, J., Stribley, K. M. (eds) (1978). *Social Research: its Principles and Procedures.* Longman, London.

Lindzey, G., Aronson, E. (ed.) (1969). *The Handbook of Social Psychology*, volumes 1 and 2. Addison Wesley. Cambridge, Massachusetts.

Oppenheim, A. N. (1966). *Questionnaire Design and Attitude Measurement.* Heinemann, London.

Treece, E. W., Treece, J. W. (1985). *Elements of Research in Nursing.* C. V. Mosby, St Louis.

Chapter 4

Providing a Safe Environment: The Patient-centred Approach

INTRODUCTION

To control infection nurses must know about the growth requirements of microorganisms and how to prevent their spread. The basis for developing this knowledge was laid in Chapter 1, where it was pointed out that development of infection is a product of the virulence of the microorganism and the susceptibility of the host. Infections develop in both hospital and in the community, but the risks are much greater following hospital admission, where they are difficult to treat because of antibiotic resistance. McNeill (1984) surveyed the incidence of infection caused by strains of *Staphylococcus aureus* resistant to methicillin in a large Australian teaching hospital over a period of 12 months; 20% of the infections reported among inpatients had developed within 2 days of admission and most of the people concerned were old. Patients from the community were sometimes infected with resistant bacteria when they presented in the outpatient or accident and emergency department. All of them, however, had recently been in hospital themselves or had been closely in contact with someone who had.

All patients who are admitted to hospital have certain risk factors in common (Table 4.1): they will share facilities like bathrooms and wash bowls to a much greater extent than at home; they will eat mass-produced food; they will be touched by many more people than usual which exposes them to other people's microbiological flora; and they will be exposed to varying amounts of physical and psychological stress (see Chapter 7). Ability to withstand these stressors is influenced by factors operating within the patient himself and his environment.

Preventing infection takes place at three different levels, as shown in Table 4.2. At the bedside, the nurse is the key person to implement

Table 4.1 Common Risk Factors Among Patients in Hospital

(1) Shared facilities
(2) Mass-produced food
(3) Contact with members of hospital staff
(4) Stress, physical and psychological

Table 4.2 Strategies for Preventing Infection

(1) *Individual patient care.* Using the nursing process to tailor the care required by a particular patient, whether in hospital or the community. Identifying factors that may increase susceptibility to infection and planning a strategy of care to reduce them as far as possible.
(2) *Hospital policies and procedures.* Using procedures and policies designed to reduce risks of infection common to every patient in a ward or hospital. All patients benefit if their nurses employ good hand-washing and sound aseptic techniques, a clean environment, hygienic catering practices and the prompt disposal of waste materials.
(3) *Community health.* Policies intended to promote the health of the entire community. These would include notification of infectious diseases to the medical officer of environmental health, immunisation programmes, provision of adequate sanitation and inspection of restaurants and factories.

safe infection control practices. To do so effectively, she must assess the risk factors operating at patient level. Ashworth (1984) argues that nurses have long used the wrong approach to infection control. Instead of taking into consideration the needs of the individual patient or situation, they view infection control in terms of 'rules, routines and rituals'. The best way is the 'hands and human beings' approach, since it is the effectiveness of simple, inexpensive measures like good hand hygiene and the way people behave that will determine whether or not the route of infection has been blocked. These factors are important at the first level, the provision of individual patient care. The nursing process is an aid to help provide the nursing care needed by a person in a particular health care situation, so that available resources will be used to the maximum advantage. This involves systematic assessment of all the factors related to the patient's needs, planning, implementation and continued evaluation. Factors relevant to infection control include all the daily activities of living; these are influenced by degree of independence, cultural and religious factors, the success or otherwise of health education, and the safety of the environment.

Environmental hazards are governed by the practices and procedures generally used throughout the hospital. Nurses in direct patient contact have an important role to play by ensuring that these are adhered to intelligently, and that the information received by learners in the school of nursing is implemented effectively. Some of the most important infection control policies that concern the nurse are discussed in Chapter 5. Nurses in managerial positions can influence the development of hospital and district-wide policies (see Chapter 10). The importance and development of community health was described in Chapter 2 (see also Chapter 5). It should be emphasised, however, that the health visitor is in a key position in raising the awareness of the family to all matters concerned with healthy living, including the prevention of infection.

Education about hygiene and preventing infection can also be provided by district and school nurses and by nurses working in certain specialist fields – for example, diabetic liaison nurses need to teach their clients about the dangers associated with infection; nurses who work in drug addiction centres must teach patients about the dangers of hepatitis B and the risks of sharing needles. In this chapter, the main focus is upon the assessment of risk factors to the individual patient.

INDIVIDUAL SUSCEPTIBILITY TO INFECTION

Over the years numerous factors have been put forward to suggest why some people fall prey to a particular infectious agent while others do not. One of the most important factors is, of course, size of the infective dose. Most healthy people do not develop clinical signs of infection unless they are exposed to a *very large* number of pathogens. Even when the size of the infective dose is relatively constant, however, some people succumb while others do not. Possible reasons are suggested below. In some cases, experimental evidence or, more often, the results of surveys and field observations, lend support to the hypothesis; in others, only circumstantial evidence suggests a link between some factor and the development of infection. Because nurses today are expected to think critically and to question the sources of information available to them (see Chapter 3), efforts will be made to provide research-based evidence wherever it exists.

Immunity

Human beings are innately immune to some infections. Canine distemper and feline enteritis, for example, have never been reported from pet owners; conversely, some animal species have innate immunity to human infections. Research on the common cold was delayed for years because the usual laboratory animals do not respond to the virus. Work began in earnest when it became known that weasels, which are not often used in the laboratory, could be infected.

As well as being inherent, immunity can be naturally developed or artificially induced. The different types of acquired immunity are shown in Table 4.3, and the schedule for immunisation in the United Kingdom and properties of the commonly used vaccines are given in Chapter 5 (p. 91).

Factors which appear to influence immunity are listed below.

- age,
- genetic factors,
- nutrition,
- fluid balance,
- immobility,
- disturbance of normal metabolic function,
- sleep and rest,
- drugs,
- invasive procedures.

Table 4.3 Innate and Acquired Immunity

Innate immunity
  present at birth;
  does not involve activity of the lymphocytes or antibody formation.
  (1) *Species immunity* – resistance of one animal species to diseases that infect other species. For example, humans are immune to canine distemper.
  (2) *Individual immunity* – resistance to infections that attack other members of the same species due to age, nutritional status, general health.

Acquired immunity
  resistance gained during the life of the individual that results from the action of the lymphocytes and antibody formation;
  antibodies may be acquired: actively or passively; naturally or artificially.
  (1) *Naturally acquired active immunity* – the immune system of the individual comes into contact with the microorganism by natural processes and the individual is stimulated to make antibodies actively against it. Examples are: measles, chickenpox, smallpox – lifelong immunity; tetanus, diphtheria – immunity lasts a few years; scarlet fever, polio – immunity may result through subclinical infections.
  (2) *Naturally acquired passive immunity* – natural transfer of antibodies from an immunised donor to a susceptible recipient via placenta or breastmilk. Immunity is generally shortlived. Examples are in diphtheria, German measles, polio.
  (3) *Artificially acquired active immunity* – a dead or inactivated microorganism or toxin (vaccine) is deliberately introduced to the recipient, where it stimulates active production of antibodies. Immunity generally lasts for years. Examples are: tetanus, measles, whooping cough, diphtheria, polio, German measles.
  (4) *Artificially acquired passive immunity* – transfer of antibodies from a donor to a recipient via an injection of serum containing antibodies. Useful when accidental exposure to an infectious agent or toxin has already occurred. Example is injection of gamma-immunoglobulins to a nurse after needlestick injury from a patient who has hepatitis B.

Age

Both the very young and the very old are particularly susceptible to infection, a reflection of the maturity or immaturity of the immune system. Babies acquire antibodies against pathogens via the placenta or in the breastmilk (see Table 4.3) but the effects are generally shortlived. Immunisation of the newborn is impractical because antibody production is not possible until at least 3 months of age. Booster doses to increase the antibody titre are usually necessary throughout childhood to provide adequate protection. Health visitors and midwives have a major role to play by encouraging mothers to breastfeed, so that some degree of protection is afforded during the first few months of life. When mothers do not wish to breastfeed or are unable to do so, it is important that they should understand the need for sterility when feeds are prepared. Vomiting, diarrhoea and failure to thrive are among the main reasons for hospital admission among young babies. Sometimes this is because parents have not reconstituted feeds correctly, but in many cases feeds have also been contaminated and made the child dangerously ill.

The problem is at its worst in crowded inner city areas, where many immigrant families live in substandard accommodation and have a poor command of English, so that they cannot understand written or verbal instructions in relation to the feeds. Continued support from the health visitor is very important – the vital role of the health visitor in relation to immunisation and the provision of information to enable the parents to make an informed choice has been mentioned in previous chapters.

With advancing age the immune system deteriorates. Ability to mount the inflammatory response and to form new antibodies both decline as the general metabolic rate slows down (Weskler, 1980; Pahwa, 1981). Epidemics of food poisoning are common in institutions which specialise in the care of the elderly, and when outbreaks of respiratory illness sweep through the community most deaths occur among this age group. Elderly people can be vaccinated against influenza, but this is usually ineffective, given the state of the immune system in old age and the large number of epidemic strains of the virus. Advice to avoid contact with infected people, to remain indoors as much as possible during cold, damp weather, and to reduce cigarette consumption is probably more helpful.

Both the infirm elderly and the newborn succumb to chest infections because they cannot move easily or cough up respiratory secretions. Physiotherapy is an important prophylactic measure in hospital; turning the patient at regular intervals will help secretions to drain, and inhalations may liquify secretions to ease expectoration. Old people should also be warned to take good care of their feet and skin, because any lesions that develop might become septic, especially in areas that do not receive a good blood supply. Pyrexia is an important warning signal, but it is unusual in the very young or very elderly, even in the presence of severe infection; so in its absence nurses may overlook the possibility of infection.

Genetic Factors

Some biologists argue that the entire length of the human lifespan appears to be under genetic control, mediated by the immune system and ability to withstand exposure to particular infective agents may be determined to some extent by genetic factors. Evidence has been obtained by studying identical twins, who are derived from the same fertilised egg and have all their genes in common. Non-identical twins grow from two separate eggs which both happen to be fertilised at the same time. Their genes are no more alike than those of other children belonging to the same family. But if one identical twin develops tuberculosis, his brother or sister will stand a greater chance of developing the infecton than a non-identical twin or another sibling (Carter, 1962). No gene responsible for 'tuberculosis susceptibility' has ever been isolated. The most likely explanation is that several genes interact with presently unknown environmental factors, predisposing an individual to susceptibility. Critics of this theory point out that identical twins often go about together and will probably be exposed to the risk of infection to a greater extent than ordinary siblings. However, in a few cases it has been possible to examine the medical histories of identical twins who have been separated at birth and brought up independently. If one twin under these circumstances has developed tuberculosis, then the other is still very likely to do so. There is also some evidence to suggest a genetic basis towards developing poliomyelitis.

Other genetically determined conditions include a rare disease called agammaglobulinaemia, the inability to make specific antibodies. With the appearance of antibiotics, more children born with these innate immune deficiency diseases have survived and it has been found that childhood immunisation is not followed by antibody production. Today, these people are kept alive by regular injections of human immunoglobulins (see Table 4.3) and antibiotic therapy, but occasionally bone marrow transplant is successful. However, normal family life may be subject to frequent disruption, and there is a need for sympathetic nursing support.

Nutrition

Antibodies are proteins, so people who are undernourished may not be able to produce these in sufficient quantities and they may become extremely infection-prone. Evidence, however, is circumstantial. People living in the third world are chronically undernourished and fall prey to infections of all kinds, such as kwashiorkor, a protein-deficiency disease which usually occurs when a child is superseded by a younger sibling so that he is no longer breastfed. Affected children cannot make antibodies in response to vaccination and they develop severe infections when exposed to ordinary childhood diseases like measles. Atrophy of the thymus gland and lymphoid tissue has been reported, and the white blood cells do not seem able to destroy bacteria adequately. Poor sanitation and the prevalence of uncontrolled pests and insect vectors in hot climates compound the problem. Nurses working in the third world have a mammoth task, instigating programmes of immunisation and teaching people about good health practice at a level feasible in relation to their living conditions (Skeet, 1981).

Malnutrition

Undernourishment, of course, is by no means restricted to the third world. Alcoholics and vagrants living in Britain do not eat properly and frequently develop infections, particularly tuberculosis. A DHSS survey in 1972 showed that a small but significant number of elderly people living in the community were undernourished mainly through poor motivation to buy food and lack of incentive to prepare meals rather than because they were genuinely impoverished. Even more alarmingly, people admitted to hospital may become deficient in protein, calories and vitamin C (necessary for tissue repair). Two reports published by the RCN, 10 years apart, have drawn attention to this situation (Jones, 1975; Coates, 1985), and it appears that many nurses consider patients' nutrition a non-nursing duty, one that is beyond their control, or one for which they receive insufficient education.

Obesity

Obesity, a common condition in the western world, also influences susceptibility to infection. Obese patients cannot expectorate or expand their lungs and their mobility may be reduced. Pressure sores may develop and become infected; surgical wounds heal slowly, for adipose tissue has a poor blood supply, and hygiene is more difficult.

A great deal has been said in recent nursing and medical publications about the need to improve patients' nutritional status. Hopefully the tide of opinion has turned, and in future clinical practice this previously neglected subject will receive all the emphasis that it deserves. It is worth pointing out, however, that nutritional status should be assessed when the patient is first admitted, or during the first visit made by the district nurse and at regular intervals afterward, so that intervention is not delayed. Sophisticated biochemical tests may be out of the question; sometimes it may not even be practical to weigh the patient. Nevertheless it is still possible to assess nutritional status: evidence suggests that when somebody appears to be the correct weight for their height and body build, then this will probably be the case; people who look either too fat or too thin would, on clinical investigation, probably be shown to be either overnourished or undernourished (Baker, 1982).

Fluid Balance

Patients who become dehydrated are at particular risk of developing urinary tract infection. If they are immobile as well, this predisposes to the formation of renal calculi (stones). Dehydrated patients develop sore, dry mouths, prone to *Candida* infection, and dry, fragile skin which easily tears, opening another portal of entry for microorganisms. Monitoring the patient's fluid balance is an important nursing task, as are mouth care, pressure area care and ensuring adequate fluid intake.

Immobility

The dangers of infection for people whose movement is impaired are urinary stasis, inadequate expansion of the lungs leading to accumulation of respiratory secretions, and pressure sores.

Metabolic Disorders

Disturbance of normal metabolic function increases the risk of infection. Patients who have diabetes mellitus, in particular, often develop infections, probably because of their high blood sugar levels and glycosuria. Malignancy is commonly accompanied by infection, either because of the patient's debility, the effects of radiotherapy and chemotherapy (see below, p. 68), deficiencies in the immune system, accompanying malnutrition, the development of fungating lesions, or a combination of all these factors.

Peripheral vascular disease, which frequently accompanies diabetes, commonly results in infection in one of the extremities, usually the toes. This may lead to necrosis, and sometimes the entire limb may be affected, often with tragic consequences. Amputation may be necessary, and in the elderly, return to normal functioning may be slow. Since cigarette smoking contributes to the development of peripheral vascular disease, by constricting the blood vessel walls, diabetics and all patients who give indication of vascular insufficiency should be advised not to smoke.

Even in healthy people rate of healing can be impaired at those sites of the body which receive a poor blood supply. Only slight trauma may result in a wound both slow to heal and easily infected. The tissues covering the tibia, for example, are poorly vasculated, so varicose ulcers commonly occur in this region.

Sleep and Rest

There is no hard evidence to suggest that adequate sleep and rest are prophylactic against development of infection, although rest has long been used to reduce the effects of harmful inflammation. The edges of wounds and fractures, for example, must be placed in close apposition before they will heal. However, the damaging effects of stress include suppression of normal growth and repair in the long term (see Chapter 7), and it is possible that tranquillity may, in future, be shown to be related to the ability to withstand infection. People who live in particularly unhappy circumstances are certainly less able to tolerate the symptoms of infection and illnesses generally.

Drugs

Antibiotics may be given prophylactically to prevent infection or to cure infection that has already become established. They destroy the normal body flora, especially in the gut, and lead to superinfection by *Candida* or antibiotic-resistant bacteria acquired from the hospital environment. Side-effects are gastrointestinal upsets, a sore mouth coated with a white layer of *Candida* or vaginal discharge. Among very sick people, urinary and respiratory infections due to *Candida* and *Staphylococcus epidermidis* are common following antibiotic therapy.

Steroid drugs suppress the normal inflammatory response that helps to protect the tissues when they are damaged and inhibit the production of white blood cells. The white cell count may also be depressed by suppression of the bone marrow after chemotherapy or radiotherapy intended to control the spread of malignant disease.

Deep X-ray therapy and anticancer drugs act by preventing cell division. Unfortunately, their effects are not limited to the target cells of the tumour they are intended to destroy, but extend to all other tissues where rapid cell divisions take place, including the red bone marrow. Protective isolation is necessary for patients whose white cell counts are likely to be severely depressed. Despite recent advances in chemotherapy, patients with acute leukaemia rarely survive for more than 2 years. Bone marrow transplantation is now an established treatment for people who have acute leukaemia, aplastic anaemia and innately acquired immune disorders. Before transplantation the patient receives very high doses of chemotherapy and radiotherapy, which eradicates all remaining leukaemia cells and produces a state of immunosuppression in order to prevent rejection of the graft; the risk of infection is profound. The transplanted marrow takes about 3 weeks to regenerate, and during this time very strict protective isolation is required.

Invasive Procedures

Invasive procedures increase the risks of developing infection because they bypass the normal protective barriers of the body. Patients who are profoundly ill are generally required to undergo the most invasive procedures, especially when their disease is in the diagnostic stages. Those who go to theatre or spend time in the intensive care unit face the greatest number of investigations and manipulations. The risks attached to some of those most commonly performed will be discussed in this section. Surgical incisions and urinary catheterisation are so commonly performed and have been the subjects of so much research that each merits a chapter to itself (see Chapters 8 and 9).

Intravenous Therapy

About 40% of all patients admitted to hospital will be given an intravenous infusion at some point during their stay. The plastic cannula (introduced in 1945), and intravenous injection as an intermittent bolus (introduced in 1948) are both techniques that contribute to nosocomial infection. According to the results of one study undertaken in 1969, contamination of the system is mainly due to bacteria of the kind which make up the normal skin flora. In this study, most isolates came from filters in the system on the side distal to the patient, suggesting entry via connections in the administration apparatus or through the air outlet (Fig. 4.1). The authors, Wilmore and Dudrick (1969), felt that contamination was most likely to occur during assembly of the equipment at the bedside, or when drugs were introduced.

The dangers attached to intravenous therapy have been examined more recently by numerous other research teams. In an extensive study of 519 cases involving the use of intravenous cannulae fitted with valved injection side ports, Cheesebrough *et al.* (1984) reported a 25.2% incidence of inflammation at the site of the cannula insertion. The longer the cannula was allowed to remain in position, the greater the risk of sepsis; after 3½ days inflammation was usually severe, and one patient developed bacteraemia. However, the bacteria responsible were never the same as those carried on the patient's skin, suggesting that they had originated from staff during handling of the system. The importance of strict asepsis when an infusion is set up and drugs added, and of changing the site of the cannula before inflammation develops, is clear.

Most hospital infection control policies forbid additives to be delivered via administration apparatus that is being used for blood transfusion or total parenteral feeding, as these fluids are full of nutrients able to support bacterial growth. Solutions used for intravenous feeding are prepared with strict asepsis under laminar air flow, either in the hospital pharmacy or on a commercial basis. On the ward, strict aseptic technique is vital whenever the feeding lines are handled. These are usually inserted in theatre, and since nutrient solutions irritate blood vessel walls, the fluid is best directed into the lumen of a large vein rather than into vessels at the antecubital fossa. Many doctors prefer to 'tunnel' the administration apparatus through the subcutaneous tissues before the cannula is allowed to enter the vein because this helps

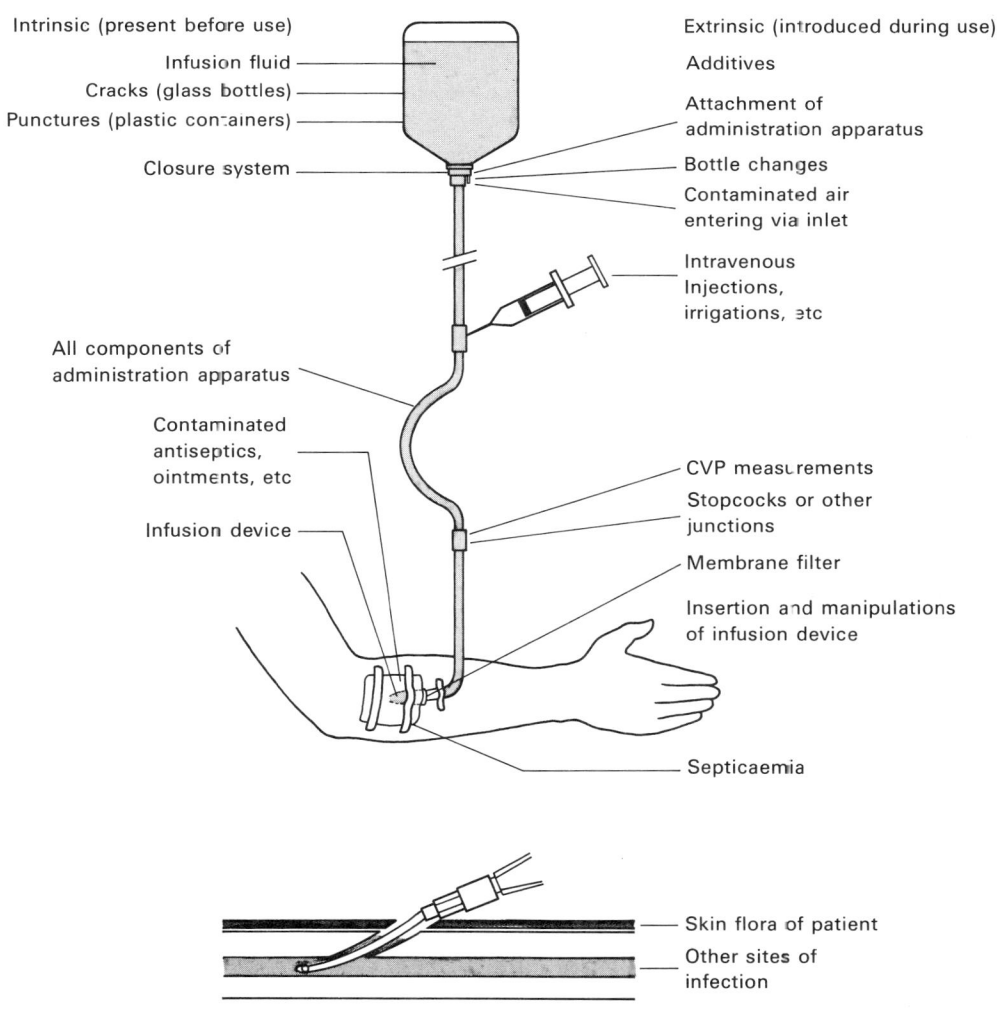

Fig. 4.1 Intravenous therapy – portals of bacterial entry.

to reduce the risk of infection. Nurses have to take great care when the entry site is redressed. Polyurethane dressings like OpSite have been found to reduce the incidence of infection (Holland, 1984), especially when they are used in conjunction with a broad-spectrum antiseptic like povidone-iodine, which can destroy spores. Polyurethane dressings, being transparent, also make good coverings for cannula sites, so inspection for early signs of inflammation is possible without disturbing the dressing.

Enteral Feeding

Increasing interest in the importance of a healthy diet, and growing awareness of the role played by nutrition in recovery, has resulted in the extensive use of nutritional supplements in hospitals. More people than ever before receive enteral feeds, usually via a nasogastric tube. Feeds may be obtained direct from the manufacturer, or they may be made in the hospital diet kitchen. The latter are exposed to the risk of contamination during preparation, so unless they are received promptly by the ward and refrigerated at once, bacteria can multiply in sufficient numbers to set up gastrointestinal infection. Gibbs (1983), an infection control nurse working in a London teaching hospital, traced an outbreak of vomiting among patients fed via nasogastric tube to the hospital kitchen. The bacteria responsible were of faecal origin, and they were isolated from a dishcloth used by the catering staff. The hospital altered its policy, so that in future all enteral feeds were purchased direct from the manufacturer. More recently, laboratory studies with *E.coli* have shown that inoculation of enteral feeds with a single bacterial cell could, within 16 hours, lead to a bacterial count sufficient to cause food poisoning among immunocompromised patients. Attaching new tubing to an infected reservoir of contaminated feed made no difference (Anderton, 1984).

If a patient nursed in protective isolation requires enteral feeding, manufactured feeds are undoubtedly the safer alternative, because the contents of each can (if marketed by a reputable company) are sterile. Cans may be opened in the patient's room after autoclaving to destroy surface microorganisms.

Mechanical Ventilation

When patients undergo assisted ventilation in the intensive care unit, the trachea rapidly becomes colonised with bacteria; and there is a good chance that they may migrate from this location further into the lungs, setting up clinical infection. Contamination of the trachea occurs by contact spread via the hands of staff. Cross-infection may occur between one patient and the next unless there is individual patient allocation. Suction via the endotracheal tube may lead to contamination of the trachea because microorganisms may be deposited in or around the lumen on the hands of staff, then transferred into the trachea when the catheter is inserted. Sterile disposable gloves should be worn, and a fresh, sterile catheter used each time suction is required. When air from the ventilator itself is likely to be contaminated, risks may be reduced by regularly checking and changing filters, adequate decontamination of equipment after use, ensuring that humidifiers are kept full of disinfectant of the appropriate concentration and stored dry after use, and that respiratory tubing is changed daily.

A leading article in the *Journal of Hospital Infection* (1983) draws attention to another possible portal of entry: contaminated secretions entering the trachea from the patient's mouth and pharynx, bypassing between the outer walls of the endotracheal tube and trachea. This possible route has received a good deal less attention, possibly because many people assume that the airtight seal afforded by the endotracheal tube cuff is sufficient to prevent the passage of secretions. However, leakage will occur whenever the cuff is deflated; possibly even when it is inflated secretions may sometimes escape due to slight movement of the patient. Bacteria of the same strain have been isolated from both the mouth and trachea of ventilated patients. Meticulous mouth care is needed to reduce this problem.

Outbreaks of infection due to mechanical ventilation can have serious consequences. Davies (1984) describes how 38 babies admitted to a special care unit developed bacteraemia due to opportunistic infection by *Staphylococcus epidermidis* soon after commencing mechanical ventilation. Gram-negative infection among ventilated adult patients can also have grave consequences (Stucke and Thompson, 1980).

Other Invasive Procedures

Endoscopy has been responsible for outbreaks of infection among hospital patients, the causative organisms including *Pseudomonas* (Earnshaw et al., 1985) and *Salmonella* (Chmel, 1976). Bacteria have contaminated peritoneal dialysis fluid (Spencer, 1984), haemodialysis fluid (Kolmos, 1984), and artificial heart valves (Newsom, 1979). *Staphylococcus epidermidis* infections of cerebrospinal fluid shunts have caused serious problems (Price, 1984).

Wherever the natural barriers of the body against infection are bypassed by some invasive procedure, the risk of sepsis increases. Both outpatients as well as inpatients may be jeopardised. For years hospital staff were happy to disinfect instruments such as proctoscopes and sigmoidoscopes, believing that since the procedure itself was not aseptic, sterilisation was not necessary. Publicity about AIDS, and the knowledge that pathogens can be transferred on these instruments, has prompted many hospital outpatient departments to use disposables or to install more autoclaves for use in outpatient clinics.

Other Factors

A patient who already has one septic focus stands a greater chance of developing further infections at other sites, caused either by the same or other microorganisms. The length of time spent in hospital is a contributory factor – the longer the stay, the greater the opportunity for infection. Patients transferred from one ward to another or between different hospitals contribute to the spread of nosocomial infection (Webster, 1986), as do shared facilities and overcrowding in old hospital wards. Patients who are elderly and lack relatives or friends have to make do with hospital soap, flannel and towels. Ideally, soap used to wash one person should never be used for another. Despite its generally good disinfectant properties, soap can still be contaminated with Gram-negative bacteria, providing a route of spread from one person to another. In hospitals where supplies of equipment can be very limited, there is some temptation to keep and reuse items that would perhaps best be thrown away. The old-fashioned trolley, loaded with soaps, lotions and washbowls played a big role in disseminating infection.

The factors that contribute to a patient's susceptibility to infection are complex, and because they interact so closely they cannot easily be quantified individually. It is fair to say, however, that the more ill the patient, the more invasive the techniques to which he is subjected and the longer he spends in hospital, the greater his chance of developing sepsis. Given the debility of some patients and the number of medical and nursing interventions that they undergo, it would perhaps be more meaningful to ask not why some people become infected, but why some people do not. Stress and personality factors have sometimes been suggested.

These ideas may not be as bizarre as they first appear. Early researchers drew attention to the relationship between cervical carcinoma in women who had unstable personality traits and unhappy childhood experiences. Gradually a picture unfolded of women who, lacking affection during the early years of life, sought it later on in the guise of multiple sexual partners. A definite link between cervical carcinoma and promiscuity is now known to exist, and a transmissible, possibly infectious agent may be responsible; many women who ultimately develop the disease have been infected with the Herpes simplex virus. Other researchers noticed that illnesses of many different kinds tended to follow periods of stress or unfavourable life events; and exacerbations of the infection followed further exposure to stress.

Some of the factors described above are open to nursing intervention. Case study 4.1 below shows how the factors which place an individual patient at risk of developing infection may be assessed, and how these risks can be minimised.

ANTIBACTERIAL, ANTIFUNGAL AND ANTIVIRAL AGENTS

This chapter closes with a description of some of the more commonly used drugs prescribed to destroy bacterial, fungal and viral infections. Nurses need to know how these drugs act, the routes by which they are best administered and their likely side-effects, so that they can provide reassurance and explanations to patients. When patients leave hospital with antibiotic tablets to

Case study 4.1

Elizabeth, aged 42, was admitted to a gynaecology ward to undergo total abdominal hysterectomy. Elizabeth told her nurse that she was relieved to have the operation because her periods had become increasingly heavy over the last 2 years, making her tired and irritable; her daughters were now aged 11 and 14, she and her husband had never wanted more than two children, and following hysterectomy there would be no further need for contraception. Several of Elizabeth's friends had had the same operation. She was reassured because they had all made good recoveries. The information pamphlet provided by the hospital had also been helpful.

In planning Elizabeth's preoperative care, her nurse took into consideration several factors that might increase the risk of postoperative sepsis:

- Possible chest infection. Elizabeth smoked an average of 20 cigarettes each day, and had not been able to cut down, although this had been suggested when she visited the outpatient department.
- Possible wound infection. Elizabeth was clearly overweight for her height and body build. Despite losing 2.2 kg (5 lb) before admission she still had a 'spare tyre' of flesh overhanging the suprapubic region, so this area would be damp and difficult to keep clean during the early postoperative days when Elizabeth's movements were restricted, and would form an ideal environment for the development of a secondary grade Gram-negative infection. Most genuine wound infections arise in theatre when the tissues are exposed (see Chapter 9). Secondary infection manifests itself several days later, and affects the superficial tissues. However, Elizabeth would also be placed at a disadvantage in theatre, because haemostasis is more difficult to achieve when there is excess adipose tissue. Obese people heal more slowly than those of ideal body weight.

  Elizabeth's combination of obesity and predisposition to chest infection could be particularly unfortunate, because coughing places additional strain on a wound, especially an abdominal wound.
- Possible urinary tract infection. Research has shown that women undergoing hysterectomy have a considerable risk of developing urinary tract infections, even though symptoms may not become apparent until the patient has been discharged (Gould and Wilson Barnett, 1985). Elizabeth told the nurse that she had had several episodes of cystitis in the past.
- Possible infection at the site of the intravenous cannula.

When she had welcomed Elizabeth to the ward, discussed the operation and recorded her vital signs, the nurse was careful to observe how her patient settled in. As she soon made friends with the other patients and appeared to be an active person, this would be an advantage during early postoperative mobilisation. It was also noticeable that Elizabeth had a pronounced smoker's cough.

There is a growing body of research evidence to suggest that surgical patients benefit if they are given information about the operation and their recovery, whether individually or in groups (see Chapter 3). On the ward to which Elizabeth had been admitted the sister explained to all the new patients what would happen on the day of operation and told them about intravenous fluids, early mobilisation and the need for adequate analgesia. However, as individual patient care was practised on the ward, the nurse allocated to each patient discussed specific issues. Elizabeth's nurse explained the need for:

- Restricting or cutting out smoking on the morning of operation, to avoid irritating the airways.
- Early mobilisation, in order to avoid complications of the lungs and circulatory system, as well as infection.
- Deep breathing exercises, which were demonstrated later by the physiotherapist.
- Adequate pain relief to permit mobilisation and physiotherapy.
- Drinking at least 2 litres of fluid daily to avoid urinary tract infection.

It was explained to Elizabeth that she was at some risk of developing an infection after the operation, but that antibiotics would be effective in treating it, and that she could do much to promote her own recovery.

The doctor arranged the following preoperative investigations:

- Full blood count, group and cross-matching 2 units of blood.
- Culture and sensitivity of a midstream specimen of urine.

Elizabeth had been taking iron supplements, so she was not suffering from iron-deficiency anaemia, and at the time of admission she did not have a urinary tract infection. However, the nurses knew that in theatre a catheter would be used to empty the bladder to avoid trauma during surgery, although it would be removed immediately.

Postoperatively, the following care was planned, including several precautions to help reduce risks of infection:

- Intravenous fluids prescribed by the doctor were discontinued as soon as bowel sounds were heard the following day.
- Sips of clear fluid were gradually increased in amount until Elizabeth was tolerating 2 litres of fluid every day.
- A light, highly nutritious diet was commenced as soon as bowel sounds were heard, because protein, calories and vitamin C are needed for tissue repair. The immediate postoperative period is not, therefore, a good time to commence a reducing diet.
- Oral hygiene was encouraged, especially when Elizabeth's diet was restricted, to prevent her developing a sore, dry mouth which could become infected.
- Early mobilisation was encouraged. Elizabeth sat out of bed on the first postoperative day, and used a commode, so that she could be wheeled to the WC where she would have privacy. The next day she walked down the ward, helped by her nurse.
- The physiotherapist visited Elizabeth each day. Between visits, Elizabeth practised chest and leg exercises. Twice daily she was given a steam inhalation to liquefy respiratory secretions and facilitate expectoration.
- Initially analgesia was provided every 4 hours, both to enable movement and for cooperation with the physiotherapist. Injections of antiemetics were given intramuscularly to avoid straining the wound by vomiting. Later Elizabeth received milder analgesia when requested.
- Maintaining an adequate standard of hygiene was an important aspect of care. It was vital that Elizabeth's skin should remain clean and dry at all times, in order to restrict the growth of bacterial contaminants. At first help was needed to wash in bed, especially when Elizabeth was restricted by the intravenous infusion. Later she was able to take a shower. Elizabeth would have preferred a bath, but her nurse explained that showering was a safer alternative in terms of preventing infection. Water lodging in a bath can support the growth of Gram-negative bacteria, which may be brought into contact with the wound.
- Wound care was tailored to fit Elizabeth's particular needs. An impermeable dressing was applied in theatre and not removed until the third postoperative day, when under normal circumstances epithelialisation should have taken place (see Chapter 9). Each day the wound site was observed for oozing, and the skin at the edges of the dressing for inflammation.

Elizabeth had a closed suction wound drain inserted through a stab wound separate from the main incision, because her obesity had impeded haemostasis. Excessive collection of blood and serous fluid may result in the formation of a haematoma, with subsequent infection. The drain was checked frequently by the nurses, to ensure that the vacuum was not lost, and to observe the quantity and quality of the fluid draining. The drain restricted Elizabeth's movements, and she was relieved when, on the third postoperative day, drainage had ceased and it could be removed. At the same time the wound was inspected and the original dressing replaced with plastic transparent spray. Elizabeth was taught to support the wound whenever she coughed.

The surgeon generally asked for sutures to be removed on the fifth postoperative day, but in Elizabeth's case alternate sutures were removed one day and the remainder the following morning to ensure that the wound edges did not gape.

Perineal toilet is an important aspect of care for patients who have had an abdominal hysterectomy, to promote comfort and minimise the opportunities for bacteria to grow, for there are two wounds: the external wound, and a sutured area at the top of the vaginal vault where the uterus has been removed. A haematoma can form in the vagina, resulting in a dark, offensive discharge. Elizabeth used the bidet after passing urine and was provided with sterile sanitary pads. Her nurse explained that some vaginal loss was normal, but that she should report any dark or offensive discharge at once.

Elizabeth's progress was monitored by:

- Bacteriological screening of sputum and urine.
- Recording temperature, pulse and respiratory rate to detect the earliest signs of sepsis.
- Observation of the cannula site for signs of inflammation.

Elizabeth left hospital on the sixth postoperative day. Her wound was oozing moderate amounts of bloodstained fluid, which required daily cleaning and the application of an absorbent dressing. The advice given to her before she left hospital and the care provided by the district nurse are discussed in Chapter 11 (case study 11.7).

take, it is very important for the nurse discharging them to explain the importance of completing the course of treatment, despite mild discomforts (such as a sore mouth). Patients feeling better may discard antibiotics before the infection has been completely destroyed. Antibiotic tablets taken at infrequent intervals will result in erratic levels of the drug in the blood, and destroy its effectiveness.

Use of the Agents

Antibacterial drugs either kill bacteria (bactericides) or prevent them multiplying (bacteriostatic agents). They may disrupt the cell wall and cause the cell to break up. Penicillins, cephalosporins and some of the more toxic drugs like polymyxin used for topical wound treatment are bactericidal because they operate in this way. Bacteriostatic drugs include tetracyclines, chloramphenicol, erythromycin and the aminoglycosides, which interfere with the replication of DNA or the manufacture of essential proteins so that the cell cannot divide. Antifungal agents appear to operate in a similar way.

The choice of antifungal agents suitable for clinical use is limited at the present time and the ones available have rather toxic side-effects. The number of antiviral agents is also small. Since viruses operate by taking over the host cell, drugs intended to damage them are nearly always harmful to the host tissues as well. Some antivirals, like amantidine, help prevent the virus entering the host cell. Others, like idoxuridine, prevent DNA replication. Acyclovir, the newest and, to date, best antiviral agent, has an ingenious mode of action: the drug itself is not active; instead it is metabolised by enzymes unique to cells that have been infected with the herpes virus, and products of metabolism then inhibit DNA synthesis; healthy host cells are not affected.

The main uses of antimicrobial drugs and nursing considerations are outlined below.

Antibacterial Agents – Antibiotics

Penicillins

Penicillins, the first antibiotics to be discovered, remain among the most effective when bacteria causing the infection are not resistant to them. They are used mainly for treating staphylococcal and streptococcal infections. Penicillin G is effective both intramuscularly and intravenously against meningitis and endocarditis. Ampicillin can be used to treat Gram-negative urinary and chest infections and otitis media. Intravenous carbenicillin is effective against serious *Pseudomonas* and *Proteus* infections. Gonorrhoea and syphilis are treated with drugs of the penicillin group, usually ampicillin.

Unfortunately, approximately 3% of the general population is hypersensitive to penicillin. Serum sickness, rashes, fever and anaphylaxis (a serious systemic shock) may result. There are also other restrictions against use. Because all penicillins operate in much the same way, bacteria resistant to one penicillin will probably also be resistant to all the others. Sensitisation may also result from handling the drug or from dietary intake, for example, in milk. Some penicillins cannot be given orally because they are destroyed by gastric secretions, and injections can be painful. Intravenous therapy has led to cases of thrombophlebitis. On the positive side, combinations of broad-spectrum penicillins such as flucloxacillin and ampillicin are effective against a greater range of bacteria.

Cephalosporins

These drugs are valuable against penicillin-resistant staphylococci and streptococci, and for treating *E.coli* and urinary tract infections caused by *Klebsiella*. Hypersensitivity may occur, especially among patients who are already sensitive to pencillins (8%), and cephalosporins may also cause disturbance of the gastrointestinal tract flora, vulvovaginitis and renal damage. Some cannot be given by the oral route and injections may be painful.

Tetracyclines

Tetracyclines can, at least in theory, be used to treat most infections because they are broad-spectrum antibiotics. In reality, many bacteria are now resistant to them. Tetracyclines alter the gut flora, leading to superinfection by *Candida* and are not suitable for pregnant women or children under

12 years of age because they may discolour the teeth of the fetus or child. Also, absorption of tetracyclines may be prevented by calcium and iron – they are ineffective if the patient is also taking antacids or mineral supplements. Some authorities also recommend restricting the intake of dairy products while these drugs are being taken.

Macrolides

The most widely used antibiotic belonging to this group is erythromycin, effective against Gram-positive infections. It is of value in people who are allergic to penicillins and cephalosporins. About 5% of the population have side-effects of nausea, vomiting and abdominal pain. Unlike most drugs, which are excreted in the urine, erythromycin is excreted in bile.

Peptides

This group includes bactracin and polymyxin, effective against Gram-negative bacteria. They are highly toxic, and this limits their clinical value, although they may be useful topically. They are not absorbed from the gastrointestinal tract and oral doses can be given against intestinal infections.

Other Antibiotics

Some antibiotics do not easily fit into the system of classification used above. They include chloramphenicol, active against enteric pathogens like *Salmonella*; fucidic acid which destroys many bacteria resistant to penicillin; lincomycin and clindamycin. These last two drugs have been used to treat bone and joint sepsis and intra-abdominal infections. However, they can depress the white blood cell count, sometimes fatally, and may cause gastrointestinal disturbances, including an inflammation of the gut wall known as pseudomembranous colitis; jaundice is also possible.

Sulphonamides

These old-established antimicrobial drugs are still valuable in the treatment of urinary and upper respiratory tract infections (such as sinusitis and tonsillitis), especially among patients sensitive to penicillins. High fluid intake should be encouraged since they may crystallise in the urine when excreted. Allergies, fever and blood dyscrasias have been reported, and sulphonamides may also potentiate the action of oral hypoglycaemic drugs. The spectrum is broader if combinations of sulphonamides are used. Co-trimoxazole is a combination of the broad-spectrum sulphonamide sulphadiazine and trimethoprim, which potentiate the action of each other.

Synthetic Antimicrobials

Trimethoprim, apart from its use as co-trimoxazole, is also used on its own against infections of the urinary, respiratory and gastrointestinal tracts and skin. Both preparations have been reported to induce folate deficiency.

Metronidazole, effective against anaerobic bacteria and *Trichomonas* is unpopular with patients because alcohol is forbidden, and adverse reactions have included fits. The drug may also cause nausea and a sore, dry mouth.

Nalidixic acid is useful in the treatment of Gram-negative urinary and gastrointestinal reactions.

Antituberculous Drugs

These drugs are not popular with patients because their side-effects are unpleasant, and as tuberculosis is a chronic infection they must be taken over a long period. Patients require supervision during therapy, and this is one reason for hospital admission. Isoniazid may cause insomnia, muscular twitching and peripheral neuropathy, which then has to be treated with vitamin B. Sodium para-aminosalicylic acid is mainly used in domiciliary treatment and can cause gastrointestinal upset. Ethambutol is used both in prophylaxis and treatment; it is effective against strains resistant to isoniazid and streptomycin, but in high doses may prompt rashes, abdominal and joint pains, peripheral neuropathy and hallucinations. Other drugs used for tuberculosis are rifampicin and streptomycin, which are often used in combined therapy with the drugs mentioned above. Patients who receive rifampicin must be warned that it turns body fluids red. Streptomycin can damage the kidneys and the eighth cranial nerve (resulting in hearing loss).

Antifungal Agents

Nystatin

This is used for vaginal, oral, oesophageal and intestinal candidosis. Unfortunately, it has a bitter taste, and for oral treatment a suspension of the drug must be held in the mouth. It is also used topically for vaginal infections.

Griseofulvin

This is used for fungal infections like ringworm that affect the scalp, nails and skin because it concentrates in keratinised cells. It potentiates the action of some anticoagulants, and its effects are reduced by barbiturates.

Amphotericin B

This is effective against most fungal infections and can be given intravenously. It has been used to treat the severe fungal infections developed by people who have AIDS. Unfortunately its side-effects include general malaise, which can be severe, and anaemia.

Antiviral Agents

Amantadine is effective against influenza, idoxuridine against herpes zoster, and acyclovir against both Herpes simplex and Herpes genitalis. Acyclovir can be given both orally and intravenously, and is the most promising drug of its kind at present.

References

Anderton, A. (1984). The potential of *E. coli* in enteral feeds to cause food poisoning: a study under simulated conditions. *Journal of Hospital Infection*, **5**: 155–163.

Ashworth, P. (1984). Infection control and the nursing process: making the best use of resources. *Journal of Hospital Infection*, **5**: 35–44.

Baker, J. P. (1982). Nutritional assessment. A comparison of clinical judgements and objective measurements. *New England Journal of Medicine*, **23**: 267–269.

Carter, C. O. (1962). *Human Heredity*. Pelican, Harmondsworth.

Cheesebrough, J. S. et al. (1984). The complications of intravenous cannulae incorporating a valved injection side port. *Journal of Hygiene*, **93**: 497–504.

Chmel, H. (1976). *Salmonella oslo*. A faecal outbreak in hospital. *American Journal of Medicine*, **76**: 203–208.

Coates, V. (1985). *Are They Being Served?* Royal College of Nursing, London.

Davies, A. J. (1984). Is coagulase-negative bacteraemia in neonates a consequence of mechanical ventilation? *Journal of Hospital Infection*, **5**: 260–269.

DHSS (1972). *Nutrition in Health and Old Age*. HMSO, London.

Earnshaw, J. J. et al. (1985). Outbreak of *Pseudomonas aeruginosa* following endoscopic retrograde cholangio-pancreatography. *Journal of Hospital Infection*, **6**: 95–97.

Gibbs, J. (1983). Bacterial contamination of nasogastric feeds. *Journal of Infection Control. Nursing Times Supplement*, **79** (7): 41–47.

Gould, D. J., Wilson-Barnett, J. (1985). A comparison of recovery following hysterectomy and major cardiac surgery. *Journal of Advanced Nursing*, **10**: 315–323.

Holland, K. T. (1984). A comparison of *in vitro* antibacterial complement activating effect of OpSite and Tegaderm dressings. *Journal of Hospital Infection*, **5**: 323–328.

Jones, D. (1975). *Food for Thought*. Royal College of Nursing, London.

Kolmos, H. J. (1984). *Klebsiella pneumoniae* in a nephrological department. *Journal of Hospital Infection*, **5**: 253–259.

Leading article (1983). Colonisation of the trachea in ventilated patients: what is the bacterial pathway? *Journal of Hospital Infection*, **4**: 15–18.

McNeill, J. J. (1984). Methicillin-resistant *Staphylococcus aureus* in an Australian teaching hospital. *Journal of Hospital Infection*, **5**: 18–28.

Newsom, S. W. B. (1979). Review of the problems of infection control. In: *Problems in the Control of Hospital Infection*, 1–4. International Congress and Symposium Series, No. 3. Royal Society of Medicine, London.

Pahwa, S. G. (1981). Decreased *in vitro* humoral response in aged humans. *Journal of Clinical Investigation*, **47**: 1094–1101.

Price, E. H. (1984). *Staphylococcus epidermidis* infections of cerebrospinal fluid shunts. *Journal of Hospital Infection*, **5**: 7–17.

Skeet, M. (1981). The science of microbiology and the art of nursing. In: *Nursing Science in Nursing Practice*, Smith, J. P. (ed.), pp. 111–113. Butterworths, London.

Spencer, R. C. (1984). Infective complications of peritoneal dialysis. *Journal of Hospital Infection*, **5**: 233–240.

Stucke, V. A., Thompson, R. E. M. (1980). Infection transfer by respiratory condensate during positive pressure ventilation. *Nursing Times*, **76** (9): 3–4 (*Journal of Infection Control Nursing Supplement*).

Webster, M. (1986). Control measures. *Nursing Times*, **82**(6): 26–28.

Weskler, M. E. (1980). The immune system and the ageing process. *Proceedings of the Society for Experimental Biology and Medicine*, **165**: 200–205.

Wilmore, D. W., Dudrick, S. J. (1969). Intravenous therapy. *Archives of Surgery*, **99**: 462–463.

Further Reading

Most general pharmacology textbooks have an account of antimicrobial drugs. Further information and dosages can be found in Mims and the British National Formulary (BNF). Useful articles are sometimes published in the popular nursing press; three recent publications are given below.

Bremner, D. H. (1981). The physiology of penicillin. *Nursing Times*, **77** (35): 1503–1505.

Hopkins, S. (1985). A new approach to combat viruses. *Nursing Mirror*, **160**(18): 28–29.

Smith, S. (1985). How drugs act, 8: antibacterial and antiviral agents. *Nursing Times*, **81** (4): 34–36.

# Chapter 5

Providing a Safe Environment: Policies and Routines

INTRODUCTION

In Chapter 4 the risk of developing an infection to the individual patient was discussed, and it was shown that although individual assessment and care planning are of key importance, many patients face similar problems because they share the same hospital environment. In this chapter ways of providing a safe environment, as free as possible of the risks of infection, are discussed.

Nurses working both in hospital and in the community need to know about decontamination and disposal procedures in order to help provide an environment that is safe for patients, visitors and all other members of staff. This is shared by nurse managers because it is part of their role to maintain overall standards of patient care, and to plan for changing needs both in the hospital and in the community. To be cost-effective, when old buildings are upgraded, new hospitals commissioned, policies changed or new equipment purchased, reputable manufacturers should be able to provide sound advice about decontaminating equipment and storage between use. Failure to ensure that equipment can be adequately maintained at reasonable cost can lead to a useless purchase and also endanger the patient.

Preventing infection for the common advantage of patients and hospital staff depends as much on cheap and relatively simple precautions as on expensive and complicated ones. Rahman (1985), evaluating the commissioning of a new hospital isolation unit and assessing its use over the first 5 years, found that much depended upon simple policies. Before the unit was open, 15 outbreaks of infection were recorded, but only one afterwards.

People are more likely to comply with procedures that do not appear to involve endless trouble. In the present cost-conscious climate of the health service there is a clear need to distinguish between those activities in which it is worth investing time and money and those in which it is not. With the correct approach, hospital infection may be controlled. Noone and Shafi (1973) reported a slight increase in the number of urinary tract infections following the appointment of an infection control nurse; probably more infections began to be detected than in the past. The following year, nurses were educated about the dangers of catheterisation and the number of reported infections declined. Further decrease followed the introduction of a policy for the use of disinfectants.

NURSING PRACTICES

Numerous nursing practices are considered to be 'good' although there is little rationale behind them in terms of infection control. For example: for years salt has been added to bath water in the mistaken belief that it would aid healing (Watson, 1984); nurses are warned not to wear uniforms in the street and to keep their hair controlled and tidy. But there is very little evidence to suggest that either of these practices has much bearing on the control of infection, either inside or outside hospital. There are, however, rational reasons for not wearing uniform outside hospital grounds, which concern litigation, should the nurse (who may be very junior) witness an incident in which medical or nursing intervention is necessary.

It has traditionally been accepted that female nurses wear hats as part of their uniform; this is a relic of the past, probably more important as a measure against infestation than to prevent the dissemination of bacteria. The question of whether or not they should continue to be worn still evokes strong feelings, but these have nothing to do with infection control.

The purpose of this chapter is not to lay down hard and fast guidelines, but to raise awareness of those activities which contribute towards cost-effective infection control, and to foster an approach that encourages the application of basic principles of microbiology to practical nursing care. Many nursing practices and procedures need to be questioned, and there is a clear need for more research in this sphere (see Chapter 8, on catheter care, and Chapter 9 on aseptic techniques).

Nevertheless, the need remains to consider the aesthetic desirability of nursing practices, irrespective of their value in terms of infection control. For instance, it is clearly not acceptable for mouthcare equipment to be stored in a sluice room, adjacent to bedpans and urinals, even though it will be handled only by nurses whose hands are socially clean. If any activity seems unpleasing in terms of social acceptability then it is not proper to expect any patient to tolerate it. Where the risk of infection is definitely known to exist, decontamination procedures must be arranged to reduce that risk.

HANDWASHING AND INFECTION CONTROL

Handwashing is the prime example of a cheap and effective infection control measure. Many infections, especially nosocomial ones, are spread by contact, and good handwashing technique is the most important method of prevention. It is important to recognise when the hands are bacteriologically contaminated. A great many infections are autogenous, bacteria being transferred from a site of normal carriage to one that is susceptible. When individual patient care is practised, this point is sometimes overlooked. There is still a need to wash hands between bedmaking for a patient and giving the same patient an injection.

Hands, like the rest of the skin, have two different microbiological flora. Those which are permanently resident stubbornly resist all attempts at removal for more than a few hours or days. Transient microorganisms, picked up and shed on skin scales during normal activities, can generally be removed by adequate handwashing, or their numbers at least reduced to a level below the infective dose.

Nurses should wash their hands:

- before an aseptic procedure,
- after handling patients,
- after handling any item that is soiled,
- before handling food,
- as soon as the hands become visibly soiled.

Adequate handwashing technique involves thorough lathering of all the hand surfaces, followed by careful drying, preferably on a disposable towel to avoid recontamination. A bar of soap kept at the side of the sink is more likely to be contaminated than liquid soap from a dispenser. The mechanical action of running water is at least as important as the detergent or disinfectant. Alternatively, an alcoholic preparation may be used. It is, however, vital that all surfaces of the hands come into contact with the water or alcohol. Taylor (1978) showed that nurses frequently employed poor handwashing techniques, the areas most commonly neglected being the tips of the fingers and the webs between them, the palm of the hand and the thumb. Other studies have shown that rings should be removed for handwashing to be effective, since bacteria tend to accumulate beneath them (Jacobson *et al.*, 1985).

Handwashing is just one important method of avoiding contamination. Other methods are now discussed.

DECONTAMINATION

Anything within the hospital environment can become contaminated with potentially infectious material: the structure, fixtures, fittings, furnishings, or the people in it. Those at risk include not only patients and their visitors, but staff, including those not directly responsible for the services provided for patients.

Decontamination can be achieved at three different levels:

- cleaning,
- disinfection,
- sterilisation.

The ultimate form of decontamination is destruction by incineration.

Each level of decontamination becomes progressively more effective at reducing the threat of infection, but also more expensive, and often more difficult to achieve and more likely to damage the item concerned. It is possible to decide the most appropriate method from a consideration of basic microbiological principles. From Chapter 1 it should be apparent that thought must be given to the likely sources and routes of infection, and the behaviour and growth requirements of microorganisms, especially the versatile opportunistic infections.

Table 5.1 summarises control measures developed from the basic microbiological principles. Table 5.2 shows situations where the risk of contamination and subsequent infection are likely to be high.

Occasionally equipment that has been in contact with a heavily infected source must be rendered safe either by disinfection or sterilisation before it can be safely handled. Cleaning will be delayed until after this has been accomplished. Other items may need sterilisation or disinfecting after use, but for the average patient (not one who is immunosuppressed) they need only be socially clean. Proctoscopes and vaginal specula fall into this category. The place of storage is also important, as mentioned above.

The different methods of decontamination are now described.

Cleaning

The purpose of cleaning is to maintain the appearance, structure, and efficient functioning of the hospital and its contents, as well as to control the bacterial population and prevent transfer of infection.

The whole issue of cleaning in hospital is a thorny one, because nurses feel, quite rightly, that their time should be spent caring directly for their patients, and that valuable resources are wasted if they are required to undertake tasks that could be performed by domestic staff.

Unfortunately there is some overlap between tasks that directly relate to patient care and are the province of nurses, and those that may be performed by domestic staff. Nurses need to know about cleaning and storage of equipment such as washbowls, soaps and flannels because they are directly responsible for the hygienic needs of the patient.

Table 5.1 Controlling Infection in the Hospital Environment: Key Factors

(1) Providing an environment hostile to the growth and multiplication of microorganisms: clean, dry, well-ventilated and with plenty of light (ultraviolet light rays destroy bacteria).
(2) Protecting susceptible patients or sites from contamination. Immunosuppressed patients may be isolated. Wounds may be dressed.
(3) Containing sources of infection wherever possible, using the appropriate isolation precautions.
(4) Decontaminating infectious material.

Table 5.2 Situations Where Risk of Contamination/Infection Is High

(1) Spillages of organic waste (blood, pus, urine, vomit, faeces) where these are not cleaned up promptly. Waste food, raw meat and fish, wet equipment and used cleaning solutions are generally heavily contaminated. In the past hospitals have often been designed so that WCs, bathrooms and sluice rooms are moist, dimly lit and poorly ventilated. Space may be at a premium, so that adequate cleaning is difficult.
(2) Materials that have had contact with an infected site. These require care when handled, stored or transported. Examples include soiled dressings, 'sharps', linen, excretion and secretions from infected patients, laboratory specimens.
(3) The immediate environment of patients who have communicable diseases or particularly virulent infections.
(4) The immediate environment of highly susceptible patients such as the immunosuppressed, special care baby units, intensive care units, theatres.

Table 5.3 Outline Policy for Good Cleaning Practice

(1) Prepare a new, correctly diluted cleaning solution for each task, using a clean, dry container; warm solutions are more effective than cold ones.
(2) Apply the solution evenly to all surfaces. Mops or wipes should be clean and dry before use. The use of excess fluid should be avoided, so that the equipment can be dried; excess fluid can seep into cracks.
(3) The cleaning solution must be changed at regular intervals to avoid a build-up of bacteria and soiled material which would lead to recontamination.
(4) Sufficient time must be allowed for the cleaning solution to penetrate the soil on the surface, but this must be tempered with the knowledge that cleaning agents can damage surfaces if allowed to remain in contact with them for too long. For example, hypochlorites corrode metal.
(5) The cleaning solution must be poured away without splashing in the sluice or a dirty utility area, not into washbasins used by patients or by nurses for clinical purposes.
(6) The clean surface must be dried as thoroughly as possible.
(7) The hands must be washed thoroughly and dried.

Principles of Cleaning

Wherever possible, nursing equipment should be stored clean and dry between use. There is no place for tanks of disinfectant containing bedpans, urinals or other items. The solution intended to disinfect rapidly becomes inactivated by organic matter coating the item (Table 5.3) and may become heavily contaminated, especially if it is not replaced by a fresh solution at regular intervals. Ayliffe *et al.* (1970) reported contamination of infant feeds in a milk kitchen where Milton was carelessly used to disinfect feeds. The authors recommended that bottles should be sterilised by heat, or that preprepared feeds should be obtained directly from manufacturers. When protective isolation is undertaken:

- soaking specific items may be necessary,
- the solution used must be at the correct dilution,
- the solution must be changed every time that it is used,
- the equipment should be reserved for the use of a particular patient,
- the time spent immersed in the disinfectant should be strictly controlled and made the responsibility of one person.

Baths should be cleaned and dried after use by *every* patient. Sheepskins, foam wedges and pillows should *never* be washed and dried on a ward, but sent to the laundry, for they dry slowly and the moisture they retain is a source of Gram-negative bacteria. Nurses are often reluctant to send such items to laundries because ward stocks run low. This situation is often made worse by 'hoarding' items, which become fomites, as they are used by several patients in succession (see Chapter 3).

Wards that specialise in care of the elderly present particular difficulties in terms of infection control, not only because incontinence is so often a problem, but because the aim of the nursing team is to enable the patient to return if at all possible to a normal life outside hospital or, if this cannot be achieved, to live as normally as possible within the confines of the hospital, wearing their own day clothes. It is highly desirable for patients to have access to a personalised clothing service, but this must be backed up with proper facilities. Clothing should not be soaked and dried on the wards, and it is not a nurse's duty to do this. Since small items of clothing are easily lost in the main hospital laundry, or damaged by harsh industrial machinery, a special small-scale laundry with its own staff is generally the best solution.

Thermometers, creams for skin treatment, eyedrops and all other items should be reserved for the use of an individual patient. Thermometers should be stored dry, not standing in solution. They can be wiped with alcoholic disinfectant immediately before use. If possible, every patient should have his/her own washbowl, stored upside down, so that any residual moisture can drain away. Flannels, soaps and towels must never be shared. One of the great benefits of individualised patient care is that it has helped to do away with communal trolleys, where equipment in short supply might sometimes be shared. Provision of unglamorous items – soaps, combs and toothpastes – cause particular difficulties when no relatives exist to supply them.

It is clear, then, that nurses rather than domestic staff are in the best position to take charge of the patient's hygiene and the equipment associated with it. Moreover, it is the nurse, and not members of the domestic service, who have been taught about the types of patient at particular risk, and who are therefore able to pay particular attention to cleaning items in immediate contact with the patient.

In hospitals most of the 'environmental' cleaning is, quite appropriately, undertaken by domestic staff, but all nurses need to appreciate the difference between good and poor standards of cleanliness. Although the nurse in charge of the ward no longer controls the activities of domestic staff, she needs to help monitor their work, and must be able to recognise activities that might jeopardise the safety of patients, staff or visitors. Many hospitals have now introduced quality assurance programmes, and the provision of a clean and safe environment comes high on the list of priorities, being one of the aspects of the hospital most immediately noticeable and important to patients and their relatives. Domestic service managers or contractors and supervisors visit wards and departments at regular intervals during the working hours of their staff, but nurses are present *all* the time, and may occasionally need to discuss routines of cleaning and other matters with the head of the department.

If spillages and other accidents happen at hours when domestic staff are not available (very late or early, or during the night) the nursing staff must clear up the soiled area efficiently and safely.

In some departments of the hospital, nurses undertake a certain amount of cleaning as a regular part of their work. In the intensive care or special baby unit, equipment that is in close contact with the patient (and usually expensive and intricate) will probably be cleaned by the nurse assigned to that patient. The entire operating theatre is washed thoroughly at least once a day, and before each list surfaces are cleaned with alcohol, beginning with high surfaces such as the lights, then working down to lower levels, such as the trolleys and stools. Nurses may help and must supervise the work of ancillary staff like operating department technicians during these procedures. Other procedures designed to reduce the risks of infection in theatre are shown in Table 5.4.

Hygiene Outside Hospital

Patients may need advice about hygiene and infection control when they go home, and a certain amount of tact is required when providing this information, as well as the imagination to foresee possible problems. Housing in inner city areas is frequently substandard. Families may live in cold, crowded rooms with shared bathroom facilities or none at all. Under these circumstances sterilising the baby's feed or emptying a colostomy bag may present insurmountable difficulties. Some people now return to the community with established infections from which other family members must be protected. The patient with AIDS or hepatitis B needs to know how to keep his environment safe for other people, and this information may be provided by the nurse in hospital before discharge. However, research has indicated that discharge-planning is one of the busy ward sister's lowest priorities (Roberts, 1978), and some people may go home with only vague instructions about what they should do. Others may never have been admitted to hospital, yet still encounter problems with hygiene and the prevention of infection. District nurses and health visitors are the key

Table 5.4 Reducing the Risks of Infection in Theatre

Maintenance of the environment
(1) Thorough washing of the theatre each day.
(2) Damp dusting of floors and surfaces between each case; visible soiling and blood should be removed.
(3) Use of a filtered ventilation system, switched on before the operating list commences each day, periodically checked by the hospital engineers. Air flows from clean to dirty areas, not the reverse, and filters changed at regular intervals moving from regions of high pressure in theatre to low pressure in the sluice. In high risk areas laminar flow is used. Air moving at high speed (approximately 30 m/min) passes through a bank of filters which takes the place of a conventional wall or ceiling in the room. It is extracted through the opposite wall or floor. The main advantage of laminar flow is the high speed at which particles can be removed from the patient's vicinity.

Precautions taken by theatre staff
(1) Protective gowns and overshoes worn by all visitors to theatre.
(2) Protective clothing worn by all members of the operating team only in the theatre area.
  (a) Filter masks.
  (b) Shoes worn only in the department.
  (e) Disposable paper hats to completely cover the hair.
  (c) Dresses or trouser suits changed at least daily. Trousers are better than dresses, as they reduce the risk of dispersal of perineal skin scales carrying staphylococci; non-woven materials also help reduce this risk.
  (e) In high risk areas a special 'body exhaust' Charnley system of ventilation may be used.
  (f) Tightly fitting disposable gloves, changed as soon as they are punctured, and a strict regime of hand disinfection by the surgeons and their assistants.
(3) Prompt reporting of infectious illnesses among staff (such as boils and stomach upsets).

Conduct during the operation
(1) Strictly observing aseptic precautions.
(2) Keeping movement within the theatre to a minimum so that the count of airborne particles is kept at a low level.
(3) Keeping as few people in theatre as possible.
(4) Reporting untoward incidents and breaches of asepsis.
(5) Monitoring the number of infections that occur in clean wounds.

people to cope with these because they see the patient in his own surroundings and can visualise the potential problems directly; they also have the opportunity to establish a relationship with the patient and family by regular visiting. Nurses working in the community are guests in their clients' houses, and it is important to bear this in mind continually when providing advice about matters concerned with hygiene; the standards of one person are not necessarily those of someone else, and may not be attainable or even considered desirable.

Nurses who work in the community need to know about services for the disposal of contaminated materials like incontinence pads, and services to which clients may be entitled, for example the incontinence laundry service. They also need to know the decontamination policies used within the hospitals which serve the community so that they can adapt these safely for the benefit of the client. Patient teaching both in hospital and the home is discussed in more detail in Chapter 11.

Cleaning Procedures

Cleaning procedures are designed to remove soiling and microbial contaminants and should be followed by safe removal and disposal of contaminated items. Inefficient practices may increase bacterial counts by redistributing microorganisms on soiled mops or cloths. In view of this, hospital domestic service managers generally choose items that can withstand autoclaving, especially if they are to be used in areas where the risk of contamination is high, such as isolation or geriatric units. Mopheads and cloths must always be stored dry between use. Disinfectant solutions may be spilt and become colonised by bacteria and they are a particular hazard on wards where children and patients suffering from dementia are nursed. The literature relating to the safe use of disinfectants is full of reports to show that solutions can become contaminated and a possible source of infection to patients. Burdon and Whitby (1967) showed that stock solutions of chlorhexidine could become contaminated with *Pseudomonas*. Such risks have been decreased since the introduction of small individual bottles and sachets containing sufficient fluid disinfectant for the treatment of a single patient on one occasion. Any unused disinfectant should be discarded and a new container opened each time. 'Topping up' small containers from a large stock one is a dangerous practice and known to increase the risk of transferring infection (Bassett et al., 1970). Cork stoppers (rarely used now) represented an infection hazard because they could harbour Gram-negative bacteria (Linton and George, 1966).

Cleaning to the required standard in hospital demands equipment, materials and methods not used in the domestic situation at home, and those people who use them must receive special training. It is important for nurses to recognise this, because the role of the domestic staff is sometimes undervalued. They have a vital part to play in maintaining a safe hospital environment and keeping morale high. Patients and staff alike feel dispirited in an environment that is neglected (Bromley, 1983).

An outline policy for good cleaning practice which needs to be recognised by nurses is shown in Table 5.3. Damp dusting is a good deal less likely to disperse microorganisms into the air than dry methods, but the cleaning solutions soon become contaminated and bacteria grow in them. Splashes and aerosols add to the risk of spreading infection and there is the problem of prompt and safe disposal. Cleaning solutions, like disinfectants, must be changed at regular intervals and, also like disinfectants, should always be used at the correct concentration. Surfaces must be dried after cleaning, because moisture will always encourage bacterial growth. A moist surface should be regarded as potentially contaminated.

Dry cleaning is used in hospitals, though not usually by nurses. Its main disadvantage is the risk of infection from dispersal of particles carrying bacteria into the air. Such particles carry chiefly skin flora, and this may, of course, include *Staphylococcus aureus*. It goes without saying that the ward routine must be organised so that dry cleaning does not occur directly before aseptic procedures take place.

Disinfection

Disinfection is the destruction of vegetative microorganisms, but not their spores. Its aim is to achieve reduction in the number of pathogens to a level not likely to result in infection. Heat and chemical methods of disinfection are both available, but chemical methods are discussed in the greatest depth here because they are most often used by nurses. It is very difficult and expensive to destroy all vegetative microorganisms, so a compromise is usually reached by attempting to destroy most of them, bearing in mind the limitations of the method chosen.

The virulence of the microorganisms likely to be present must be taken into consideration, for some are destroyed more readily than others. The susceptibility of the patient must also be borne in mind; a level of bacteria that would not be harmful to a healthy person might cause a fatal infection in a leukaemic child. Another important point is the nature of the equipment being disinfected. Some areas, for example, ward floors, drains, sluice hoppers and WCs become recontaminated so readily that it is wisest to regard them as permanent sources of potential pathogens (Ayliffe et al., 1967). Hill (1984), working as an infection control nurse, provides some evidence to suggest that nurses' knowledge of disinfectant properties may be incomplete.

The ideal disinfectant should not damage surfaces, or harm the people who use it, and should remain in contact with the surface long enough to exert its effects. It should be possible to achieve all this at minimal cost price. Unfortunately, the ideal disinfectant does not exist, so compromise is necessary. Misuse may result in serious and detrimental effects to the environment for which protection was intended. Reliance upon an unsuitable disinfectant can increase the risk of infection.

Most chemical disinfectants are applied as liquids, but gases such as formaldehyde vapour, used mainly in specialist departments and CSSD, are more penetrative. However, nurses often handle disinfectant solutions, and Table 5.5 gives a checklist to show their effectiveness. Some of the more commonly used liquid disinfectants are discussed below.

Table 5.5 Factors Which Determine the Effectiveness of Chemical Disinfectants

(1) *Satisfactory contact.* Disinfection cannot be achieved unless the solution has contact with all the contaminated surfaces. This is not always easy to ensure because grease, trapped air, or protein may form a film between the solution and surface.

(2) *Neutralisation.* A wide range of substances may neutralise disinfectants, reducing their effectiveness. Common examples include: hard water, soaps, detergents and many types of plastic, including plastic buckets.

(3) *Concentration of the disinfectant solution.* It is fairly obvious that a solution made up below the recommended dilution will not destroy microorganisms efficiently. It is generally less well appreciated that disinfectants may also be inefficient if their concentration is too high. This is because stabilisers or 'wetting agents' are incorporated into the solution. Dilutions should always be made accurately.

(4) *Stability.* Some disinfectant solutions are not stable, especially when dilutions are made, and they may deteriorate with storage. Solutions should never be used after the expiry date, and if further dilution is necessary before use, the solution should be prepared freshly before use.

(5) *Speed of action.* Disinfectants destroy microorganisms at different rates. Some may act slowly, yet be suitable for a particular task because they have other advantages. Although alcohol acts rapidly it penetrates poorly. Hypochlorites are rapid, very cheap, and can be effective at low concentrations, but they are corrosive and easily neutralised. Glutaraldehyde acts slowly and is expensive, but is often chosen because it will destroy spores and does not damage costly equipment.

(6) *Range of action.* Disinfectants are not equally effective against all types of microorganism. Cetrimide, hexachlorophane and, to a lesser extent, chlorhexidine, are able to destroy Gram-positive bacteria better than Gram-negative ones. Hypochlorites are preferred when there is a risk of hepatitis B or AIDS, since they effectively destroy these viruses.

(7) *Cost.* Expensive disinfectants purchased for special purposes are uneconomic and unsuitable for general-purpose disinfection. Disinfectants that can be safely used on human tissue must be non-toxic, non-allergic, and non-corrosive. These properties are costly to achieve and are generally obtained at the expense of some other desirable property.

Disinfectants

Clear Soluble Phenolics

These include Clearasol, stericol and hycolin, which at 1–2% concentrations are commonly found as environmental disinfectants in hospitals. They are toxic and corrosive, but suitable for surface use because they are stable in solution, not easily neutralised (see Table 5.5), cheap and able to destroy a wide range of microorganisms, although not spores or viruses.

Hypochlorites

This group of chemicals, the bleaches, is sold under many different names and at different dilutions. These are usually expressed as parts per million (ppm). Solutions like Domestos have gained wide popularity within the home. Hypochlorites are very active against a wide range of microorganisms. If present in high concentrations, they will destroy spores and viruses, including the hepatitis B and HIV virus (the AIDS virus), but toxicity declines with increasing dilution. Neat bleach contains 100 000–150 000 ppm and is suitable for environmental use at dilutions of 1:100, although it will still be corrosive. The considerably more dilute solution of Milton (125 ppm) can safely be used in food preparation, but is unstable and readily neutralised by organic matter. It is essential to use the precise dilution of hypochlorite recommended for effective disinfection.

Glutaraldehyde

Glutaraldehyde, also marketed as Cidex, is used as a 2% alkaline solution, either to disinfect or to sterilise expensive or complicated equipment liable to be damaged by heat or stronger chemicals. It is generally allowed a contact period of 20 minutes, which is sufficient to destroy vegetative microorganisms. After prolonged contact (3 hours) spores will be destroyed.

Alcohol

This is probably the most familiar disinfectant of all to nurses; 70% solutions (often impregnated into swabs) are used to rapidly disinfect physically clean surfaces such as thermometers and catheter outlets before emptying. Alcohol evaporates swiftly, leaving the surface dry, but it is a fire risk when used in large quantities and it penetrates poorly. Although it is suitable as a hand disinfectant it will dry the skin unless combined with emollients, and does not destroy spores or every type of virus.

Diguanides

This group includes chlorhexidine (Hibitane), a complex chemical disinfectant that has been formulated specifically to disinfect human tissue, and been developed as a non-toxic, non-corrosive, non-allergic fluid. Its major drawback is that these important and necessary properties have been achieved only with the sacrifice of some loss of activity against certain types of microorganisms; Gram-positive bacteria are destroyed by chlorhexidine much more readily than Gram-negative ones. Activity against acid-fast bacilli is slight and spores are not destroyed. Chlorhexidine is seriously inactivated by organic matter and neutralised by many different substances. It should be apparent that this agent is highly unsuitable as an environmental disinfectant, and despite its pleasing odour, it does very little good when poured down drains, used to soak thermometers or to wash the underwear of patients who have been incontinent. Its other drawback is that it is far too expensive.

Iodophors

Although iodophors like povidone-iodine compounds (such as Betadine and Disadine) have a broader spectrum than chlorhexidine, they have not achieved such widespread use because they discolour the skin brown. Betadine has found favour in the operating theatre because it can destroy spores.

Quaternary Ammonium Compounds

The most widely used member of this group is cetrimide, which has natural detergent properties and is often used as a wound disinfectant. It destroys Gram-positive bacteria well, and has fair activity against Gram-negative bacteria, but will not destroy acid-fast bacilli or spores and is inactivated rapidly by organic matter and neutralised by many substances.

Cetrimide and chlorhexidine are marketed in combination as Savlon which is frequently used to disinfect wounds (see Chapter 9).

Principles of Disinfectant Use

In hospitals the use of disinfectants is strictly controlled according to the policies developed by members of the infection control team, and all members of the domestic staff should be trained in their use. A typical policy would prescribe the use of one hypochlorite and one phenolic solution for 'heavy' cleaning, with hypochlorites specifically for use when hepatitis B or AIDS may be a risk, and 70% alcohol for cleaning equipment such as thermometers and wound dressing trolleys. Chlorhexidine and perhaps an alcoholic hand rub will usually be prescribed for skin disinfection, with glutaraldehyde reserved for use mainly in theatre and CSSD. The number of compounds used is best restricted in order to reduce confusion and because there are financial advantages if large quantities can be purchased from suppliers on contract.

Advertisements in this sphere can be very persuasive. Not every hospital has developed or reviewed its cleaning and disinfection programmes as satisfactorily as it might, and every year thousands of pounds are poured, literally, down the drain. Sometimes this happens despite good policies and well-trained domestic staff, because nurses are using products for purposes for which they were never intended. This may happen in the home too. A team evaluating the effectiveness of different disinfectants in the domestic situation found that phenolics and hypochlorites marketed under familiar brand names could produce substantial reductions in the bacterial counts of kitchens, bathrooms and WCs, but that their effects were generally shortlived, mainly because householders used the solutions incorrectly. Dishcloths and other utensils were not washed frequently enough and tended to disseminate infection throughout the rest of the kitchen. Disposable cloths would have been far more effective. Sinks and WCs become recontaminated so rapidly that disinfection achieved no more than aesthetic cleaning. The authors felt that most of the problems stemmed from the public's ignorance of general hygiene (Scott et al., 1984). Given the number of babies admitted to hospital every year with gastrointestinal upsets, and the susceptibility of elderly people to food poisoning, this should be a matter of concern for all nurses who work in the community.

Ideas about matters relating to hygiene are not always fully appreciated by the general public. For example, it is considered socially acceptable to cover the mouth when coughing or to sneeze into a handkerchief, to protect others from the infectious aerosol of droplets generated by a cough or sneeze. Perhaps less well appreciated is the fact that toilet paper is permeable to bacteria, while faeces are full of bacteria, including many potential pathogens. When a WC is flushed, the fine spray of contaminated water that results is comparable to a sneeze. Bacteria of faecal origin can be isolated from the surrounding walls and ceiling. Here they do no harm; but others, located on door handles and beneath the seat, represent a greater health hazard. It is obviously best if facilities for handwashing are available in the same area as the WC, but this is not often the case in public facilities, including British hospitals.

Before reaching for the disinfectant, all nurses should consider the type of bacteria they are trying to eradicate, their properties and the numbers in which they are likely to be present. The concentration of the disinfectant solution is just as important as its chemical properties and spectrum. In hospital, this rarely presents a problem since most disinfectants are provided from the pharmacy or stores in the concentration recommended for a specific purpose. In cases where dilution is necessary, graduated containers are usually available. In the community, the nurse has to know the likely properties of the disinfectant that the patient has chosen to purchase, the dilution at which it is supplied and is most likely to be effective, and the damage it may cause to surfaces in the patient's home, where she is a guest. Those who have to contend with an infection control problem (AIDS, hepatitis B, carriers of gastrointestinal pathogens) need to be provided with information about suitable disinfectants, disposal and mopping up spills before they leave hospital, told about the effectiveness of hypochlorites, and warned about the damage that this disinfectant can cause, particularly if it is splashed into the eyes. Some disinfectant solutions are marketed without information of their chemical composition, and these are best avoided.

Heat Disinfection

Heat is the cheapest method of disinfection, but not the one most commonly used by nurses, unless they work in clinics or departments where they are required to operate hot air ovens, pasteurisers or autoclaves (which sterilise, *not* disinfect). This may be the case in general practitioner surgeries, outpatients and family planning clinics, isolation units and wards where immunosuppressed patients are nursed.

Although the ability of microorganisms to withstand heat varies considerably, nearly all those of medical significance are destroyed after exposure to moist heat at 50–70°C for between 20 and 30 minutes. Some species, like *Streptococcus faecalis*, are more resistant, and bacterial spores are very heat-resistant indeed.

Heat is less selective in its action than the majority of chemical disinfectants, but more penetrative and much more easily controlled. The simplest method is, of course, boiling. Diabetic patients who feel happy with their own glass syringes need to be taught to immerse the equipment completely in water, and keep it in the saucepan, still immersed, until it is required. Nurses who work overseas will fall back much more heavily on this method than those who work in developed countries.

The biggest drawback of heat disinfection is the damage that it can inflict, related to the time and temperature required to destroy the target microorganisms. Fortunately, it is often possible to disinfect heat-sensitive materials at a lower temperature over a longer period of time. Since rapid heat penetration reduces the time required to achieve disinfection at any given temperature, the more rapidly penetrating methods of applying heat are preferred. Steam penetrates more rapidly than hot water, but the latter is more effective than hot air.

The method of moist heat disinfection used most widely by nurses is the bedpan washer. The length of time of the cleaning and disinfecting cycle must be kept as short as possible, since no patient or nurse would be prepared to wait for more than a few minutes. Mechanical bedpan washers are available that clean bedpans and maintain them at 80°C or more for at least a minute in order to achieve disinfection. Some bedpan washers are still manufactured that do not disinfect, since the temperature achieved is below 65°C. When new machines are installed, these products should be avoided, and their inadequacies borne in mind by the nurses obliged to use them.

In some hospitals, macerators are used in conjunction with disposable bedpans and urinals. There is a danger that contaminated aerosols can be produced when the door of the machine is sealed (Collins *et al.*, 1980). Nurses who have used this system soon observe that overloading the machine can lead to the system becoming blocked and breaking down.

Sterilisation

Sterilisation is necessary when the small number of bacteria that would survive disinfection processes might result in infection. This could happen either because they were exceptionally virulent, or because they might be given the opportunity to reach an unusually susceptible site of the body or a particularly vulnerable patient. The main requirements for sterilisation are shown in Table 5.6. Different methods used to achieve sterilisation are outlined in Table 5.7.

Table 5.6 Situations When Sterilisation Is Necessary

(1) All items of equipment that will break the natural barriers of the body to infection (surgical instruments, urinary catheters, injection needles, intravenous fluids).
(2) Dressings and topical applications that will be in contact with broken skin or areas of the body that are normally sterile.
(3) Where contamination with resistant bacterial spores in large numbers is likely (for example, *Clostridium tetani*, *Clostridium welchii*, *Bacillus anthracis*).
(4) To treat equipment that has been in contact with pathogens that are extremely virulent and life-threatening, for example, viral haemorrhagic fever.
(5) In situations where ordinary disinfection procedures are not sufficient owing to the extreme susceptibility of the patient. Patients who have leukaemia or who have undergone organ transplant and are immunosuppressed fall into this category.

Except when they operate small autoclaves, usually in clinics, or sterilise delicate equipment by chemical methods, nurses do not use sterilisation techniques to any great extent, and for this reason they are described only briefly. It is important to point out, however, that although the term sterilisation is commonly taken to imply the destruction of all microorganisms, including spores, this is misleading. In practice, it is never easy to determine when destruction has been absolute, although methods of quality control are employed both in the hospital CSSD (where most sterilisation is achieved by autoclaving controlled by ancillary staff), or commercially.

Table 5.7 Methods of Sterilisation

Heat
(1) Dry heat
   incineration
   hot oven air ovens
   infrared convectors
(2) Moist heat under pressure (autoclaving) in hospital CSSD or theatre departments for surgical supplies and commercially

Radiation – used commercially, such as in syringes, needles destroyed by heat
(1) Ultraviolet radiation
(2) X-rays
(3) Gamma-radiation

Chemical – for delicate items
(1) Ethylene oxide gas
(2) 40% formaldehyde gas
(3) 2% gluteraldehyde solution

} usually undertaken in CSSD, or theatres for delicate equipment like endoscopes, destroyed by heat. For the gases, special equipment is necessary and care must be taken as they are toxic and highly resistant

Filtration (applicable to fluids) – undertaken commercially; 0.2 mm filters can remove all vegetative bacteria, spores and viruses

Microorganisms will be destroyed at relatively low temperatures in the presence of moisture; an exposure of 60 minutes at 160°C is necessary for sterilisation under dry conditions, but only 15 minutes at 121°C when using steam under pressure. Steam also has the advantage of rapid penetration of porous objects and fabrics. In the autoclave, air is removed by suction to create a vacuum before the steam enters, to ensure that penetration of the steam and contact with every surface is complete. Failure of contact means failure to sterilise.

The care of sterile equipment such as CSSD packs is of central importance to nurses. Packs must be kept dry and the paper covering undamaged, or their contents can no longer be regarded as sterile (Alder, 1961). Cupboards are better than open racks because they offer protection from dust. Packs that are not often used may be further protected by storage in plastic bags.

DISPOSAL OF WASTE MATERIALS

Nurses need to know how to dispose of waste materials safely because the problem begins in the ward. Any large institution is bound to generate a great deal of waste material, and hospitals are no exception. Any waste material that has been in contact with human or animal sources will contain potentially pathogenic moisture and organic matter. Although this will also apply to domestic waste, the sheer bulk of waste from a big hospital will give rise to major problems of safe and efficient disposal. Inappropriate handling by nurses and other members of staff may lead to contamination of the environment and a reduction in socially acceptable and aesthetic standards. The way in which waste materials are sorted will also influence infection control, outside as well as inside the confines of the hospital. Although some wastes are incinerated within the hospital, others are removed by local authorities or by contractors.

The DHSS has recently introduced a system for colour-coding the different categories of hospital waste and these are shown in Table 5.8. The disposal of waste from infectious patients, including urine, faeces and vomit, is discussed in Chapter 6 in conjuction with isolation procedures.

'Sharps'

In the past there has been a great deal of controversy regarding the safe disposal of needles, syringes, intravenous administration equipment, and other sharp, non-usable instruments (all known as 'sharps'). According to some authorities, the risk of puncture wounds ('needlestick injuries') and thus the spread of parenteral disease, was likely to be increased if needles were routinely separated

Table 5.8 Colour-coded Bag System for the Disposal of Waste in Hospital

Colour of bag	Contents	Destination
Red, with alginate-stitched liner	Foul/infected linen	Laundry
White	Soiled linen	Laundry
Yellow	Clinical waste, including all infectious waste	Incinerator
Green	Waste from offices, non-clinical areas	Incinerator

after use. Others worried that aerosols containing virus particles could be produced if a needle was left in position while blood obtained from venepuncture was transferred to a collecting bottle. The rising incidence of hepatitis B, followed by AIDS, has helped to focus more attention upon the safe disposal of 'sharps'. Research findings from the United States have now shown that virtually all puncture injuries result through resheathing needles after use (Wormser et al., 1984). Most people now agree that needles, syringes and other sharp instruments should be handled as little as possible once they have been used. The needle and syringe are best left unseparated and unsheathed and should be placed in a 'sharps' box as soon as possible by the person who has used them. Sharp instruments left on bedside tables, hidden in bedclothes or allowed to fall on the floor are a great danger to ancillary staff and are responsible for a considerable number of accidents each year. Cost-conscious hospital managers may be aware that 'sharps' boxes will fill up very rapidly if they are used in this way, but trying to avoid this expense is false economy. The cost of inpatient care, treatment and litigation against a hospital that proved negligent in its disposal policies, resulting in a member of staff developing hepatitis B or AIDS, would be very much greater. The cost in terms of human suffering could not even be measured.

'Sharps' boxes that have become full should be sealed and sent for incineration. They should be constructed of material thick enough to resist wetting from any fluid released inside the box, or penetration from a sharp object inside or out. Boxes made of thin cardboard present a risk that hospital staff (porters as well as nurses and doctors) should not be prepared to accept.

Precautions When Handling Blood and Blood Products

A discussion of the disposal of 'sharps' leads naturally to the safe handling of blood and blood products. It is a peculiarity of western society that whereas most bodily secretions and excretions are considered to be contaminated almost by instinct, blood is not. Yet disease can be spread parenterally by at least two viruses: HIV (the AIDS virus), and to a lesser extent hepatitis B, have achieved notoriety. But there may be other blood-borne viruses whose route of spread have yet to be determined. *All* blood and blood products should be regarded as potentially contaminated and *never* handled unless the individual wears gloves and then washes the hands thoroughly. Neither HIV nor the hepatitis B virus is very robust, and rely heavily on spread by parenteral and sexual routes precisely because they *cannot* survive for long outside the body. Both are readily destroyed by hypochlorites and by heating to 80 °C. Dilutions of Domestos at a ratio of one measure of disinfectant to nine measures of water can be used safely in the home.

Bedclothes from patients who have active hepatitis B or HIV or who are carrying these viruses, must, like all bloodstained laundry, be placed in the appropriately colour-coded laundry bag (see Table 5.8) and subjected to a temperature of 98 °C for 1 minute.

All dressings and other waste materials must be placed in a yellow bag and sent promptly for incineration. This procedure does not differ in any respect from the disposal of contaminated waste from any other patient. Much distress can be spared patients and their families if precautions taken for parenterally spread infections can be approached rationally, bearing in mind the principles of microbiology. Some of the patients concerned may be terminally ill; all will be in great distress. Exaggerated and unnecessary precautions are no help to the patient, his family or the nurses caring for him.

Precautions for staff working in theatre are shown in Table 5.9 (overleaf).

Table 5.9 Theatre Precautions When a Patient Is a Hepatitis B Carrier (or Has Another Parenterally Spread Infection)

General principles

Avoid accidental inoculation with blood or blood-contaminated instruments.

Choose equipment which can easily be decontaminated.

Whenever possible use disposable equipment, linen and drapes.

Arrange for the surgery to be performed at the end of the operating list.

Obtain adequate supplies of a disinfectant known to destroy the virus, such as sodium hypochlorite 1% solution (10 000 ppm available chlorine).

Dispose of all waste materials carefully, according to hospital policy.

In the anaesthetic room

Only essential staff should be present.

All non-essential equipment should be removed.

Have a 'sharps' box available.

Fill the suction bottles to be used with 100 ml sodium hypochlorite 1% solution.

If a ventilator is to be used, the anaesthetist or his assistant should make sure that it is fitted with a detachable autoclave circuit and autoclavable filters.

Protect the patient's trolley and the theatre table with a water-repellent laminate material or equivalent.

During the operation

Keep movement in the theatre to a minimum.

Make sure that a runner is available in the theatre corridor so that no member of the operating team needs to leave during the course of the operation.

Wipe up blood spillages as soon as they occur, using sodium hypochlorite 1% solution.

Handle all bloodstained swabs with forceps, and put them into a yellow plastic bag for incineration as soon as they have been counted.

All members of the operating team should wear disposable gowns gloves and hats; goggles should be available if needed.

After the operation

Handle the instruments as little as possible

    Autoclavable instruments should be returned unwashed to CSSD in a container marked with a 'Danger of infection' or 'Biohazard' label if a tray service exists; the instruments must be cleaned in theatre, under gently running water, before they are autoclaved. Protective clothing must be worn. Brushes used for cleaning must be discarded after use. Instrument trolleys must be wiped with 1% sodium hypochlorite solution and allowed to dry. Corrosion can be avoided by rinsing with warm water and detergent.

Non-autoclavable instruments must be washed in gently running water, then chemically disinfected.

Empty suction bottles into the sluice hopper.

The person responsible must wear protective clothing. The bottles can then be autoclaved. Containers in which urine and other body fluids have collected must be treated in the same way.

Wipe down anaesthetic equipment with sodium hypochlorite solution, allow it to dry, then rinse thoroughly. Wash all connections before autoclaving. Discard endotracheal tubing, airway and face mask. Discard the rebreathing bag unless it can be autoclaved.

The closed circuit of the anaesthetic machine and the ventilator must be decontaminated in accordance with manufacturer's instructions.

COMMUNITY HEALTH: IMMUNISATION

Introduction

The purpose of this chapter has been to show how nurses working at different levels of seniority in the hospital and community can help to prevent the spread of infection. It is vital for nurses to learn about the basic principles of microbiology so that they can apply these to different working situations, whether in a high dependency unit, in a client's home or overseas, irrespective of the facilities available. Many of the most effective infection control measures are simple and inexpensive. If high technology equipment like positive pressure ventilation, laminar air flow and bodily exhaust systems are available, then of course they should be used, but even when they are not nurses can do a lot to break the chain of infection, providing a happier and safer environment and preventing undue discomfort and distress.

Infection control falls into two categories: firstly the everyday precautions that have been described in this chapter, which should form part of the education and practice of all nurses; and secondly, untoward events like outbreaks, that need the attention of infection control experts. Nurses must be able to recognise unusual and potentially dangerous situations, so that they know when to call a member of the infection control team (described in Chapter 10). In the next chapter, the principles of isolation nursing will be discussed, completing the theme of infection prevention. Before turning to this, however, it may be valuable to reflect how the spread of infection in the community can be prevented by a planned programme of immunisation.

Vaccines and Immunisation

The way in which infection has influenced the lives of ordinary people was described in Chapter 2, which showed how vaccines were discovered and how their use became widespread. Here, the term vaccine is defined, and different programmes of immunisation discussed.

A vaccine is a suspension of microorganisms that is able to induce a state of immunity in the host. They are either suspensions of microorganisms that have been killed (by heat or chemical treatment) or attenuated so that their virulence is reduced, but not their ability to stimulate antibody production by the host. Exceptions are vaccines that consist of microbial exotoxins; these are called *toxoids*.

Older children respond better to immunisation: 3–6 months is an acceptable time, but 6–12 months is better because the immune system matures

Table 5.10 Immunisation Schedule Recommended in Britain

3–6 months	Diphtheria, tetanus, whooping cough*, oral poliomyelitis
6–9 months	As above*
12–18 months	As above*
2–4 years	Measles
4–5 years	Diphtheria, tetanus boosters
10 years	Tetanus booster
13+ years	BCG, rubella

*Given as triple vaccine

Table 5.11 Commonly Used Vaccines

Diphtheria	Toxoid, 80% immunity, probably lifelong, after three doses Side-effects – minor local reactions Contraindications – severe previous reaction
Tetanus	Toxoid, 5–10 years immunity after three doses Side-effects and contraindications – as above
Whooping cough	Killed bacteria, probably lifelong immunity Side-effects – minor local reactions. Very rarely fits and encephalopathy have been reported after immunisation, for which no other cause has been found. Contraindications – family history of epilepsy or febrile fits.
Poliomyelitis (1) Oral (Sabin)	Live, attenuated virus. Side-effects – one individual in a million will develop paralysis. Contraindications – should not be given in cases of diarrhoea, because it will have no effect. Should not be given to patients with hypogammaglobulinaemia.
(2) Inactivated (Salk)	Killed virus, good protection when the oral suspension is contraindicated.
Measles	Live, attenuated virus, immunity for many years. Side-effects – mild rash resembling measles and fever, appearing about a week after vaccination. One case in 100 000 will develop encephalitis.
Rubella	Live, attenuated vaccine, good protection for many years. Contraindication – pregnancy at the time of administration or possible within the following 3 months.
Bacille Calmette Guérin (BCG)	Live attenuated vaccine. Side-effects – local reactions if given by subcutaneous injection, intradermal injections are preferred. Contraindication – severe eczema, generalised vaccinia may result.
Typhoid	Dead bacteria, primary vaccination – 4–6 week intervals, with booster doses at 3 year intervals. Side-effects – local and generalised reactions with subcutaneous and intramuscular injection, but not if given intracutaneously.
Influenza	Killed virus given in one dose; exact content of vaccine depends upon the current strain of influenza, but there is no proof that it can help control epidemics; it is recommended only for groups at high risk: the elderly, those with chronic respiratory or cardiovascular disease, health care workers.

gradually. Treatment with live vaccines generally requires only one dose. For dead microorganisms or toxoids, three doses are usually necessary. Booster doses may be needed, initially at intervals of 3 or 6 months, eventually at intervals every few years. Immunisation schedules for children vary around the world, depending upon the particular diseases that are endemic. The recommended schedule for children in the United Kingdom is shown in Table 5.10. Details of commonly used immunisations are shown in Table 5.11. Pregnancy, febrile illness, malignancy, and immunosuppression are contraindications against all immunisation.

International certificates of vaccination are required by some countries. Since WHO reported the eradication of smallpox from the world, fewer countries require vaccination against the disease; one injection, effective for about 8 years, is necessary. Yellow fever vaccination is required for travellers within 15° north and south of the equator; again, one injection is necessary and effects last about 10 years.

Cholera vaccination is still recommended for most hot countries, though generally insisted upon only when there is an epidemic. Two injections are necessary, at least one week apart. Immunity lasts for 6 months.

Immunisation against rabies, plague, typhus and anthrax are precautions necessary only for visitors to remote parts of the world, or for those who, through the nature of their work, may be exposed – for example, laboratory workers, customs and excise officers.

References

Alder, V. G. (1961). Preserving the sterility of surgical dressings wrapped in paper and other materials. *Journal of Clinical Pathology*, **14**: 76–78.

Ayliffe, G. A. J. *et al.* (1967). Ward floors and other surfaces as reservoirs of hospital infection. *Journal of Hygiene*, **65**: 515–520.

Ayliffe, G. A. J. *et al.* (1970). Contamination of infant feeds in a Milton milk kitchen. *Lancet*, **1**: 559.

Bassett, D. C. V. *et al.* (1970). Wound infection with *Pseudomonas multivorans* as a waste-borne contaminant of disinfectant solutions. *Lancet*, **1**: 1188–1189.

Bromley, D. (1983). Psychological factors in hospital infection. *Nursing Times Journal of Infection Control Nursing*, 79 **(23)**: 11–14.

Burdon, D. W., Whitby, J. L. (1967). Contamination of hospital disinfectants with *Pseudomonas* species. *British Medical Journal*, **2**: 153–154.

Collins, B. *et al.* (1980). A survey of the use and abuse of bedpan macerators. *Nursing Times Journal of Infection Control Nursing*, 76 **(8)**: 4–5.

Hill, S. (1984). Which disinfectants do nurses use? *Nursing Times Journal of Infection Control Nursing*, **80** (7): 60–61.

Jacobson, G. *et al.* (1985). Handwashing: ring wearing and number of micro-organisms. *Nursing Research*, **3**: 186–187.

Linton, K. B., George, E. (1966). Inactivation of chlorhexidine by bark corks. *Lancet*, **1**: 1353.

Noone, P., Shafi, M. S. (1973). Controlling infection in a district general hospital. *Journal of Clinical Pathology*, **26**: 140–145.

Rahman, M. (1985). Commissioning a new hospital isolation unit and assessment of its use over five years. *Journal of Hospital Infection*, **6**: 65–70.

Roberts, I. (1978). *Discharged from Hospital*. Royal College of Nursing, London.

Scott, E. *et al.* (1984). Evaluation of disinfectants in the environment under 'in use' conditions. *Journal of Hygiene*, **2**: 193–203.

Taylor, L. J. (1978). An evaluation of hand-washing techniques. *Nursing Times*, Part I **74** (2): 54–55; Part II **74** (3): 108–109.

Watson, M. (1984). Salt in the bath. *Nursing Times Occasional Paper*, **80** (19): 57–59.

Wormser, G. P. *et al.* (1984). Needle stick injuries during the care of patients with AIDS. *New England Journal of Medicine*, **310**: 1461.

Further Reading

Lowbury, E. J. L. *et al.* (eds) (1983). *The Control of Hospital Infection: A Practical Handbook*. Chapman and Hall, London.

Maurer, I. M. (1986). *Hospital Hygiene*. Edward Arnold, London.

Royal College of Nursing (1986). *Guidelines for the Care of Patients with AIDS*. Royal College of Nursing, London.

Chapter 6

Isolation Nursing

INTRODUCTION

The purpose of this chapter is to draw attention to those activities that are particularly useful in helping to prevent the spread of infection and to cut out unnecessary procedures, wasteful of time and resources.

Chapter 1 described the routes of transmission of microorganisms; Chapter 2 showed how precautions have been taken since biblical times to prevent spread from people with communicable diseases. These, however, were often useless because they did not succeed in blocking the *route* of spread. Fumigation, incarcerating the unfortunate victims in 'pest houses', and the use of primitive disinfectants like vinegar sometimes worked, but they were applied indiscriminately on a trial-and-error basis.

However, understanding of hospital infection developed during the 1950s, and it is now possible to design the care of infected patients to suit their needs and to provide a safe environment for others. Success depends upon two factors:

(1) Effectively blocking the route of transmission of the microorganism responsible for the infection.
(2) Paying attention to those factors known to block the route of transmission, and ignoring useless measures.

HOSPITAL FACILITIES FOR NURSING INFECTIOUS PATIENTS

First a description is given of the facilities available for nursing infectious patients within British hospitals. These are: cubicles in ordinary wards; separate isolation wards, and specially designated units organised mainly on a regional basis.

Cubicles in an Ordinary Hospital Ward

The facilities available vary enormously according to when the hospital was built. Modern hospitals, of course, are designed with the problems of nosocomial infection in mind (see Chapter 5). Cubicles may have airlocks or laminar air flow systems and a separate bath and WC. But in older hospitals the cubicles used to isolate infectious patients lack these refinements, are cramped and often depressing, and may open directly into the main ward corridor.

Isolation Wards

Some hospitals, though perhaps no longer many, reserve particular wards for infectious patients. Ayliffe *et al.* (1979) believe that, owing to their tedious nature, isolation precautions are seldom conducted effectively on ordinary wards. This view is shared by Bagshawe *et al.* (1978), who advocated nursing infectious patients on special wards. These recommendations were made on the grounds that nurses working on isolation wards would develop special expertise in caring for infectious patients and preventing the spread of infection. However, isolation wards in ordinary hospitals present a variety of problems:

- The patient is moved from the ward which specialises in treating his particular condition. Some procedures (such as renal dialysis or mechanical ventilation) may be difficult to arrange outside a particular hospital unit.
- The number of beds on an isolation ward is limited. Sometimes patients are isolated when management on the ward of admission would have been feasible or more desirable; at other times the number of infectious patients may exceed the isolation beds available. Priorities may be difficult to determine, leading to conflict among staff.
- Isolation wards are often difficult to staff, and few centres run the English National Board course for the care of patients with communic-

able disease, so the 'expertise' envisaged by Bagshawe *et al.* (1978) is not easily provided.

Special Isolation Units

A number of specialist units have been set up throughout the country, with wards categorised according to the stringency of precautions available.

Most of the beds provided are for low or medium grade isolation, and the facilities available may differ little from those that can be achieved in a modern hospital. In older units, relatively unsophisticated conditions prevail, emphasising that the control of infection depends more upon careful nursing procedures than on environmental refinements.

However, staff who work in special units generally have more experience with a wide range of highly infectious and potentially dangerous diseases than nurses who work in ordinary hospitals, and they are usually more confident in their approach. There is greater recognition of the psychological needs of isolated patients and the extra demands made upon nursing time. In purpose-built units patients may benefit from rooms fitted with speak-through channels and glass partitions.

The Trexler Isolator

The ultimate form of isolation is the Trexler isolator, consisting of a plastic tent surrounding the bedframe, to provide an impermeable barrier between the patient and the environment (Fig. 6.1). Half suits and invaginations into the plastic permit nursing procedures without entry into the tent. Inflow of air is carefully controlled, and air coming out of the isolator is filtered. All items are wrapped in plastic film before they come out of the isolator, and are incinerated. Despite its cost, the plastic of the tent itself is destroyed once the patient is no longer infectious. But few diseases demand precautions this stringent. Trexlers are used mainly for cases of viral haemorrhagic fever (Ebola, Lassa and Marburg fevers) which are brought to this country by travellers from parts of Africa where these viruses are endemic. They are carried chiefly by rodents, but may spread to people who have been living in the bush. The

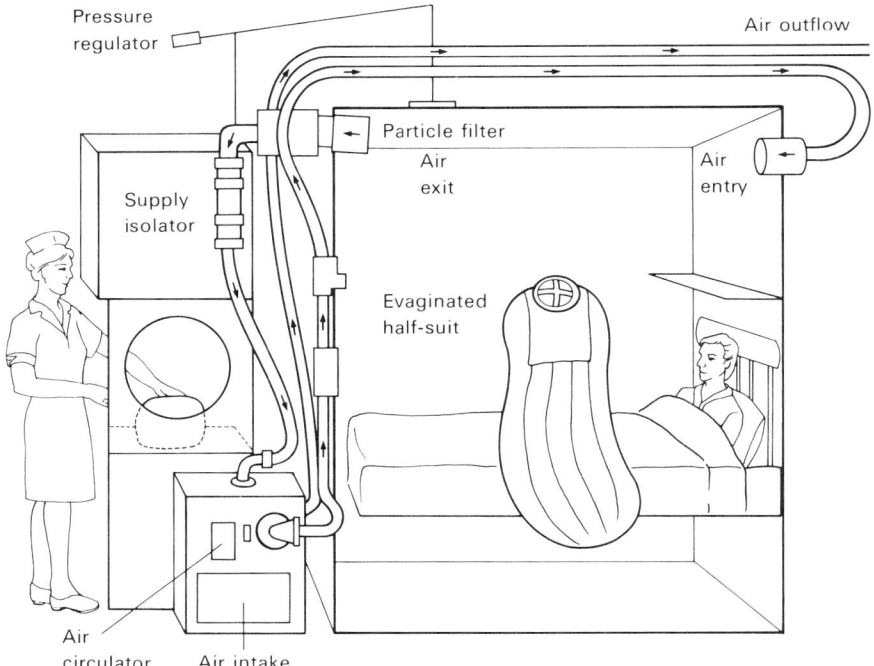

Fig. 6.1 A Trexler isolator (adapted with permission from Brettle and Thompson, 1984).

associated rate of mortality among western people is estimated at about 50% for Lassa fever; Ebola and Marburg fevers are nearly always fatal.

Isolation in a Trexler places a great deal of stress on the patient (who is usually severely ill), his family and the nurse. The patient is never left unattended, and may experience the same problems of sensory deprivation faced by people nursed in intensive care units (ICU). All his personal possessions must be incinerated when he leaves the isolator. Relatives have to contend with the interest of the press, and they need support because they may have had contact with the patient during the incubation period of the disease, and will need to be placed under surveillance by the public health authorities. The fire hazard of nursing someone beneath a sheet of plastic cannot be dismissed lightly. Cigarette smoking must be forbidden.

Care Policy for Isolation Units

In the past, many hospitals developed guidelines for isolation by assigning patients to a particular category of infection in relation to the mode of transmission (Table 6.1). These have often been helpful to staff, but they are of limited use when the mode of transmission is not really clear (as in the case of an unusual infection), or when different precautions may be required for patients who have the same underlying infection. For example, a chronic carrier of hepatitis B who is in hospital for the assessment of rheumatoid arthritis will require very different care from one who has undergone major surgery, and has blood and serous fluid draining from the wound.

When a patient is isolated according to the old system, a card with predetermined instructions is commonly placed on the door of his room, and nurses are encouraged to apply a blanket policy of care rather than use a problem-solving approach to develop a care plan which depends on:

- the individual needs of the patient,

Table 6.1 Isolation According to Category of Infection

(1) *Strict isolation* Lassa fever
multiresistant staphylococcal infection
Marburg fever
anthrax
diphtheria
rabies
  Aim to prevent aerosol and contact spread; patients are nursed, if possible, in special regional units

(2) *Respiratory isolation* measles
whooping cough
meningococcal infections
legionnaire's disease
  Aim to prevent aerosol and secretory spread

(3) *Enteric isolation* enteric fevers (typhoid)
Salmonella gastroenteritis
cholera
dysentery (*Shigella*)
viral meningitis
diarrhoea of unknown origin
  Aim to prevent spread by direct and indirect contact

(4) *Secretory or exudate precautions* mumps
venereal disease
infectious mononucleosis (glandular fever)
  Aim to prevent spread of infectious agents found only in saliva or sputum and not airborne

(5) *Wound/skin precautions*
  Aim to prevent spread of infection from wounds or infected skin lesions

(6) *Protective isolation* immunosuppressed patients (leukaemia, organ or bone marrow transplant)
  Aim to prevent spread of microorganisms from the environment or other people to highly susceptible patients

- the nature and virulence of the causative agent,
- the stage of the infection (acute, chronic),
- the period of infectivity.

If the old system of categorising infection is used, nurses will not be encouraged to work from microbiological principles, and vague, unhelpful suggestions may become incorporated into the care plan. For example: 'The articles that have been in Mr Brown's room and which may be contaminated must be disinfected or destroyed.'

This aim can never be fulfilled because it is not explicit. A better approach would be the problem-solving one suggested by Ashworth (1984) (see Chapter 4) geared to:

- the individual needs of the patient,
- the nature and virulence of the infectious agent,
- the route of transmission.

BLOCKING THE ROUTE OF TRANSMISSION: A PROBLEM-SOLVING APPROACH

In this section, methods of blocking the route of transmission are discussed, illustrated by outline care plans.

When planning the precautions which should be taken to limit the spread of a particular infection, the points shown in Table 6.2 should be considered.

Principles for Preventing Spread

(1) *The causative organism if yet known.*
(2) *The reason for the precautions.* Is the aim to protect both other patients and the nurse, just other patients or the nurse herself? The aim of

Table 6.2 Principles for Preventing the Spread of Microorganisms from Infected Patients: the Problem-solving Approach, Key Factors (see text)

(1) The causative organism if yet known
(2) The reason for the precautions – *who* are they designed to protect?
(3) Mode of transmission
(4) Articles likely to become contaminated, and appropriate methods of decontamination
(5) Need for a single room

isolation precautions is sometimes not made clear. In an outbreak of food poisoning, for example, nurses and patients are both at risk, although frail elderly patients will be more susceptible. Open pulmonary tuberculosis threatens infirm patients and any visitors to the ward who have escaped the net of immunisation (Table 6.3). Tuberculosis, however, is a disease of elderly, frail, poorly nourished people; young, fit people are not likely to catch it, especially nurses who must have immunity before they are allowed to work on the wards.

But in the case of hepatitis B, it is the nurse rather than the other patients who is placed at greatest risk (Table 6.4). She is exposed to the patient's secretions, but hygienic precautions alone should ensure that other patients are not (Table 6.5). Cytomegalovirus can cause severe congenital malformations, but is otherwise responsible only for mild, often subclinical infections, except among patients who are immunosuppressed; these people and nurses

Table 6.3 Outline Care Plan for Open Pulmonary Tuberculosis

(1) Causative organism: *Mycobacterium tuberculosis*.
(2) Reason for precautions: to prevent other patients, visitors and staff developing tuberculosis
(3) Transmission: droplets, dust
   route: mainly airborne (but also touch, handling sputum).
(4) Items contaminated, to be handled with special care
   - Sputum
   - Clothes/bedclothes
   - Every item in contact with the patient's exhaled secretions; those nearest to the patient will be the most heavily contaminated
(5) Need for a single room: essential, door shut; if the patient leaves the room for treatment or special investigations he must wear a mask
(6) Protective clothing: gloves, aprons, masks
(7) *Special points*: in most cases tuberculosis is treated initially with three drugs (triple therapy) because the bacteria rapidly become resistant if single drugs are used. When the sensitivities are known, usually after 1 or 2 months, one or two drugs are given for 9–12 months. When treatment has been started, or when *Mycobacterium* is no longer present in three consecutive specimens of sputum, isolation can be discontinued. However, tuberculosis is a chronic disease, and the bacteria may persist for a long time.

who may be pregnant should never be allowed contact with patients carrying cytomegalovirus.

(3) *Mode of transmission.* The problem-solving approach demands that the nurse has an appreciation of the basic principles of microbiology (see Chapter 1). Gould (1985) found that nearly every nurse who participated in a research study designed to reveal knowledge and attitudes about isolation procedures knew the mechanisms of dissemination for open pulmonary tuberculosis and hepatitis B. However, their knowledge of the methods designed to *prevent* spread were often poor.

Questions were not asked about other microorganisms in this study, and it is possible that for bacteria and viruses encountered less frequently knowledge of transmission may be less complete. Most nurses recognise that *Salmonella* is spread by the faecal–oral route, but they may be unaware that contact spread of this Gram-negative bacillus is also possible. Herpes zoster, the virus which causes shingles, a painful infection of the nerve ganglia, is present in the exudate of the weeping lesions that form over the skin. Unlike many other viral infections, there is no droplet spread; when the lesions become dry and crusted, they are no longer infectious.

(4) *Articles likely to become contaminated and appropriate methods of decontamination.* These must be recognised so that they can be handled with the proper precautions and either destroyed or decontaminated when the patient no longer needs them (see Chapter 5). For patients with airborne infections, every item in the room will be potentially contaminated, although those nearest to the patient will probably receive a larger infective dose. The nature of the article must be taken into consideration; bacteria will not remain in a viable state for very long if they settle on a hard, cold, clean surface and spores will not germinate. A television in the far corner of the room will be a less important reservoir than warm, damp bedclothes, for example. A hepatitis B carrier is unlikely to contaminate his surroundings providing that he is continent, not bleeding, and his personal hygiene is of a high standard. Most hepatitis B carriers are young, and soiled bedclothes are not a problem.

(5) *Need for a single room.* If an infection is spread

Table 6.4 Outline Care Plan for Hepatitis B Carriers

(1) Causative organism: hepatitis B surface antigen remaining from the virus in the patient's blood; the titre will vary, depending on when the patient was infected, and whether it was acute or subclinical
(2) Reason for precautions: to prevent members of staff acquiring the virus. Transmission to other patients or to visitors is unlikely in modern hospitals
(3) Transmission: blood. Virus particles are probably present in secretions derived from blood (saliva, urine, semen, tears, etc.), but probably in smaller numbers than in blood
(4) Items contaminated
 • Blood
 • Visibly soiled items like bedclothes
 • Possibly items soiled with perspiration, saliva, urine and other secretions, depending on the length of time since infection. This may be difficult to determine because of the high incidence of subclinical infections
(5) Need for a single room: desirable, but not essential unless the patient has a respiratory ailment, is likely to lose blood or serous fluid, or is incontinent. A separate WC is desirable
(6) Protective clothing: aprons and gloves for contact purposes; masks only for patients who have copious respiratory secretions, or who require suction

Table 6.5 Outline Care Plan for Shingles

(1) Causative organism: Herpes zoster virus
(2) Reason for precautions: to prevent spread of the virus to susceptible people; other patients (especially the immunosuppressed, who may develop severe infection), visitors and staff. People who have had chickenpox are generally immune
(3) Transmission: exudate from weeping lesions; dry, crusted lesions are not infectious
(4) Items contaminated
 • Weeping lesions and exudate
 • Soiled dressings
 • Soiled bedclothes
(5) Need for a single room: desirable. Occlusive dressings prevent the escape of virus particles, but they may be difficult to apply if the lesions involve the eye, or if the edge of the dressing would encounter the hairline. Patients are frequently in a great deal of pain or visibly disfigured; they often appreciate the peace of a single room
(6) Protective clothing: aprons and gloves

by the airborne route, a single room with the door kept shut will be necessary to contain it, although absence of an airlock may limit its usefulness (see Chapter 1).

In other cases a separate room may be desirable, but not essential. For example, a patient who has profuse diarrhoea due to *Salmonella* food poisoning may be grateful for the privacy of a single room, and the nurses may be prompted to maintain high standards of hygiene because the infection has been regarded as sufficiently serious to warrant the use of one (Table 6.6). However, the bacteria are disseminated on hands and other fomites, so a single room in itself does not guarantee that the infection will be contained. Many people who develop *Salmonella* food poisoning are elderly, and isolated in a single room they may be anxious that they will be unable to call a nurse quickly enough in an emergency; starved of human contact in an unfamiliar environment they may become disorientated.

When an extensive outbreak of food poisoning occurs, sufficient cubicles may not be available on one ward, or even in one hospital. So rather than have ten infectious patients each occupying a cubicle, on ten different wards, with the risk of spread correspondingly multiplied, it would appear more logical to nurse them altogether on the same ward, closed to new admissions and non-infected patients.

Patients with wound infections need not be incarcerated in single rooms provided that the site of infection is completely occluded with a dressing impermeable to bacteria (Geelhoed, 1978). Polyurethane dressings (OpSite) are ideal for this purpose providing that they are carefully applied so that no infected material can escape from the edges (see Chapter 9). Disposable drainage systems are also available, but they may be prohibitively expensive.

Similarly, a patient with a urinary tract infection caused by a multiresistant bacterial strain need not be nursed in a single room provided that great care is taken when handling him or her. The bacteria may be present on the patient's skin, or the bedclothes, so correct handling and disposal of fomites is vital. Nevertheless, isolation of the source of infection and contaminated articles does not necessarily imply shutting the patient in a cubicle if he is too unwell, or would become depressed. Outline care plans can be designed to show how to break the chain of infection. Several factors must be taken into consideration when deciding whether isolation in a cubicle would be desirable, including:

- priority,
- facilities available,
- susceptibility of other people.

Priority is a vital consideration. Only one cubicle may be available, and another patient may need it at least as much, or more. A terminally ill person may require privacy with his family, or there may be a noisy, disoriented patient who persistently disturbs the ward.

The facilities that a particular ward can offer must be considered, particularly those available for handwashing. It may be possible for an infected patient to be allocated his own bathroom and WC. If the source of infection is a wound, the decision of where to undertake the dressings is more difficult, especially if the bacteria are spread by the airborne route.

If an infected wound is dressed at the bedside and the other patients' wounds receive

Table 6.6 Outline Care Plan for *Salmonella* Gastroenteritis

(1) Causative organism: *Salmonella* sp.
(2) Reason for precautions: to protect other patients, visitors, staff
(3) Transmission:
  faecal–oral route
  contact spread
  environmental reservoir where conditions are damp
(4) Articles contaminated
  - Bedpans, faeces
  - Bedclothes, especially if visibly soiled
  - Crockery, cutlery
  - Patient's hands
(5) Need for a single room: recommended. The door may be kept open. When outbreaks occur infected patients may be nursed together on the same ward, but the same nurses should not care for non-infected patients
(6) Protective clothing: aprons, gloves

treatment in the ward treatment room, provided one is available, this could result in contamination of the ward environment, and it might not be possible for all other wounds to be dressed away from the bedside. Inspection during the doctor's rounds could present difficulties, and if a wound needed attention at night it might not be feasible to transfer a patient to the treatment room.

Alternatively, the treatment room could be reserved for the infected patient, although this would expose all the patients to the bacterial counts prevailing on the ward at each dressing change. Fortunately, there is evidence, discussed in Chapter 9, to indicate that surgical wounds rarely develop infection on the ward.

The susceptibility of other patients must also be taken into account. Decisions must be taken according to the circumstances prevailing at the time. For instance, a patient with herpes zoster will represent far less threat on an orthopaedic ward, occupied by young men who have fractures but who are otherwise fit, than on a ward where immunosuppressed patients are nursed. A child who has developed cytomegalovirus because of immunosuppressive chemotherapy will not only need continued protection from the environment, but may represent a threat to young, possibly pregnant mothers visiting other children on the ward. Clearly decisions need to be collectively based on the interests of the individual patient, other patients on the ward, visitors and members of staff.

GENERAL PRINCIPLES OF ISOLATION NURSING

It should be possible to design care plans to suit patients individually and to treat each episode of infection as a unique event. Care plans can be updated with the progression of the infection and the condition of the patient. This is not possible when standard categories of isolation are used; for this reason, collaboration between nurses directly responsible for patient care and the infection control experts in the hospital is vital (see Chapter 10).

Handwashing

The hands should be washed before and after attending to any patient, using a skin disinfectant like chlorhexidine or 70% alcohol (see also Chapter 5). But should this take place before or after leaving the cubicle? In Gould's (1985) study most nurses said they would wash their hands before leaving the cubicle, thus regarding the inside doorhandle as a conventionally 'clean' area. In the case of airborne dispersal, the handle may already be contaminated, although the number of bacteria might not be very great, and they might not be able to survive for very long. Nurses who wash their hands outside the cubicle could risk transmitting infection outside the immediate environment of the patient. The safest approach is probably to wash hands inside the room so that they are 'socially' clean, then wash or treat them with 70% alcohol rub after leaving. Doorhandles should be cleaned thoroughly every day.

Protective Clothing

Basic protective clothing should include plastic disposable apron and gloves. Gould (1985) found that nurses were aware that they should wear protective clothing with isolation of patients with tuberculosis and hepatitis B, but were often vague about which garments were actually required. Some wanted to wear masks, headgear or overshoes, although they were not usually appropriate. The use of protective clothing is discussed below.

Aprons

Transmission of bacteria from the clothing of staff is a theoretical possibility, but in practical terms it seems slight. Ayliffe et al. (1982) cite evidence to show that only small numbers of *Staphylococcus aureus* and Gram-negative bacilli have been obtained from the clothing of staff who work on isolation wards. It is, however, rational to protect clothes when infected material is handled. A plastic disposable apron is preferable to a cotton gown, because bacteria can pass through fabric weave, especially if it becomes wet. Staff often state a preference for gowns, particularly among nurses who work on paediatric wards. In these circumstances a gown can be worn over a plastic apron to prevent a child from slipping. Although the areas most frequently contaminated on clothing are above the waistline, they do not include the shoulders. Gowns therefore offer no advantage over aprons in terms of the greater surface area covered.

Plastic aprons can be worn on more than one occasion when attending to the same patient, provided that they are kept inside the cubicle and the outer surface of the apron is marked (some manufacturers make the sides of the apron of different colours). The chief objection to this practice is the clutter created in the patient's environment.

There has been very little evidence to document the spread of infection from clothing, except staphylococci from people who disperse heavily. However, protective clothing draped outside a cubicle seems generally undesirable. In fact, most nurses in Gould's (1985) study considered that protective clothing should not be taken outside the cubicle unless sealed into a bag ready for incineration.

Gloves

When contaminated items must be handled, gloves are worn to prolong the effects of hand disinfection and to help prevent them becoming grossly contaminated. The number of microorganisms that must be removed by handwashing is therefore reduced, but need for this is still necessary because recontamination can occur if gloves are carelessly removed or punctured.

Plastic disposable gloves must be well-fitting, so that manual dexterity is not sacrificed. Exasperated nurses are more likely to tear the gloves off if they do not fit properly.

Masks

Masks are now thought to contribute very little towards the safety of either patients or staff on the wards, and they have no value in the prevention of wound sepsis (Ayliffe *et al.*, 1977). Ill-fitting and damp masks offer no protection at all, and may contaminate the hands when they are touched or removed. Filter masks are desirable only when patients have infections spread by the airborne route, for example, meningococcal meningitis. Masks need not be worn for patients with AIDS or hepatitis B, unless they are expectorating, need suction, or have another airborne infection that merits protection.

Overshoes

Overshoes are worn in theatre because patients are particularly vulnerable and there is a need to keep overall contamination to a minimum. They have no place on the ward. The floor is not a source of infection under normal circumstances, and overshoes may increase the risk of spread from contaminated hands when the shoes are put on. Microorganisms may not be removed by adequate handwashing afterwards.

Headgear

Headgear is not justified for any isolation procedure intended to prevent the spread of infection on an ordinary hospital ward. *Staphylococcus aureus* acquired from heavy dispersion by a patient may be carried transiently in the hair, but provided it is otherwise clean and controlled, the risk attached is slight.

Infected Wastes

All waste materials except sharp instruments should be placed in a bag that can be sealed and incinerated. A colour-coded scheme for different categories of waste materials has recently been introduced by the DHSS (see Chapter 5, p. 89).

In Gould's (1985) study, nurses' knowledge of safe disposal procedures was found to be unsatisfactory. In this study 60 subjects, some qualified, some learners, were asked questions about isolation precautions in a non-threatening interview which took place on the wards. According to their self-reported behaviour, they would have placed themselves and others at risk.

In some hospitals infected waste is enclosed in a second bag for extra protection, but provided that the original bag is of the correct gauge and will resist perforation and leakage, this should not strictly be necessary. A bag that can easily become perforated, or cannot effectively be sealed, should not be used for the purposes of disposal in hospital. If spillage does occur, it should be cleared away with a disposable cloth and an appropriate disinfectant (see Chapter 5) by a responsible person wearing gloves.

Needles and Sharp Instruments

These should be placed in a 'sharps' box immediately after use. The box may be stored in the room of an adult patient, provided that he has no psychiatric history, and is not disoriented or a drug abuser.

Linen

Linen from infected patients must not be hand-sorted by laundry staff. It should be placed inside water-soluble linen or alginate bags with dissolvable stitching, which can be transported to the laundry in the appropriate colour-coded nylon bag, but tipped without sorting into the washing machine. During the ordinary wash cycle, infected linen should reach a temperature of 65°C for 10 min, then 71°C for 3 min. Linen from patients who have hepatitis B should reach at least 93°C for 10 min (Ayliffe and Collins, 1974).

Bedpans and Urinals

Special provision must be made for handling infected excreta. If the room contains a WC and the patient is independent there is no problem. If the patient is confined to bed, bedpans and urinals *could* be emptied into the WC, but every care should be taken to avoid splashing. The alternative is for the bedpan to be carried to the sluice by a nurse wearing plastic apron and gloves. If disposables are not used, the bedpan must be reserved for the patient alone. The bedpan washer or macerator should be checked by the engineer to ensure that it is in good working order.

Bedpans and urinals should always be removed from the cubicle as soon as they have been used. As well as cluttering the space occupied by the patient, their accumulation is aesthetically undesirable and increases the risk of spillage.

In Gould's (1985) study, nurses often worried about discarding infected faeces and urine into the bedpan washer without first soaking them in disinfectant. Efficient decontamination is not possible unless the disinfectant is left in contact with the infectious material; but in the case of large solids this is not likely to take place for hours because of poor penetration. Soaking is always inefficient because disinfectants are inactivated by organic materials.

As with all infection control procedures, it is vital to keep a sense of proportion. Large numbers of the general population become infected with enteric pathogens and many excrete them with few symptoms or none at all. Even if the public health authorities could identify them all (which they do not; mild symptoms may not merit medical consultation), disinfection before discharge into the sewage system would be impossible. It would be illogical, expensive and extremely difficult to decontaminate excreta from the relatively few people admitted to hospital with enteric pathogenic illness. However, bedpan washers should always be checked regularly to ensure that they are in good working order. They must have a heat disinfection cycle (Ayliffe *et al.*, 1974), and where a macerator is used, it must have a reliable door seal and lock. Regular maintenance is necessary to ensure that aerosols are not produced (Gibson, 1973; Collins *et al.*, 1980).

Crockery and Cutlery

Lack of evidence for spread of infection on cutlery and crockery may indicate that they are relatively unimportant as fomites. However, in the case of severe enteric, blood-borne and droplet-spread infections, precautions seem advisable. Virus particles from patients with hepatitis B and AIDS have been detected in saliva, but it is not known whether infection is actually transmitted by this route. For severe infections where washing by hand is inadequate, the method of choice is either pasteurisation or decontamination in a dishwasher where the final rinse temperature reaches 80°C. Where these facilities are unavailable, patients may have to use cardboard and plastic disposables, though this should be avoided wherever possible.

Cleaning

When isolation nursing is necessary, battles are fought in some hospitals because ancillary staff have exaggerated fears about the danger of infection. As soon as a patient is isolated the domestic services manager must be informed, so that explanations can be given and arrangements made for cleaning the room. As a general rule, equipment that has been in closest contact with the patient will be the most heavily contaminated, a point to be considered when arrangements are made for terminal cleaning.

Cleaning equipment must be kept separate from that used for the rest of the ward, and spillage of bodily fluids should be attended to by people who are most aware of the risks attached to them (this is usually the nurse).

Specimens

Laboratory specimens must be specially marked with yellow 'Biohazard' or 'Danger of infection' labels so that laboratory staff are warned of their special risk. The accompanying request form should also be labelled and, as with all specimens, both should be sealed in a plastic bag.

Visitors

In many hospitals a card bearing isolation instructions is displayed on the door of the patient's room. Some warning is obviously necessary, but a better system would probably involve a simple request to obtain further information from the nurse looking after the patient before entering. A list of instructions is a reflection of the attitudes held before attempts to individualise care.

Visitors to infectious patients require careful explanations and may need supervision to ensure that they comply with the procedures necessary. This may be difficult in cubicles separated from the main ward area. The extent to which visitors should be enforced to adopt the same procedures required by hospital staff will vary. If the patient has developed an enteric infection that other members of his family have managed to escape, there is a clear need for them to adopt full precautions. However, it is obviously illogical to impose a regime of gloves and aprons upon the wife of a hepatitis B carrier, who has been exposed to his secretions everyday for years.

Every case needs individual assessment. Visitors are more likely to comply with isolation procedures if the demands made are reasonable, uncomplicated and comprehensible. Visitors can do much to help alleviate the boredom of patients who require isolation, and they should be welcomed by nurses (see Chapter 11).

Last Offices

If the patient dies, last offices can be performed in much the same way as usual, but *it must be remembered that anyone who has been infectious during life will remain so after death.*

Protective clothing must be worn and the cadaver must be protected so that it does not contaminate other people or the environment. In some hospitals it will be placed in a large polythene bag which must be sealed. In others, special 'cadaver bags' are available. In either case, the bag must be labelled to indicate the risk of infection and the mortuary staff should be warned that they are about to receive an infected patient. It is advisable for relatives to see the patient *before* the polythene bag is in place because the mortuary staff may feel reluctant to handle an infectious patient more than absolutely necessary.

PROTECTIVE ISOLATION

Protective isolation is a reversal of the methods used for isolating infectious patients, and is necessary for people whose disease or treatment has made them unusually susceptible to infection. They may fall prey to endogenous infection, so that the normal body flora presents a grave hazard. Bacteria and viruses from other people may easily set up infections in these immunocompromised patients, so they must be offered protection by isolation from both other people and environmental contaminants. Sometimes nurses become confused about the purpose of protective isolation; it is designed to promote the safety of someone who is himself not infectious, and not a threat to others.

Some centres specialise in the care of immunosuppressed patients and protective isolation units have been set up in these. The patients, who are often undergoing treatment for neoplastic disease or immunosuppressive therapy to prevent tissue rejection after organ transplants, are all nursed in single rooms. Special ventilation systems (laminar flow), filters and airlocks are necessary. The protective clothing required will vary according to the particular unit. In some, staff are required to wear masks, headgear, overshoes and theatre clothing. However, Ayliffe *et al.* (1982) demonstrated a lack of evidence to suggest that infection is transferred to patients from shoes or hair, so that other units have now adopted a more moderate policy. In units where patients who have had cardiac or bone marrow transplant are nursed, however, very strict precautions are taken. The patients occupy plastic Trexler isolator tents (see p. 94, and air is always filtered before it enters the isolator.

Patients who require protective isolation must use disinfected crockery, cutlery and bedpans. In most units, this is achieved by autoclaving. Food may have to be sterilised, so the diet becomes restricted and monotonous. Salads and other uncooked dishes are not permissible because bacteria will always be present on them. If possible, linen should be sterile. Flowers must not be brought into the isolated area and visitors who have infections may not enter the unit. Because items like razors and flannels carry a risk of infection, sterile disposables should be used whenever possible.

These patients, often children and young adults, require a great deal of nursing support, as do their families. Further discussion of the psychological and social implications of isolation for patients can be found in Chapters 7 and 11.

References

Ashworth, P. (1984). Infection control and the nursing process – making the best use of resources. *Journal of Hospital Infection*, 5: 35–44.

Ayliffe, G. A. J., Collins, B. J. (1974). Control of infection in hospital laundries and kitchens. *Health and Social Services Journal*, **February**, p. 230.

Ayliffe, G. A. J. *et al.* (1974). Tests of disinfection by heat in a bedpan washing machine. *Journal of Clinical Pathology*, 27: 760–764.

Ayliffe, G. A. J. *et al.* (1977). Surveys of wound infection in the Birmingham area. *Journal of Hygiene*, 79: 299–313.

Ayliffe, G. A. J. *et al.* (1979). A unit for source and protective isolation in a general hospital. *British Medical Journal*, 2: 461–463.

Ayliffe, G. A. J. *et al.* (1982). *Hospital-acquired Infection: Principles and Prevention*. Wright, PSG, Bristol and London, p. 60.

Bagshawe, K. D. *et al.* (1978). Isolating patients in hospital to control infection. *British Medical Journal*, 2: 609–612.

Brettle, R. P., Thompson, M. (1984). *Infection and Communicable Disease*. Heinemann, London.

Collins, B. J. *et al.* (1980). A survey of the use and abuse of bedpan macerators. *Nursing Times Infection Control Supplement*, **76** (8): 4.

Gibson, G. L. (1973). Bacteriological hazards of disposable bedpans. *Journal of Clinical Pathology*, 26: 146–150.

Geelhoed, G. W. (1978). Isolate the infection, not the patient. *Association of Operating Room Nurses*, **28**: 54–61.

Gould, D. J. (1985). Isolation procedures in one health district. *Nursing Times Occasional Paper*, **81** (7): 47–50.

Chapter 7

Response of the Body to Infection

INTRODUCTION

The term 'stress' is heard a great deal in relation to nursing and ill-health. Nursing is a stressful occupation, and stress is commonly thought to result in disease. Much has been written about the stress associated with hospitalisation, although a universal definition for the term has never really been accepted despite its widespread use. However, all recent research on the subject has emphasised the inseparable nature of both physiological and psychological stress. The concept of stress, the models which various authors have developed to illustrate its relationship to disease and its influence upon recovery, may be used to demonstrate the effects of infection on the tissues and the psychological response of the individual.

In recent years nurses have become increasingly concerned with the overall effects of ill-health on the individual and the impact of disease on psychological and social welfare, as well as on physical well-being. A holistic model has been suggested for the study of recovery in order to describe their impact (Wilson-Barnett, 1981). In this chapter the physiological response to infection is discussed together with its psychological and social implications for people both in hospital and in the community. A framework for helping patients to cope with the problems of infection and the role of teaching and counselling is presented in Chapter 11.

STRESS AND INFECTION

The term homeostasis was introduced in Chapter 1, where it was used to describe the ability of living organisms to maintain internal stability despite continuous environmental change. Disease can be regarded as a disturbance in homeostasis (Montague, 1981), and stress as a harmful environmental stimulus that disrupts homeostasis, resulting in disease (Cannon, 1935; Selye, 1956). This model may be extended, so that pathogenic microorganisms are seen to constitute a threat from the environment which alters homeostasis if they are able to overcome host defences. Disease in the form of infection will become established (Fig. 7.1).

The experimental work of Hans Selye, published in 1956, has influenced contemporary ideas about stress. Selye documented a syndrome of reactions when laboratory animals were exposed to a wide range of harmful stimuli. Subsequent work has shown that the physiological response to stress involves three interconnected processes:

(1) increased activity of the sympathetic nervous system, often described as the 'flight–fright' response;
(2) endocrine response mediated by the pituitary gland;
(3) increased secretion of glucocorticosteroid hormones from the adrenal cortex.

Glucocorticosteroids stimulate the breakdown of large protein and fat molecules from stores in the liver, raising the blood glucose levels. Additional glucose provides the energy required for tissue metabolism to fuel the flight–fright response of the sympathetic nervous system. People who are unable to secrete normal levels of glucocorticosteroids cope poorly even with relatively low levels of stress. Increased levels of these hormones may therefore be regarded as an adaptive response. Nevertheless, glucocorticosteroids may exert a deleterious effect upon the tissues, and their secretion in large quantities can be considered maladaptive: the inflammatory response is suppressed; formulation of granulation tissue in healing wounds is inhibited; and the production of white blood cells in lymphoid tissue is depressed. Very large quantities of glucocorticosteroids appear to enhance the blood clotting mechanism and induce formation of ulcers in the gastrointestinal tract.

The effects of stress on the brain are mediated by the hypothalamus, which controls endocrine and

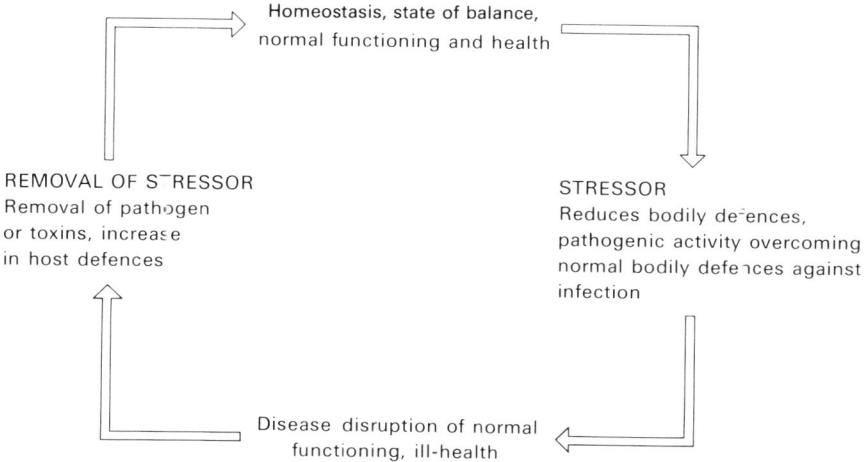

Fig. 7.1 Stress, homeostasis and infection.

sympathetic nervous activity. Information about emotional state *may* also be relayed to the hypothalamus. The limbic system in the brain is thought to be important in the interpretation of emotions; a few nerve fibres run between the hypothalamus and the cerebral cortex. The psychologist Lazarus (1966), who has written extensively upon the theme of stress, has suggested that the body may respond both physiologically and psychologically to stress, and that adaptation to its effects may take place at either of these levels. Invasion by a pathogen, for example, may involve the inflammatory response and the production of antibodies at the physiological level. Overwhelming stress, however, may reduce antibody production because of its inhibitory effects on the lymphoid tissues. At the behavioural level the individual might respond by resting until the symptoms associated with infection subside. Changes at the cognitive level may also take place: an individual may learn from previous experience activities that have resulted in stress and try to avoid them in future. A model to show the effects of stress on normal homeostatic function is shown in Table 7.1. Selye (1956) believed that exposure to stress is part of everyday life, and that the stress reaction should be viewed

Table 7.1 Stress, Homeostasis and Infection: The Action of Physical and Psychological Stressors

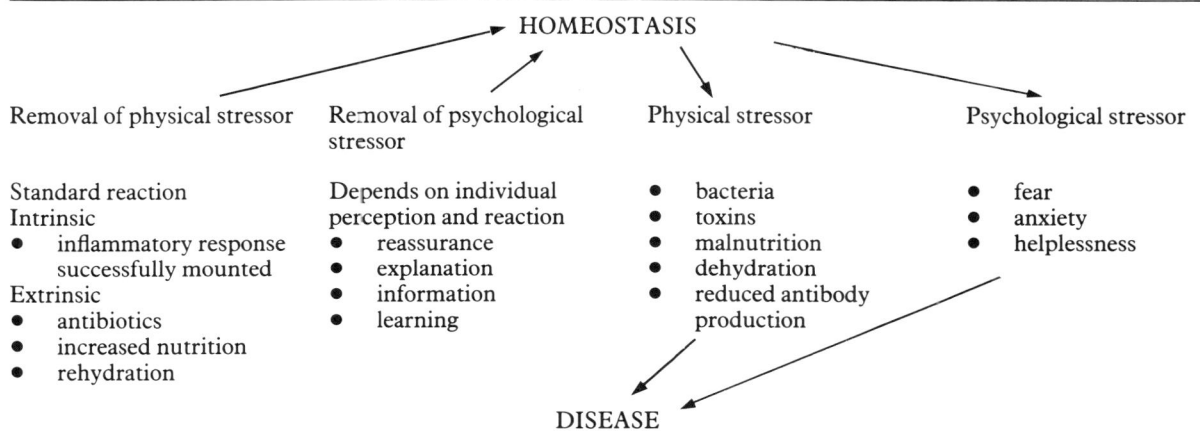

primarily as beneficial, although he agreed, on the basis of his more extreme laboratory findings, that stress could also be harmful.

The work of later authors like Lazarus focused more closely on the maladaptive effects of stress, suggesting that some of the responses inherited from animal ancestors may no longer be regarded as appropriate. Animals run away from threatening stimuli, but an examination candidate or a nurse faced with a worrying situation on the ward cannot hope to achieve anything by the flight reaction; they may, of course, respond in the same way, with racing heartbeat, dilating pupils and glucocorticosteroid release.

The way in which stress is perceived varies in human beings. Factors likely to influence individual perception include personality and previous experience. Lazarus (1966) postulated different 'coping mechanisms' that an individual might employ at the behavioural level to mediate the effects of stress. Two patients who have both developed the same infection might respond quite differently: one may cope by denying the existence of the problem, refusing to cooperate with the nurse responsible for designing a care plan to avoid transmission of the infectious agent; the other might cope by learning everything possible about his condition and participating actively in his care. From these examples, it may be inferred that although the physiological responses to a given stress stimulus are probably quite similar at the tissue level, according to age and general physical condition of the subject, response at the behavioural level is open to many different interpretations and variations.

Various models have been developed to suggest how social and psychological stimuli may be interpreted as stress. Currently it is thought that exchange of information may take place between the cerebral cortex, hypothalamus and the limbic system, and that if the event is seen to be distressing, the stress response will be initiated in the hypothalamus, sparking off endocrine and sympathetic nervous system activity.

Burchfield (1979) emphasised that in the course of everyday life people are more likely to be subject to chronic or intermittent stress than to the acutely stressful situations analogous to those created under laboratory conditions by researchers like Selye. Chronic stress may cause both physiological and psychological damage. Excessive cigarette smoking by an anxious person will damage the endothelium lining the respiratory tree and predispose him to chronic respiratory disease. Infection may thus be regarded as both a possible cause or a product of stress. Tissue damage may make an individual particularly vulnerable to invading pathogens. Once the infection has become established, it may pave the way for further stressful experience, such as isolation or prolonged hospital stay. At the tissue level, septicaemic shock may follow. This chain of reactions is illustrated in Table 7.2.

Table 7.2 Chronic Stress and Health Problems

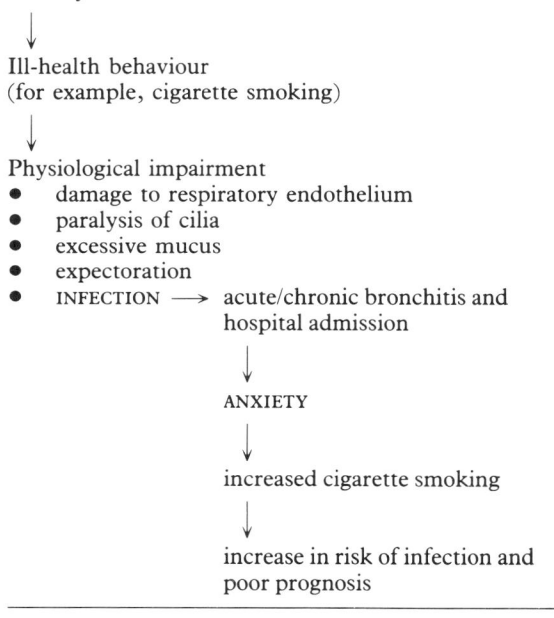

PSYCHOLOGICAL AND SOCIAL FACTORS

Although everybody is an individual and will respond to the effects of stress in his/her own particular way, there remain certain situations in which the vast majority of people are likely to feel insecure. One of these events is represented by coming into hospital. Illness itself is highly stressful, whether it is experienced in the community or necessitates hospital admission. Unpleasant symptoms and the side-effects of treatment, separation from the family, loss of status, function and financial remuneration, loneliness and other unforeseen events all help to make the situation worse. Someone who has been admitted to hospital with an infection, or who has developed infection during their stay will probably feel additional apprehension, an anxiety shared by their family and friends, and probably by the nurses and doctors responsible for their care. Even if the infection does not merit time spent in hospital, it may be intensely worrying, especially in the case of a chronic or recurrent infection.

The degree of psychological stress experienced as a reaction to infection will depend on:

(1) *Severity of the symptoms experienced.* Some infections are so mild that the patient, remaining asymptomatic, will never know about them. Others, like influenza, are unpleasant and may be debilitating, but generally offer no lasting threat to a person who is fit. At the other end of the spectrum, fear of AIDS, for example, may paralyse an individual and his family.

(2) *Need for hospital admission.* There is a great deal of evidence from nursing researchers and psychologists to suggest that coming into hospital generates anxiety (Wilson-Barnett, 1979). If the patient can be cared for at home, among familiar surroundings, his progress may be speedier and his anxieties fewer, provided that he has adequate support from his family and from health care professionals, who include the district nurse and general practitioner.

Recovery from illness depends on the stage in the life cycle. Old people who live neglected and alone still die needlessly from conditions like pneumonia and influenza. Recovery from otherwise mild infections may take place slowly if an individual feels unhappy or lacks social support (Imboden, 1972).

(3) *Need for isolation.* There has been little systematic research into the effects of isolation on infected patients, but case study reports suggest that it is a lonely and distressing experience. Forcing a patient to endure his own company needlessly is cruel; it induces boredom, exacerbates fears and leads to much added inconvenience. Elderly patients, or the very sick may become disoriented. Accidents may happen when the patient cannot be observed.

(4) *Whether the infection is acute or chronic.* Most people think of infection as an acute episode, and even when patients have to endure hospitalisation and isolation, they can usually be reassured that the precautions necessary will not last forever. Sometimes, however, the period of infectivity is protracted and the danger of infection to other people will be prolonged. This may happen when enteric pathogens may be carried asymptomatically throughout convalescence (see case study 1.2, p. 14); the sputum from a patient with open pulmonary tuberculosis may contain acid-fast bacilli sometimes for months after a course of chemotherapy has begun. Patients who have had hepatitis B may carry antibodies in their blood for years.

(5) *Need for change in lifestyle.* In cases where it is likely that the patient may remain infectious over a long period of time, or perhaps for ever, certain changes may be inevitable in the lifestyle. The degree of stress experienced by the patient and his family will be reflected according to the nature of the precautions considered necessary and the length of time over which they must continue. A nurse or a chef will be suspended from work (on full pay) if they are carrying an enteric pathogen, and will not be allowed to return until several consecutively negative stool specimens have been obtained even though they feel physically fit. Some people enjoy the unexpected holiday. Others worry endlessly about loss of earnings that inevitably result when a shift worker is placed on the basic rate of earning.

At the other end of the spectrum, someone who is positive for the HIV antibody is under an enormous amount of stress. The individual has to reconsider his entire lifestyle, not least his sexual behaviour, bearing in mind the possibility of developing the full syndrome of AIDS.

Even when the possibility of infecting others ceases to exist, the episode of infection may leave unwanted side-effects. A wound that has been infected is likely to result in unsightly scarring; contractures with loss of function may result. Leprosy is still a disfiguring disease, gonorrhoea may end in infertility. Regret may persist for a lifetime, even though the individual may not have been aware of the infection when it occurred.

(6) *The stigma attached to the infection and the reaction of other people influence the amount of stress perceived.* Infections commonly look and smell offensive. Distaste on the part of other people is hurtful, and the effect is compounded when carers wear protective clothes and take precautions. When these are clearly exaggerated, or, as in the case of viral haemorrhagic fevers, very stringent precautions are deemed necessary, the patient may feel 'unclean'.

Sexually transmitted diseases still retain their stigma; in the clinic patients are issued a number and in some centres may not even be addressed by their name. The need for contact tracing may be resented and regarded as an infringement of privacy. Syphilis is a chronic disease, victims being followed up annually for years, so that they are reminded at intervals about their infection. Syphilis, like hepatitis B, often accompanies homosexuality. The fact of developing the infection at all reflects on the private life of the individual and may lead to searching questions by professionals as well as stereotyped responses from lay acquaintances. The stigma attached to AIDS is greatest of all. At least the emergence of this condition has, if nothing else, drawn the attention of health care professionals to their own attitudes towards people of differing lifestyles and caused them to question the approaches they take to these groups. Even before AIDS hit the headlines, people were made to feel uncomfortable if they developed an infectious illness. Case study 7.1 is a case in point, describing the experiences of a patient who had hepatitis B, and felt she must communicate them to the medical profession (Personal paper, 1984).

The care that can be given to infected patients will never be good unless health care professionals

---

Case study 7.1

The patient received a blood transfusion in 1958. In 1974 she was admitted to hospital for routine cholecystectomy but found to be a hepatitis B carrier immediately before the operation, and sent home again. She understood that surgery was now impossible. Her symptoms became worse and she required pethidine and diazepam. Her husband and general practitioner tried to find someone willing to perform surgery; and 2 years later the operation took place in a disused theatre due for demolition in a hospital over 30 miles from home.

Some months later the patient's dentures required attention. After several months spent fruitlessly on the trail of an understanding dentist, she was treated in a local mental institution. She was never given the reason for this (but there is a high incidence of hepatitis B among mentally subnormal people). Four years later, and now living in another part of the country, the patient went to a dental hospital, to be warned by the nurse on each visit of the risk faced by staff attending her, and how the room would be thoroughly disinfected after her departure. Later, the same hospital required a blood specimen and the patient was amazed when her general practitioner sent it by post, taking no special precautions.

The patient acknowledges that the situation for hepatitis B carriers has eased with the passage of time. Since 1976 she has been in hospital for surgery on a number of occasions. Once she was isolated in a room that seemed to have been a broom cupboard. During a subsequent admission her cubicle was bright and modern, but the precautions taken were extreme. Purchasing items from the hospital trolley shop was forbidden, meals were served on lukewarm plates, disposable bedpans were allowed to accumulate and the patient's husband received a lecture for sitting on a chair that she used.

Case study 7.1 illustrates many of the distressing problems associated with infection, isolation and hospital admission. It does little credit to the obviously intelligent and articulate recipients of care. Nursing knowledge of hepatitis B is poor (Ho Yen *et al.*, 1985) and followup studies of patients found to be carriers of the infection by the Blood Transfusion Service have found gross misunderstandings among medical staff in both hospital and the community.

---

succeed in replacing fear, ignorance and intolerance with a more rational approach based on epidemiological knowledge of the particular infectious agent and the risks attached (see Chapter 6). The degree of risk is generally overestimated. Patients react to stress by repression, rationalisation, denial and a variety of other defence mechanisms which may represent unhealthy methods of coping. Cooperation in limiting the spread of infection is not likely to be enhanced by this kind of behaviour, and the psychological stress experienced may have an adverse effect on physical defence mechanisms used to fight infection. Chapter 11 explores in detail how nurses can reduce the amount of distress experienced by patients who have infections and positively help adjustment and return to normal levels of functioning. In the meantime, the physiological response to infection is described.

PHYSIOLOGICAL RESPONSE TO INFECTION

The body is protected against pathogens by both specific and non-specific defence mechanisms.

Inflammation is a non-specific defence mechanism which the tissues evoke against any invading pathogen. The mechanical barriers of the body against infection discussed in Chapter 1 may also be regarded as non-specific defence mechanisms. Immunological defence mechanisms are specific; antibodies are stimulated by the presence of foreign substances (antigens) and once produced they will attack only that particular antigen. Invasion by the measles virus will stimulate the formation of antibodies specific only for that virus, and they will not exert an effect on any other organism. Scientists have never successfully found any effective artificial immunisation against the common cold because the infection is due not to one distinct type of virus, but to many different ones all capable of reproducing the same symptoms, and each destroyed by a particular antibody.

The following sections deal with inflammation, and specific bodily defence mechanisms.

Inflammation

Inflammation is the tissue response to damage, and it is identical, irrespective of the nature of the injury. Chemicals, cuts, or pathogenic invasion will all evoke the same inflammatory response. This is an important point, because nurses sometimes fail to appreciate that infection does not inevitably accompany inflammation.

The classical features of inflammation are:

- redness,
- swelling,
- pain,
- heat.

Depending on the extent of the injury, some loss of function may occur.

The inflammatory response is beneficial and has been adapted to destroy the agent responsible for injury or, failing this, to remove its effects from the tissues. Toxins secreted by bacteria may be neutralised or 'walled off' to prevent them spreading, followed by repair or replacement of the damaged tissue.

Before the process of inflammation can be described in detail, it is necessary to give an account of the white blood cells which contribute to it.

White Blood Cells and Inflammation

An adult has approximately 7000 white blood cells per cubic millilitre (cm^3) of blood, differentiated into five different types according to their staining properties, and the presence of granules in the cytoplasm. Their relative proportions in human blood are shown in Table 7.3.

Polymorphonuclear granulocytes (polymorphs) contain big lobed nuclei. Within their cytoplasm there are large, granular inclusions. Monocytes and lymphocytes may be distinguished by their clear cytoplasm and simple nuclei (Fig. 7.2). Polymorphs and monocytes are discussed here because of the role they play in the inflammatory response. A description of the lymphocytes is given below, in relation to the specific defence mechanisms (p. 119).

Polymorphs

Polymorphs develop in the bone marrow from large precursor cells called megakaryocytes. In childhood all the bone marrow helps to make polymorphs, but in healthy adults polymorphs develop only within the flat bones of the axial skeleton and

Table 7.3 Types of Leucocytes and the Normal White Blood Cell Count

Normal total white blood cell (WBC) count:
5000 – 10 000/cm^3 blood (average 7000)

Polymorphonuclear granulocytes
Formed in the red bone marrow.
Characterised by large-lobed nuclei and cytoplasm with granular appearance due to cytoplasmic inclusions containing lysozymes and other bactericides.
Three types, according to staining properties with microscope dye
1. *Neutrophils*
   Stain purple. Phagocytic, 60–70% total WBC count.
2. *Eosinophils*
   Stain red. Kill parasites, important in allergic reactions, 2–3% total WBC count.
3. *Basophils*
   Stain blue. Contain heparin, 0·4% total WBC count. Function obscure. Mast cells are very similar to basophils, but are naturally present in the tissues.

Agranulocytes
Cells with clear cytoplasm and nuclei without lobes
Two types
1. *Monocytes* – large cells with characteristically shaped nuclei. Formed in red bone marrow and carried by blood to the tissues where they mature into phagocytic macrophages, 4–8%* total WBC count
2. *Lymphocytes* – large active nuclei, 25–40% WBC count
   (a) T cells
   (b) B cells
   Look alike, but have separate origins and functions

*Count is difficult to estimate, because the number in the tissues cannot be assessed

---

skull. Three types of polymorphs can be distinguished by their microscopic reactions: neutrophils, basophils, and eosinophils (see Table 7.3 and Fig. 7.2).

The term *leucocytosis* is used to describe the appearance of large numbers of white blood cells, mainly neutrophils (when the count exceeds 10 000/cm^3 of blood). It occurs in response to acute infections and in other conditions which induce inflammation. Myocardial infarction, which causes inflammation and death of cardial muscle, leads to leucocytosis. Metabolic conditions, drug therapy and strenuous exercise spark off the same response.

Leucopenia is the reverse condition, when the white cell count becomes depressed. People who have developed leucopenia are highly susceptible to infection, which may be acute, even fatal, or chronic and recurrent. Deficiency may arise through damage to the bone marrow by irradiation, or by treatment with drugs like chloramphenicol, which suppress the activity of the megakaryocytes. Large quantities of alcohol inhibit release of neutrophils from bone marrow. In leukaemia white blood cells are released into the circulation when they are too immature to be of much use in defending the body against infection. Leucopenic patients require protective isolation (see Chapter 6).

The physiological properties of neutrophil polymorphs (Fig. 7.3) enable them to reach and destroy foreign materials in the tissues. These properties include:

- mural flow,
- diapedesis,
- chemotaxis,
- phagocytosis.

Bacteria which have been ingested by neutrophils are digested by lysozyme, an enzyme released from the cytoplasmic inclusions. Sometimes bacteria survive and continue to multiply after they have been ingested. The neutrophil eventually explodes, releasing lysozyme, and digestion continues extracellularly. Pus is formed from the remains of exploded neutrophils, their contents and breakdown products of tissue that have been destroyed.

Monocytes

Monocytes are distinguished from polymorphs by their clear, inclusion-free cytoplasm and horseshoe-

Response of the body to infection 111

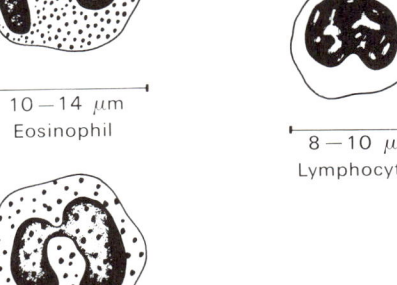

Fig. 7.2 White blood cells.

shaped nuclei. Like polymorphs, however, monocytes are manufactured in bone marrow and share the properties of mural flow, diapedesis, chemotaxis and phagocytosis. When monocytes leave the blood vessels they sometimes become 'fixed' within the tissues, and are then referred to as *macrophages*. Because so many monocytes are present as macrophages in the tissues, their count per cm^3 of blood is not really an accurate representation of the total number present in the body at any one time. Macrophages which move about freely in the tissues are called *wandering macrophages*, and play an important role in inflammation, especially during the later stages. They are larger than polymorphs and have a greater capacity for phagocytosis. This means not only that they can engulf larger particles, including fragments of dead tissue, but also polymorphs that have been destroyed.

The Process of Inflammation

For the sake of convenience, inflammation may be divided into three stages:

(1) vasodilatation with increased permeability of the blood vessel walls,
(2) migration of polymorphs and macrophages to the site of damage,
(3) repair.

Vasodilatation

Immediately after injury the blood vessel walls dilate and become more permeable. These changes occur very rapidly in response to tissue damage. Dilated capillaries are able to carry more blood to the injured area, and account for the redness and sensation of heat that accompany inflammation.

Increased permeability allows greater quantities of fluid to move from the capillaries into the extracellular space, hence the oedema associated with inflammation. Increased amounts of extracellular fluid help to dilate the toxins released by invading pathogens. The pain of inflammation is caused by nerve damage, pressure exerted by oedema on the nerve endings and by the irritant effect of bacterial toxins.

Vasodilatation and increased blood vessel permeability are due to the release of locally acting hormones: histamine, kinins and prostaglandins. Histamine is released by many tissues in response to damage, and during the inflammatory response it is liberated mainly by basophils and thrombocytes (platelets). Kinins originate from polymorphs attracted to the injured site, and by stimulating the nerve endings they contribute to the pain experienced during inflammation.

Another function of vasodilatation is the transport of large numbers of clotting factors to the site of injury. Blood clots 'wall off' microorganisms and their toxins which limits spread to other parts of the body. Pimples and boils are really small abscesses (see p. 113).

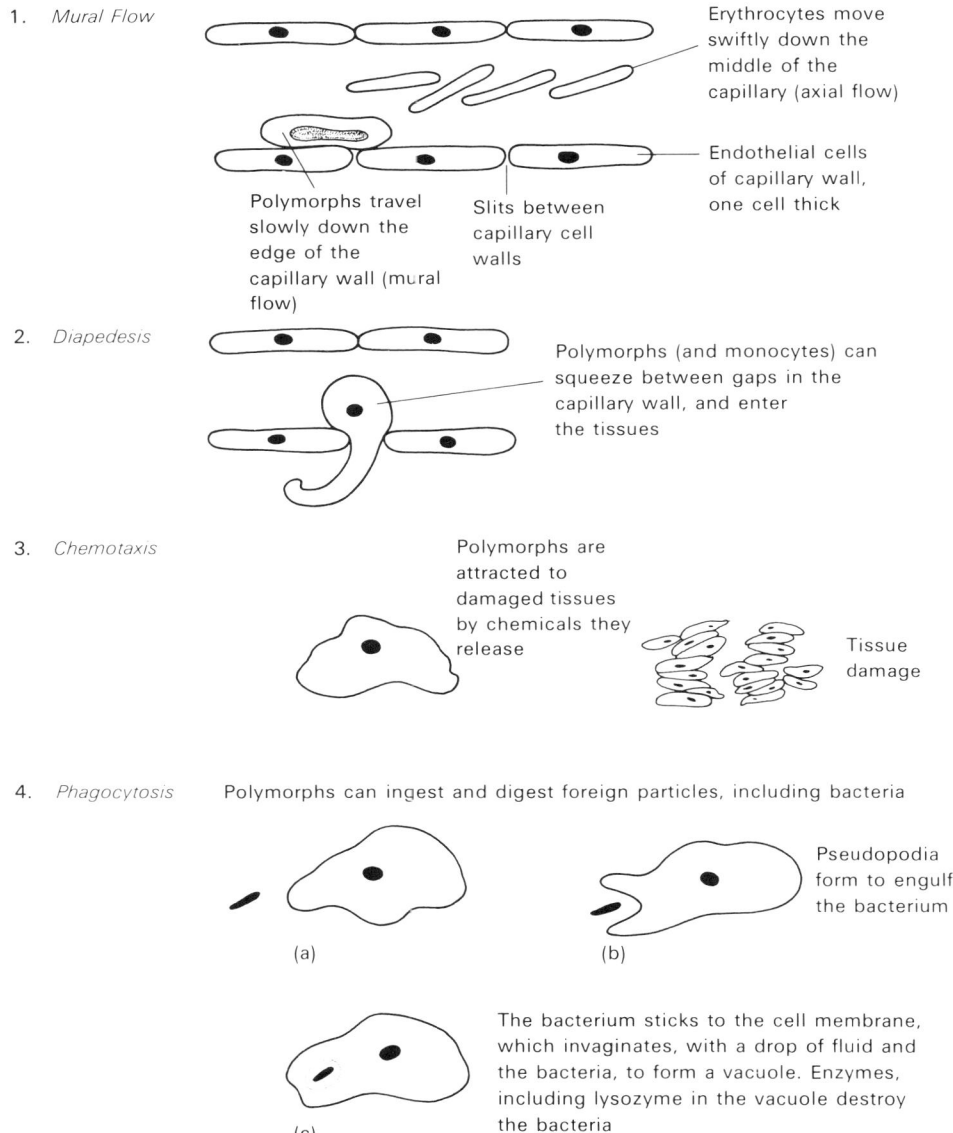

Fig. 7.3 Physiological properties of polymorphonuclear granulocytes.

Migration

Polymorphs begin to appear locally at the damaged area about an hour after the inflammatory response has been initiated. Inflamed tissue liberates a substance called *leucocytosis releasing factor* which stimulates increased activity of the bone marrow. Diapedesis and migration can take place in less than 2 minutes. As the inflammatory response progresses, monocytes enter the tissues and wandering macrophages become activated to 'angry macrophages' which have a higher metabolic rate. Fixed macrophages in the tissues begin to reproduce, become mobile and also migrate to the site of injury.

Having engulfed large numbers of microorganisms and fragments of dead tissue, neutrophils and macrophages eventually die. After a few days a pus-containing cavity forms within the tissues, and continues to accumulate until the infection has subsided. Common sites of abscess formation are shown in Table 7.4 Abscesses may 'point' on to the external or internal surfaces of body, eventually discharging their contents. Alternatively, pus may remain enclosed in the tissues. It may be gradually destroyed and absorbed over a period of days or surgical intervention may be required to drain it (see Chapter 9).

Table 7.4 Sites of Abscess Formation

Site	Kind of abscess
Appendix	Appendix abscess
Brain	Cerebral abscess
Fallopian tube	Pyosalpinx
Gallbladder	Empyema
Labia	Bartholin's abscess
Liver	Liver abscess
Lung	Lung abscess
Renal pelvis	Pyonephrosis
Pericardium	Purulent pericarditis
Peritoneal cavity	Subphrenic abscess
Pleural cavity	Empyema
Surgical wound	Wound abscess

Repair

Although divided into three stages for the convenience of discussion, separation of the inflammatory response is artificial, since each of the stages really overlap. Tissue repair commences during the active phase of inflammation, but it cannot be completed until all the microorganisms and their toxins have either been destroyed and removed from the body, or their effects neutralised. Some tissues have a greater capacity for regeneration than others, depending upon their degree of specialisation and differentiation. Cells covering the external and internal bodily surfaces (skin epithelium and gut endothelium) are subject to a great deal of wear and tear, but damage is readily repaired. The most extreme contrast is afforded by nerve cells which have become so highly specialised during the course of differentiation that they are unable to regenerate. In compensation, they are protected deeply within the body, for example, the spinal cord within the vertebral column, and the brain within the skull. Tissue regeneration is discussed further in Chapter 9, together with wound infection.

Pyrexia

Pyrexia (fever) is a systemic reaction of the body to infection, provoked by microorganisms and their toxins. In man and higher animals temperature is controlled by the hypothalamus, and the temperature regulating centre is often compared to a thermostat. Human temperature is fixed at about 37°C (98.6°F). Deviations detected by receptor cells in the skin are relayed to the hypothalamus along nerve fibres (Table 7.5). If temperature falls below 37°C, heat-conserving mechanisms are initiated. Arterioles in the skin constrict so that blood is diverted more deeply into the body, reducing heat loss by conduction and convection from the surface. Shivering generates heat by muscular activity when the temperature is very low. Muscles attached to the shafts of the hair follicles contract, an important mechanisms in animals, which results in the hair standing on end so that a layer of warm air is trapped next to the skin. In man, this causes 'gooseflesh'.

If the temperature rises above 37°C, the hypothalamus relays impulses to the rest of the body so that heat loss is promoted. Arterioles in the skin dilate. Heat is lost by conduction, convection and evaporation as the rate of perspiration is increased.

When infection occurs, antigens on the bacteria cause the hypothalamic thermostat to 'reset' at a higher temperature until the foreign antigens have been eliminated from the body. During the inflammatory response, polymorphs, especially neutrophils, release a protein called *leucocytic pyrogen* (Atkins, 1972). It is the diffusion of this substance into the bloodstream, and its subsequent carriage to the hypothalamus, that causes the thermostat level to rise. Mild infections raise the temperature by only a fraction of a degree, but some pathogens, for example, *Salmonella typhi* (causing typhoid) can cause the thermostat to reset at 39°C or higher.

Once the thermostat is reset above 37°C, the body responds by vasoconstriction, shivering, and an increase in metabolic rate in order to achieve the new level. But despite the increase, the patient feels

Table 7.5 Temperature Regulation

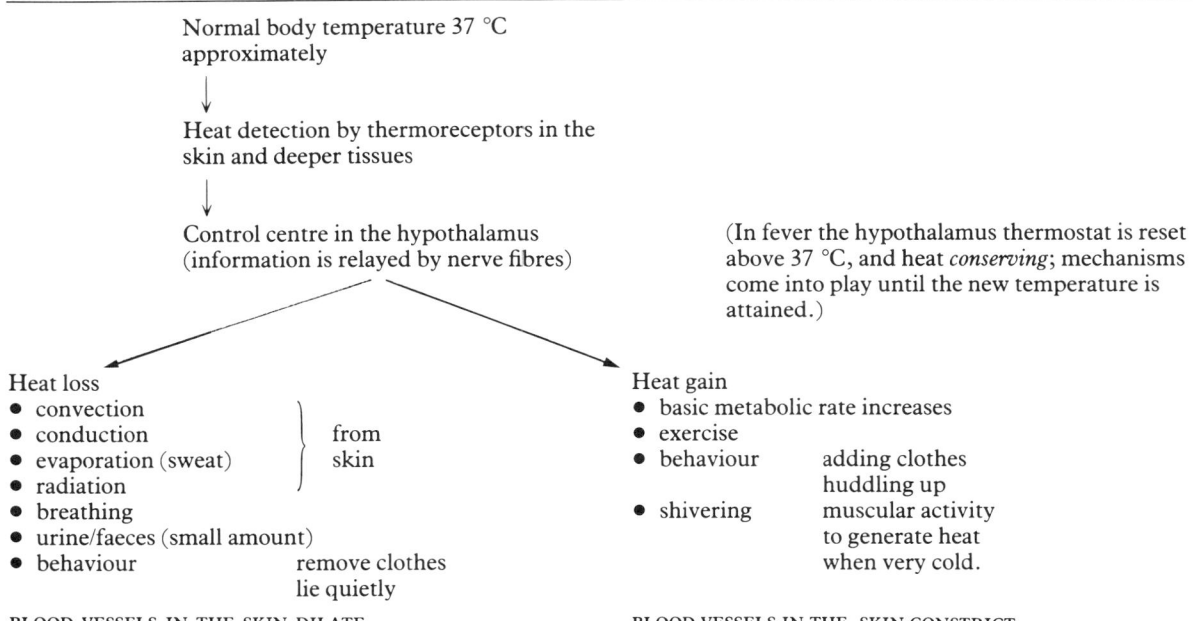

cold, experiencing a chill. When bodily temperature eventually reaches the new, elevated level, it will be maintained until all the foreign antigens have been neutralised or removed from the body. As the infection subsides, mechanisms to reduce temperature such as vasodilatation and perspiration come into operation.

Pyrexia is presumed to be of some benefit, since it accompanies infection in all higher animals, but at the present time its value is obscure. Most bacteria of medical significance thrive better at 37 °C than at the higher temperatures attained during fever, but human enzymes also have optimal activity at 37 °C. Higher temperatures may possibly help to speed tissue repair by increasing general metabolic rate, or foreign antigens may be destroyed more easily.

As far as the patient is concerned, fever has a number of disadvantages. The rise in metabolic rate can be exhausting; for every 1 °C rise in temperature above normal, the adult pulse increases by about 20 beats per minute and the respiratory rate by about 7 breaths per minute. The bodily stores of glycogen become depleted, leading to nitrogen wastage as proteins are used to provide energy, and possibly causing negative nitrogen balance. If this situation continues for long the patient will become debilitated and healing will be impaired due to tissue damage.

Rigors may occur. These are uncontrollable attacks of violent shivering, often associated with the presence of bacteria or toxins in the blood. As well as being extremely distressing, rigors contribute to debility, increased fever and exhaustion. Febrile convulsions may occur in young children (1–6 years) or patients who have a history of epilepsy. They are usually transient, but are dangerous because they can lead to trauma or aspiration of secretions and asphyxia.

Delirium is another unwanted effect of fever, most often seen in the very young or elderly. It is a serious nursing problem because the patient becomes confused and restless, endangering intravenous infusions, urinary catheters and hurting himself as he attempts to resist treatment. The nursing care of a pyrexial patient is discussed in case study 7.2.

In addition to its mechanical barriers against invading pathogens, the inflammatory response and the questionable benefits of pyrexia, the body

Case study 7.2

Mark, aged 20, was a full-time student. His grant was modest and the best accommodation that he could afford was a bed-sitting room. The bathroom and kitchen, which he shared, were situated on another floor.

Throughout the winter months there was a considerable amount of sickness in the college, mainly due to influenza, and one afternoon Mark developed a headache and sore throat. The next morning he awoke with a severe headache, shivering with cold. Although he did not feel hungry, Mark was very thirsty and the day spent alone in his room seemed endless. It was not possible to make an appointment with Mark's general practitioner at short notice, so when he returned from college, Mark's friend drove him to the accident and emergency department of the nearest hospital.

When Mark arrived in the department he was greeted by a staff nurse who provided extra blankets because he was shivering with cold. The doctor took a careful history which established that:

- Mark had not been abroad since the previous summer and that he had not had any contact since that time with anyone returning from abroad.
- He had not recently been vaccinated.
- He had been in contact recently with several people who had influenza.

In view of this it did not seem necessary to undertake stringent isolation precautions. These might be necessary if a patient was suspected to have a tropical fever (see Chapter 6).

The nurse recorded the following vital signs:

- Temperature: 38.9°C (102°F)
- Pulse: 96 beats/min
- Respirations: 26/min
- Blood pressure: 120/70

Mark felt hot to touch but complained of cold. His lips looked sore and dry and he said that he had not eaten anything since the previous day. He had a harsh non-productive cough and was clearly feeling very unwell. No rash was apparent.

The doctor confirmed a diagnosis of influenza. He explained that most young, fit people recover within a week, but that in the middle of the city, where so many people lived alone, admission to hospital could be arranged, especially if home circumstances were difficult. Mark was surprised, but the nurse pointed out the advantages of being in warm surroundings with no need to worry about shopping and other domestic arrangements. Eventually Mark was admitted to a side room in a general medical ward, where the nurse allocated to look after him planned the following care to meet his needs:

- Extra bedclothes, since Mark still felt cold.
- At least 3 litres of fluid daily, to balance the water vapour lost with his heightened respiratory rate; warm and cool drinks were provided as desired.
- Encouragement with oral hygiene; Mark was able to brush his own teeth and was grateful to be offered mouthwashes.

Regular recordings of temperature, respiration and pulse were maintained. Pressure area care was not necessary since Mark could move freely, although he felt unsteady when he got out of bed. The nurse noticed that his urine was dark and concentrated, so she observed fluid intake and output carefully. A throat swab ordered by the doctor was sent to the laboratory, but no bacteria were cultured. Lying in bed, pyrexial, Mark had a headache and felt stiff and sore. The doctor prescribed soluble aspirin as a simple analgesic. The nurse knew that at this stage Mark's temperature would continue to rise until it reached the new 'set point' of the hypothalamus, and that until this happened the aspirin would not help to reduce pyrexia.

During the night Mark's temperature reached 39°C (102°F). When he woke he complained that he felt hot and his skin was flushed and clammy. The group of viruses responsible for influenza (myxoviruses) do not remain in the body for long and it was apparent that Mark's normal defence mechanisms were overcoming the infection, so that the thermostat in the hypothalamus was being reset at a lower level. It was now important for the nurse to promote Mark's comfort and to help reduce his temperature as fast as possible.

- The bedclothes were removed, leaving Mark covered with one sheet.
- He was helped to wash, using tepid water, his skin was gently sponged and patted dry at regular intervals.
- A fan was provided, making sure that it was positioned sufficiently far from the bed to avoid disordering the bedclothes. Many patients feel that the air from a fan increases their discomfort if it is placed too close to them. The window was not opened, thus avoiding making the ward too draughty for other patients.
- Cool drinks were encouraged.
- Aspirin was given every 4 hours; this drug helps to reduce temperature in pyrexia because it interferes with the formation of prostaglandins, hormones released locally in the tissues that appear to have a role in the generation of pyrexia.
- Mouthcare was encouraged.
- Vital signs and fluid intake and output were recorded.

cont.

> Mark was not subjected to isolation precautions because influenza is a very difficult infection to contain, and most of the patients admitted to the ward from the neighbourhood and the nurses had already been exposed to the virus.
>
> Mark left hospital 5 days later, feeling rather shaky. His nurse advised him to eat nourishing, high-calorie meals. Infection increases the metabolic rate and the body may wastefully burn proteins to provide energy if insufficient carbohydrates have been included in the diet. In the case of a young man ill for only a few days this should not really be a problem – but Mark's nursing history had suggested a poor standard of living overall, and it was evident that facilities for preparing food were not good.

produces several other chemicals that are able to exert non-specific effects against microorganisms: interferons that destroy viruses, and the proteins that make up the complement system.

Interferons

Interferons are proteins released by host cells in response to viral infections. They prevent the multiplication of virus particles by halting the synthesis of viral nucleic acids (DNA and RNA) and their effects spread to neighbouring cells by diffusion in the extracellular fluid. The effectiveness of interferons appears to be limited because they are shortlived proteins, released only in small quantities. Moreover, their clinical application is restricted because they are specific to the host species which produces them. Although they will destroy a range of different viruses, they will operate in human cells only. Interferons obtained from animals cannot therefore be used to treat human infections.

Until recently, interferons for clinical use could only be obtained from human tissue culture. Genetic engineering has now made possible the artificial synthesis of interferons from bacteria (the genes controlling interferon protein have been isolated from human cells and inserted into those of bacteria). Interferons have been used to treat a variety of malignant conditions including AIDS, but they are still very expensive, and the results are often disappointing. Work in this field has really only just begun, and it is becoming apparent that the action of interferons is more complicated than scientists believed at first.

The Complement System

The complement system is another of the body's non-specific defence mechanisms, since it is active against a whole range of different invading microorganisms, not against specific types. Its function is to increase the efficiency with which bacteria are phagocytosed. 'Complement' is a series of proteins which are activated one after the other (in a way reminiscent of the blood-clotting mechanism). The final protein released by the chain binds to the surface of the pathogen, encouraging it to stick to the surface of the phagocytic cell. This process of attachment is called *opsonisation*.

Complement seems to be particularly effective in destroying Gram-negative bacteria responsible for enteric diseases (such as *Salmonella* and *Shigella*), and defects in the system can predispose to severe infections.

The complement system consists of about 15 different proteins which circulate in the blood. Their molecules account for 10% of all plasma proteins, and activation can proceed by two distinct routes:

- The classical pathway (the first to be described), initiated when a specific antibody of the IgG or IgM class binds to the surface of a specific antigen.
- The alternative pathway, initiated by a variety of polysaccharides including those present on bacterial cell walls.

The cascade of complement activation is illustrated in Table 7.6. This shows that whichever pathway operates, the result is cleavage of C3 protein into two fragments called C3a and C3b which destroy pathogens in three different ways.

- C3a contributes to the inflammatory response by increasing permeability of the capillary walls and attracting neutrophils by chemotaxis.
- C3b activates all the remaining proteins in the complement system from C5 to C9. C9 des-

troys bacteria by puncturing holes in their cell membrane. Lysis of bacterial cells in this way is called *complement fixation*, and it forms the basis of an important diagnostic laboratory test (see Chapter 10).
- C3b is the agent responsible for opsonisation, enhancing phagocytosis.

The effects of the complement system are shortlived. Activated complement proteins are rapidly destroyed by enzyme inactivators present in the extracellular fluid. This is an important protective action on the part of the host tissues, whose own cells might otherwise be destroyed. Activation is generally restricted to the immediate vicinity of the damage. In cases where complement activation is stimulated on a very large scale, acute widespread damage of the blood vessels will result. This condition, called diffuse intravascular coagulation (DIC), results in blood clot formation and haemorrhage. It is a very serious but rare complication of severe bacterial and viral infections.

The Specific Defence Mechanisms

Antigens

An antigen is any chemical substance which causes the body to respond to its presence through the production of specific antibodies. Most are large molecules containing at least some protein, for example,

- bacterial cells,
- pollen grains,
- foreign cells (from tumours, transplanted organs, or mismatched blood transfusions).

The surfaces of all these structures are covered with protein molecules and, not surprisingly, the antibodies which form are always specific for the antigens which stimulated them. Fig. 7.4 shows a typical antigen.

Most antibodies do not form against the whole antigen, but against specific surface sites called antigenic determinant or binding sites. Combina-

Table 7.6 The Complement Cascade

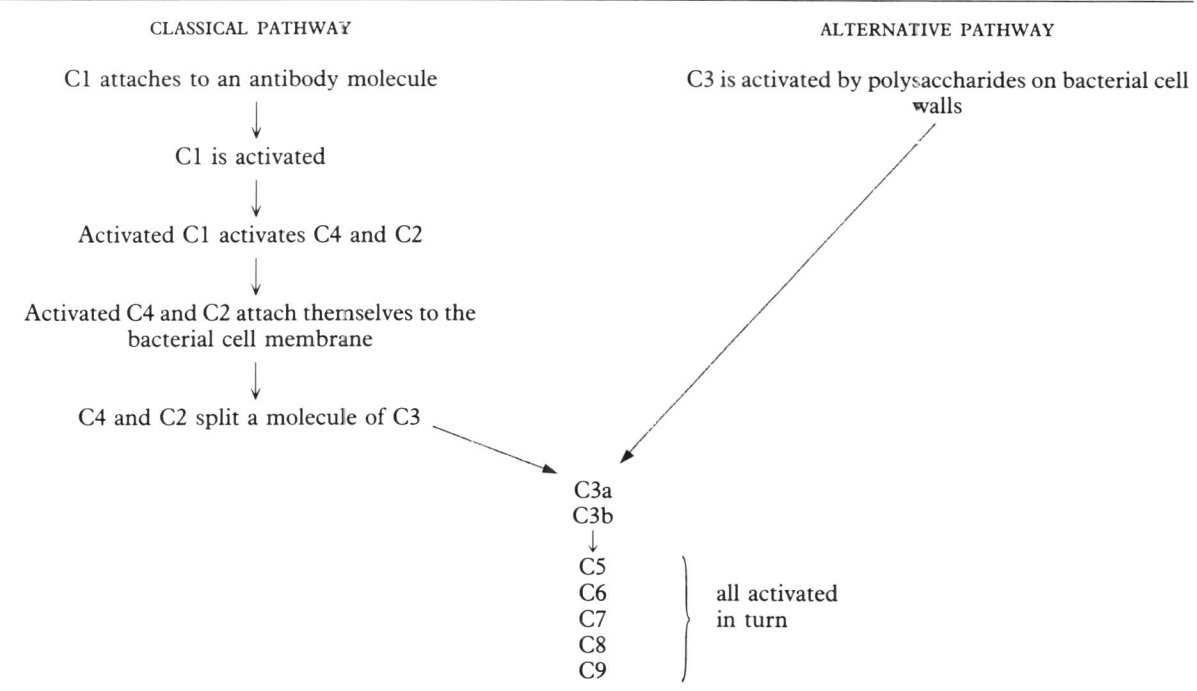

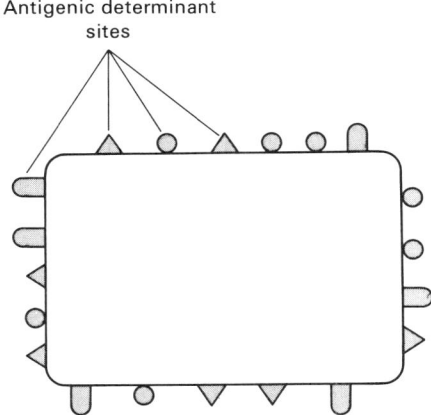

Fig. 7.4 A typical antigen.

Antibodies

Antibodies may be defined as proteins synthesised by the body in response to the presence of specific antigens. Antibodies are always specific to their stimulating antigens, and like antigens have one or more binding sites on the molecular surface. However, there is an important difference between the two. All antibodies will combine with one specific antigen; but antigens, having more than one kind of binding site, may be able to combine with one or more specific antibody.

All antibodies belong to the class of plasma proteins called *globulins*, and because of the role they play in immunity they are often referred to as *immunoglobulins*. Their structure is unique. Each immunoglobulin molecule is made up of one or more basic units, and each of these units consists of four protein chains. Two of the proteins are identical, and because of their size they are called heavy chains; the other two units, also identical to one another, are called light chains. This is illustrated in Fig. 7.6, which shows that the light

tion of antigen and antibody occur at these sites; comparisons have been made to interlocking jigsaw pieces and lock-and-key mechanisms (see Fig. 7.5). Combination will either destroy or inactivate the antigen. Some antigens contain only a few binding sites of the same type, others contain many sites. The antigen–antibody complex, like all foreign materials entering the body, is phagocytosed (or engulfed), usually by a macrophage.

The immune system is able to identify cells of the host tissues and will not produce antibodies against them (except in autoimmune diseases).

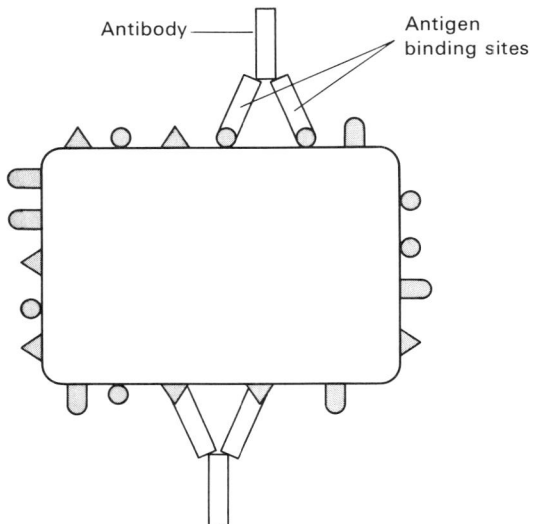

Fig. 7.5 Combination of antigen with antibodies.

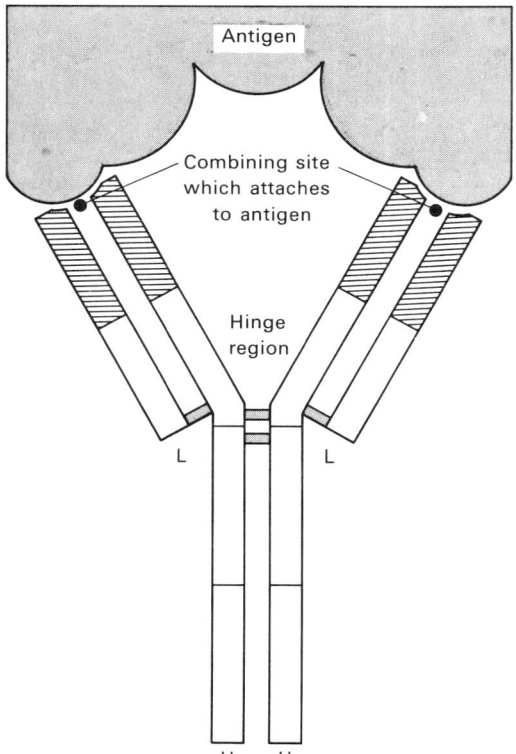

Fig. 7.6 An antibody molecule shown in detail (adapted with permission from Staines *et al.*, 1985).

and heavy chains join together in a Y shape. The two 'arms' of the Y have the same structure, and it is here in the molecule that combination with the specific antigen occurs.

The most abundant immoglobulin is IgG, which illustrates the basic structure as it consists of only one unit, with two heavy and two light chains. Table 7.7 and Fig. 7.7 show the structure of all five different types of immunoglobulin and their main functions.

The Lymphocytes: Humoral and Cellular Immunity

The lymphocytes are the cells of the immune system which react to antigens. Referring back to Fig. 7.2 (p. 111) shows that lymphocytes are distinguished from granulocytes by their clear cytoplasm and from monocytes by their large, dark nuclei which occupy nearly all the cellular space. The size and appearance of these nuclei indicate that lymphocytes are some of the most active cells in the entire body. They are present throughout the body, in blood, lymph and in the specialised lymphoid tissues. Their distribution is shown in Fig 7.8. Like the other blood cells, lymphocytes develop from stem cells in the red bone marrow, then enter the bloodstream, and circulate throughout the body, travelling through the lymph nodes.

Lymph nodes are lymphoid tissues encased in a connective tissue membrane; their structure is shown in Fig. 7.9. They filter tissue fluid and lymph as it travels through the body's network of lymph vessels, so that antigens become trapped close to the regions where the lymphocytes are stored. Lymph nodes are positioned strategically in the tissues, at points where bacteria may enter; the tonsils and adenoids respond to antigens from the nose and throat, while Peyer's patches up and down the gut respond to antigens that have been swallowed. Lymph from most parts of the body drains through a series of nodes before emptying into the thoracic duct in the neck. Here lymph re-enters the general circulation via the jugular vein, allowing the lymphocytes to recirculate again via the blood.

There are two types of lymphocytes, called T and B cells, which look identical, but which behave quite differently. They are both derived from the same stem cells, but in order to fulfil their active roles they are 'programmed' by different mechanisms, at different sites in the body. *T cells* migrate to the thymus gland in the neck to be activated, then move to the lymphoid tissue. There is

Table 7.7 The Immunoglobulins

Class of immunoglobulin	Per cent total plasma antibody	Location	Length of time active	Function
IgG	80	Blood Lymph	50 days	Protects the tissue from microorganisms and their toxins; produced in response to acute infection
IgM	5	Blood Lymph	10 days	The main first-line defence against microorganisms once they have invaded the blood stream
IgA	14	Secretions: mucus, tears, breast milk, blood, lymph	12 days	Protects mucosal surfaces
IgD	0.2	Blood Lymph Surfaces of B lymphocytes	6 days	Helps B lymphocytes to manufacture antibodies
IgE	0.002	Blood Mast cells	4 days	Protects against intestinal parasites (worms, protozoa) Responsible for many of the symptoms of allergy

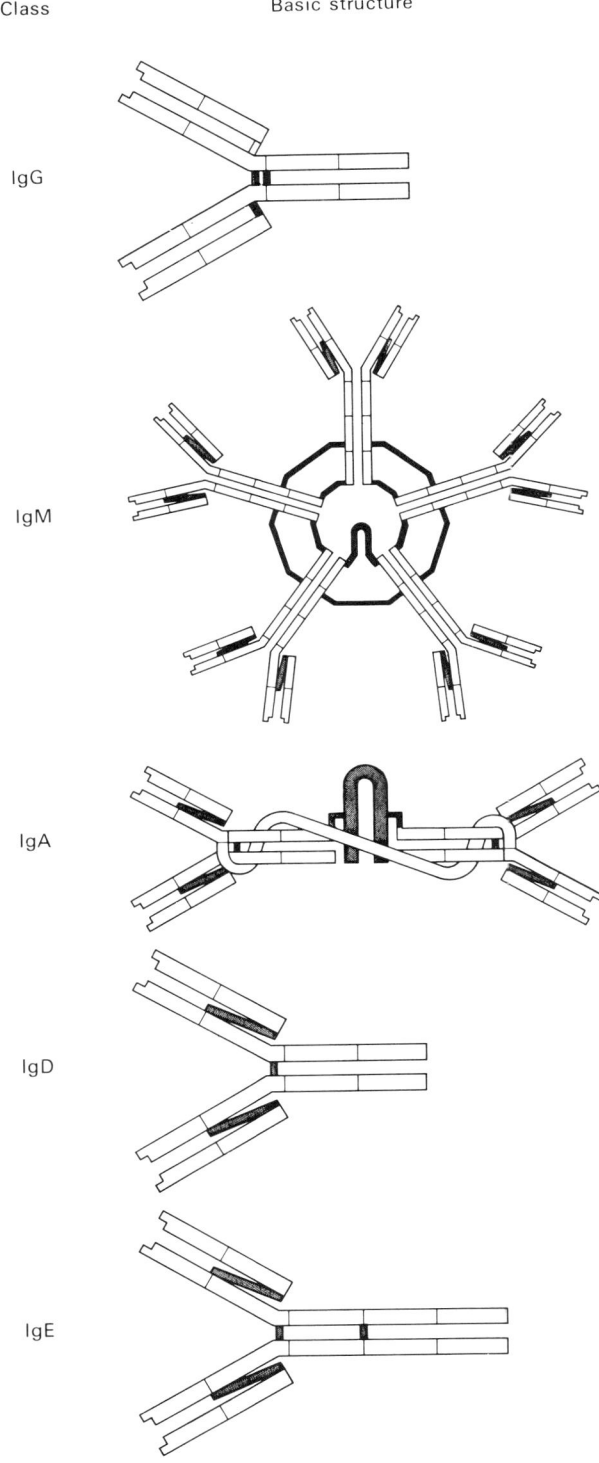

Fig. 7.7 Immunoglobulin class and basic structure.

evidence that this occurs before and soon after birth; the thymus regresses during childhood, and if it is removed at an early stage of development, the immune mechanism is damaged. The B cells are activated in the bone marrow itself, and in the lymphoid tissue and spleen, without migration through the thymus.

B cells are activated to produce specific antibodies in response to antigens. Since antibodies travel in the bloodstream and lymph, they are sometimes said to provide humoral immunity. T cells, which have numerous complex functions described below, are responsible for cellular immunity. Both systems must operate if the individual is to remain healthy and infection-free.

The human body contains not just one type of B or T cell, but thousands of different ones; for every specific antigen that the individual has ever encountered there will be a corresponding B and T cell. When an antigen enters the tissues it ultimately contacts a B cell specific for it, and this becomes activated. During this process the cell enlarges, dividing many times to form a clone or colony of identical daughter cells called plasma cells. Throughout the activation period, the B cell nucleus is making large quantities of new DNA and cell proteins. This is why the nuclei, the distinguishing feature of these cells, are so large and so reactive with microscope dyes. It is, however, the plasma cells which actually synthesise antibodies. Rate of production is enormous; up to 2000 antibody molecules can be released per second from every plasma cell over a period lasting 4 or 5 days. The plasma cells then die, with the exception of just a few, retained in the body as 'memory cells'. If the same antigen ever enters the tissues again, the memory cells will still be there, ready to divide even more rapidly, to form a large clone of cells all able to make the necessary antibodies.

The Physiological Basis of Immunisation

Types of immunity were described in Chapter 4. Here it is time to explain the physiological basis of immunisation. Antibody production by the B cells is more intense after a second exposure to an antigen, and this can be demonstrated by measuring the titre (concentration) of the antibody in the plasma. When the antigen enters the host tissues

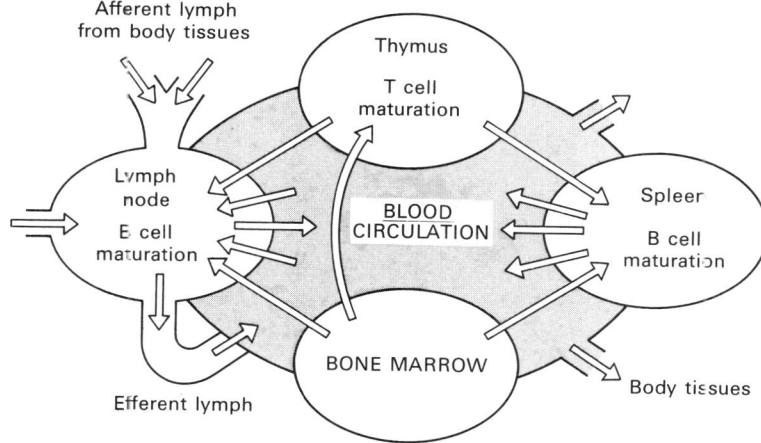

Fig. 7.8 Development of lymphocytes and release into the circulation (adapted with permission from Staines et al., 1985).

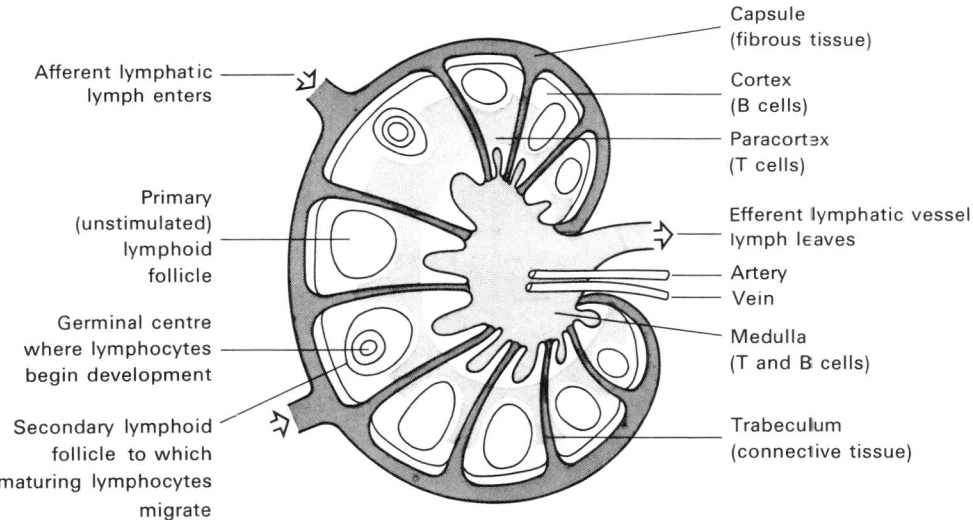

Fig. 7.9 Structure of a typical lymph node.

for the very first time there is a period of several days before antibodies are formed, followed by a slow rise, then a decline in titre. This is the primary response, coinciding with the cloning of the B cells and their eventual synthesis of antibodies. On a second, or any subsequent exposure to the same antigen, the antibody titre rises much more rapidly, because the memory cells which have survived from the initial exposure have cloned and released the antibody more promptly. This is the secondary response (Fig. 7.10). Booster doses given to enhance artificially induced immunity stimulate the antibody titre to reach a higher level.

T cells do not make antibodies, although they form clones on exposure to their specific antigens and a few survive as memory cells, to help promote a more rapid secondary immune response. Immunologists have discovered that several kinds of T cells exist, able to perform different functions.

- Regular T cells control antibody production by B cells.

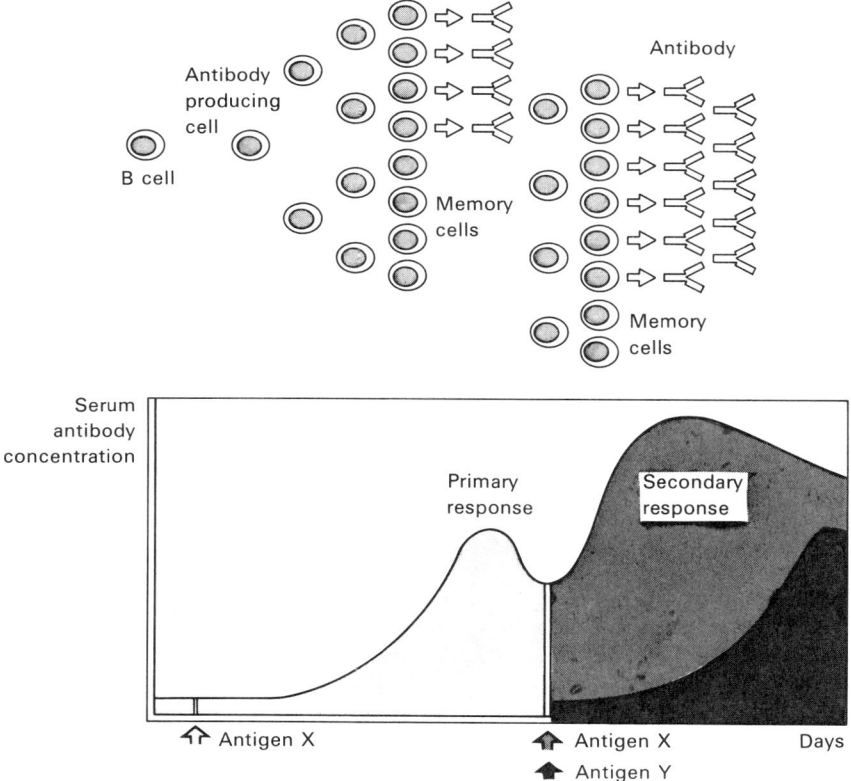

Fig. 7.10 The basis of immunity; primary and secondary responses (adapted with permission from Staines *et al.*, 1985).

- T helper cells help initiate the immune response.
- T suppressor cells inhibit the T helper cells when the tissues no longer require protection by antibodies.
- T cytotoxic cells destroy host cells that have become infected with particular types of virus, including those of the influenza group. Although these host cells are sacrificed, further replication of the virus is prevented in compensation.
- T death (Tdth) cells make cytotoxic factors called lymphokines, which seem to be important in controlling the activities of many of the white blood cells, as well as being important in cell-mediated immunity. They destroy those bacteria that manage to grow inside cells of the host tissues, by activating macrophages through the action of the lymphokines. Apart from their important function in combating infection, T cytotoxic cells also do a certain amount of damage; they promote hypersensitivity reactions, some autoimmune diseases and rejection of organ transplants.

Because T cells control cellular immunity, they are particularly important in controlling chronic, slowly developing infections, like tuberculosis and virus infections, since organisms responsible tend to survive intracellularly. They are also effective against certain types of cancer, and fungi. This helps to explain the nature of the typical opportunistic infections developed by people who have AIDS, (see p. 46), for the cells affected by the HIV virus are the T helper cells. In contrast, complement and antibody are most active against microorganisms freely present in the blood, and they operate faster to eliminate them.

Recent research has shown that T cells which perform different functions can be categorised into groups which immunologists called subsets. Each subset appears to protect the body against different kinds of antigens, and will contain T helper and suppressor cells, Tdth cells and T cytotoxic cells.

To summarise: lymphocyte activity is initiated by immunological events within the body which are always specific. Some lymphocytes synthesise antibodies, while others destroy virally infected cells or serve regulatory functions. A particular immune response will involve some, or perhaps all of these cells, which must interact together in a highly complex way. Type and strength of the immune response will depend on:

- dose of the antigen,
- route of entry into the body,
- previous exposure to the same antigen,
- factors like age and general health status.

Lymphocytes do not merely cooperate with one another; their process of activation and subsequent functioning depends on other cells, particularly macrophages and neutrophils. It has already been pointed out on p. 116 that phagocytosis is enhanced if bacteria or other foreign particles are first opsonised. Opsonisation occurs through activation of the complement system, and also because foreign particles may become coated with specific antibodies. This covering facilitates the attachment of phagocytic cells because they have receptors for the Y-shaped part of the antibody on their cell surfaces. Uncoated bacteria are cleared only slowly from the bloodstream; opsonised ones are removed swiftly. Phagocytic cells also have receptors for the C3b complement protein, so bacteria that have been covered with complement are engulfed quickly too.

Very few antigens bind directly to T or B cells. Instead they are presented to them on the surfaces of phagocytic cells placed strategically in the tissues. Some of these cells are always present in the lymph nodes, others are in the tissues, for example, the cells of Kupffer in the liver and the mesangial cells in the kidney (see Chapter 1). These migrate to the lymph nodes once they have trapped antigens, and when they arrive the T and B cells in the node become activated to form a clone. The types of T cell which become activated vary according to the antigen concerned and the duration of the immune response. Surprisingly, the antigen-presenting cells, which are only weakly phagocytic, are more effective at trapping antigens than macrophages, although macrophages do have a limited capacity to behave in this manner. Ability to present antigens, like many other cellular functions, appears to be related to the structure of the cell concerned. The amount of available surface area on the cell membrane appears to be important. Kupffer and mesangial cells have much bigger surface areas than macrophages, which have specialised much more in efficient phagocytosis and destruction.

The immune system is highly complicated but it is worth the effort of trying to understand because developments in this field are rapid and have already shown that when the functioning of the immune system goes awry, disease results. The immune system is most efficient at recognising foreign substances which have invaded the tissues, but its means of determining whether they are actually dangerous is not infallible. Most of the time the system operates well to control infection, but there can be unfortunate side-effects like the violent immune response against foreign yet harmless pollen grains in some people (hay fever), and the rejection of much needed tissue grafts, which the body identifies as 'not-self'.

There is evidence that many diseases of previously obscure aetiology could have their basis in a damaged or defectively functioning immune system. For example, rheumatoid arthritis seems to be caused by the activity of factors (called autoantibodies) which destroy IgG. It is an autoimmune disease and the damage to the joint may be caused by the formation of immune complexes.

Successful pathogens are those which can evade, resist or inhibit the immune system. Many cause tissue damage directly, usually by toxin formation, a feature of the most virulent microorganisms. A good deal of the tissue damage which accompanies infection and inflammation, especially that of a chronic nature, is however due to the host response, as in the case of chronic wounds, like pressure sores (see Chapter 9). The well-adapted pathogen only moderately damages the host, so that the immune response it provokes is not severe enough to eradicate it from the tissues before it can multiply, disseminate and perpetuate the species.

References

Atkins, M. D. (1972). Fever. *Physiology in Medicine*, **286** (**1**): 27–35.

Burchfield, S. (1979). The stress response. A new perspective. *Psychosomatic Research*, **41**: 661–672.

Cannon, W. B. (1935). Stresses and strains of homeostasis. *American Journal of Medicine*, **189**: 1–14.

Ho-Yen, D. O., Crossan, M. N., Walker, E. (1985). Nursing knowledge of hepatitis B infection. *Journal of Advanced Nursing*, **10** (2): 169–172.

Imboden, J. B. (1972). Psychosocial determinants of recovery. *Advances in Psychosomatic Medicine*, **8**: 142–155.

Lazarus, R. S. (1966). *Psychological Stress and the Coping Process*. McGraw-Hill, New York.

Montague, S. W. (1981). The contribution of the biological sciences to nursing. In *Nursing Science in Nursing Practice*, Smith, J. (ed.) Butterworths, London, pp. 133–151.

Personal paper (1984). The hepatitis carrier. *Lancet*, **1**: 332.

Selye, H. (1956). *The Stress of Life*. McGraw-Hill, New York.

Staines, N., Brostoff, J., James, K. (1985). *Introducing Immunology*. Gower Medical, London.

Wilson-Barnett, J. (1979). *Stress in Hospital*. Churchill Livingstone, Edinburgh.

Wilson-Barnett, J. (1981). Assessment of recovery with special reference to a study with post-operative cardiac patients. *Journal of Advanced Nursing Studies*, **6**: 435–445.

Further Reading

Playfair, J. H. L. (1984). *Immunology at a Glance*. Blackwell Scientific Publications, Oxford.

Chapter 8

Care of the Patient with an Indwelling Urinary Catheter

INTRODUCTION

Years ago, catheters were allowed to drain into glass bottles, with a stopper preventing the contents being spilled. The closed, sterile system of drainage was introduced by Dukes in 1928, but its value in the prevention of urinary tract infection was not appreciated until the 1960s, when two independent teams (Gillespie *et al.*, 1960; Sandford, 1964) identified that a closed system of drainage could reduce the incidence of sepsis following catheterisation from 80% to about 10%. However, the incidence of urinary tract infection in hospital still remains extremely high, and it appears that despite the development of new, improved drainage systems, either fresh problems have arisen or standards of catheter management remain poor. Of course, 'closed' systems are not really closed at all; they are certainly an advance on the old stoppered bottle, but they must be opened to empty the urine away, and disconnected when the drainage bag is changed.

Urinary tract infection has been the subject of numerous research studies, but many of the findings are questionable, either because the studies themselves have been poorly controlled, or because researchers have tried to compare patient samples which are dissimilar. It is not meaningful to compare modern rates of infection with those obtained years ago, when the risks were less fully appreciated and precautions against urinary tract infection less stringent. Factors such as age, sex, length of time that the catheter has been *in situ*, reason for catheterisation and medical diagnosis all influence individual susceptibility to infection (see Chapter 4). This means that when prospective, controlled trials are undertaken to compare the effect of a particular method of catheter management with a control population, the lack of homogeneity between the two groups will almost certainly interfere with the interpretation of the results. The findings of any one particular research study reflect the method used to conduct the investigation (see Chapter 3), and all too often samples used to examine the problems associated with catheterisation have been small, or have consisted of patients belonging to a particular medical specialty (often genitourinary, geriatric or intensive care patients). The results, therefore, cannot be generalised to the entire patient population of a hospital or community, and it is important to remember the shortcomings when reading these studies.

Despite the restrictions of the information available from research, it is fair to say that nurses' knowledge of urinary tract infection and catheterisation is generally not good. In 1982 a nurse and a geriatrician (Kennedy and Brocklehurst, 1982) highlighted many examples of poor catheter management among 107 elderly people in hospital and the community who had been catheterised for longer than 3 days. In the study 25 nurses were interviewed, and knowledge of catheter care was found to be inadequate, with very little appreciation of the patient's need for dignity, or the hazards of infection. In 1985 Gould undertook a similar, though not an identical, study since she investigated patients admitted to a district general hospital in which a high proportion of patients were elderly. Her findings were not quite so disappointing, but it was apparent that nurses still did not appreciate the dangers associated with urinary tract infection, experienced considerable difficulty interpreting microbiology report findings, and on ten of the 19 wards to which learners were allocated did not attempt to teach the principles of catheter management believing erroneously that this took place in the school of nursing.

These findings are worrying because prevention of urinary tract infection and safe catheter management are important nursing responsibilities. A careful nursing assessment will reveal the extent to which each patient is likely to be exposed to risk, and if this is significant preventive measures should be included in the care plan.

The problems associated with indwelling urinary catheterisation are discussed in this chapter in terms of frequency of occurrence, epidemiology, factors which predispose to the development of urinary tract infection, and bacterial virulence. Guidelines for safe catheter management will be provided, although it should be recognised that these can only be suggested in the light of the research evidence currently available.

INCIDENCE

The National Prevalence Study (Meers *et al.*, 1981) revealed that 10% of inpatients in the hospitals visited had developed a nosocomial infection; 30% of these were urinary tract infections. These results are broadly in agreement with the results of an earlier survey conducted by Ayliffe (1971), in which 11.2% inpatients had developed an infection during hospital stay, 26% of these being of the urinary tract. However, this problem is not unique to British hospitals; data provided by the National Nosocomial Infection Study in America (Clifford, 1982) reporting throughout the years 1971 to 1974, revealed that 40% of all hospital acquired infections affected the urinary tract.

The risk of urinary tract infection is much greater following catheterisation and increases with the length of time that the catheter remains *in situ*; much will depend upon the original reason for catheterisation (Table 8.1).

In 1966 it was estimated by Kunin that 10% of all people admitted to an acute general hospital ward would be given an indwelling urethral catheter at some point during their stay. This proportion has undoubtedly increased since the 1960s, owing to the growing numbers of elderly and critically ill patients admitted to acute wards.

Stamm (1978) estimated that approximately 75% of all hospital acquired urinary tract infections were associated with episodes of catheterisation, although other urethral manipulations have been implicated, mainly cystoscopy.

A small proportion of those patients who develop

Table 8.1 Reasons for Catheterisation

Short-term (a few hours or days)
(1) To empty the bladder during a surgical procedure where there is a risk of trauma to a full bladder, for example, for rectal and gynaecological operations, caesarean section
(2) To determine residual urine where it is suspected that the bladder may not be emptying properly
(3) To measure urinary output accurately as part of critical fluid balance estimation, for example, following major surgery, intensive care
(4) To relieve acute urinary retention, for example, benign enlargement of the prostate gland in elderly men or following vaginal surgery where the insertion of a pack to prevent bleeding may inhibit micturition
(5) During urological investigations and operations

Long-term
(1) Unconsciousness
(2) Chronic inoperable obstruction, for example, advanced malignancy of the prostate, or benign protastatic enlargement in a patient too frail to withstand anaesthesia
(3) Urinary incontinence

nosocomial urinary tract infections (possibly between 1% and 3%) will develop secondary bacteraemia, a grave condition, carrying a mortality rate of 30%. In her extensive review of urinary tract infection, Clifford (1982) estimated that approximately 500 000 patients in the United Kingdom will be catheterised per annum. Assuming that between 8% and 10% develop a urinary tract infection, then between 40 000 and 50 000 may go on to develop septicaemia. For a small number (500) the consequences will be fatal.

The main reason for inserting a long-term indwelling catheter is still urinary incontinence (see Table 8.1) even though it is now generally accepted that this condition is neither incurable nor an inevitable consequence of growing old, but more often the result of poor management or inadequate diagnostic investigation (Report of the Association of Incontinence Advisers, 1984). Several alternatives to the use of long-term indwelling urinary catheters are now available, including electronic devices, condoms and drainage systems for men and intermittent self-catheterisation. Adults and children have been taught successfully to catheterise themselves (Deegan, 1985). Suprapubic catheterisation offers another possible alternative;

it has been associated with lower levels of urinary tract infection than those reported for urethral catheters, and has gained some degree of acceptance, chiefly among those whose bladder dysfunction has resulted from neurological disorders. The formation of an ileal conduit is a more drastic approach for patients who have this problem.

The best way to prevent urinary tract infection is clearly to avoid the use (particularly long term) of indwelling urinary catheters, wherever possible. However, for some people there is still no suitable alternative at the present time, and for these catheterisation may be welcomed with resignation and a certain amount of relief. Applying a condom and self-catheterisation both demand a certain amount of manual dexterity, as well as perseverance until the individual is sufficiently confident to venture into society. Unfortunately, many people who become incontinent are either paralysed or their movement has become restricted as part of their general incapacitation.

The care of catheterised patients within the community is a major part of the district nursing work load (Wastling, 1978). Although the risks of cross-infection are generally considered to be much lower in the community than in hospital, catheter care is still known to be the source of much discomfort among patients, especially problems associated with blockage and bypassing (Kennedy et al., 1983).

EPIDEMIOLOGY

Endogenous infections are caused by microorganisms which form part of the patient's own microbiological flora. Exogenous infections are derived from other people, or from the hospital environment (see Chapter 1). Although urinary tract infections acquired in hospital may be either exogenous or endogenous, the majority fall into the second category. Bacteria most commonly implicated are Gram-negative bacilli such as *Pseudomonas*, *Proteus*, *Klebsiella* and *Serratia*. *Escherichia coli* is reported on more single occasions than any other bacteria. *Streptococcus faecalis* is responsible for a high proportion of urinary tract infections, probably because like *E. coli* it is part of the normal bowel flora. Until recent years other Gram-positive bacteria were considered to be responsible for relatively few urinary tract infections. However, *Staphylococcus epidermidis* is now believed to cause up to 30% of nosocomial urinary tract infections, usually in combination with *Candida*. These occur most frequently among patients who are immunocompromised. *Staphylococcus aureus* is not a common urinary pathogen, and if it is reported from the urine its presence is nearly always due to contamination (see Chapter 10).

Hospital-acquired urinary tract infections tend to be more serious and more intractable than those acquired by patients in the community. Evidence discussed in previous chapters has suggested that people in hospital are much more susceptible to infection and those who have urological problems are at particular risk. Opportunities for cross-infection via the hands of staff are much greater among inpatients. Early research by Dutton and Ralston (1957) implicated hand contamination as a major contributory factor in the spread of urinary tract infection. This has since been verified by Casewell and Phillips (1977) who identified the hands as the main source of infection in an outbreak of *Klebsiella*. Other risk factors are the invasive procedures that urological patients may undergo in addition to catheterisation. These further traumatise the urethral mucosa and provide additional opportunity for microorganisms normally inhabiting the urethra to be thrust in a large inoculum into the bladder. The normal gut bacteria of hospital patients rapidly become resistant to antibiotics, probably because food from hospital kitchens is contaminated with resistant bacteria.

FACTORS PREDISPOSING TO URINARY TRACT INFECTION

Early research by Turck (1962) showed that the risk of urinary tract infection among elderly hospital patients was greater than among younger, ambulant subjects following a single episode of urethral catheterisation. Johanson et al. (1969) demonstrated that the skin and mucous membranes of older and debilitated people were more likely to become colonised with Gram-negative bacteria, while Chin and Davies (1976) showed this to be particularly true of the hands of paraplegics. It is therefore not surprising that Garibaldi et al. (1974) were able to demonstrate high rates of nosocomial urinary tract infection among elderly people, especially when they were very ill. The bacteria responsible were nearly always the same as the skin flora.

In the early study by Turck (1962) the incidence of urinary tract infection increased from 1% for a single episode of catheterisation to nearly 100% when the catheter was allowed to drain for several days. In more recent studies, like Garibaldi et al.'s (1974) (when closed systems of drainage replaced the stoppered glass bottles used at the time of Turck's research), the risk of infection continued to rise to between 5% and 10% for each day that the catheter was allowed to remain in situ. Garibaldi concluded that despite the development of modern drainage systems, half the patients making up any sample will show evidence of urinary tract infection 14 days later if the catheter has not been removed.

Bacteria may gain access to the urinary tract via four different portals of entry (Fig. 8.1):

(1) The most obvious of these is carriage on the top of the catheter when it is inserted, through faulty aseptic technique; this danger is heavily emphasised when nurses are taught about the catheterisation procedure.
(2) Once the catheter has been inserted, however, bacteria may still gain access if the drainage bag and catheter tubing are ever disconnected – modern drainage systems are fitted with a special sleeve so that urine specimens can be withdrawn without the need for disconnection.
(3) Bacteria may also enter the system in the thin film of moisture always present between the outside of the tubing and the urethral mucosa.
(4) They may migrate from a contaminated drainage system along the lumen of the catheter, and ultimately into the bladder.

Enormous emphasis is placed upon good aseptic technique during the catheterisation procedure, but the third and fourth portals of entry mentioned above tend to be overlooked by nurses, who are often much more relaxed about the management of the catheter once it has been inserted. Unfortunately, there is evidence to suggest that the majority of hospital-acquired urinary tract infections result from the migration of bacteria along the

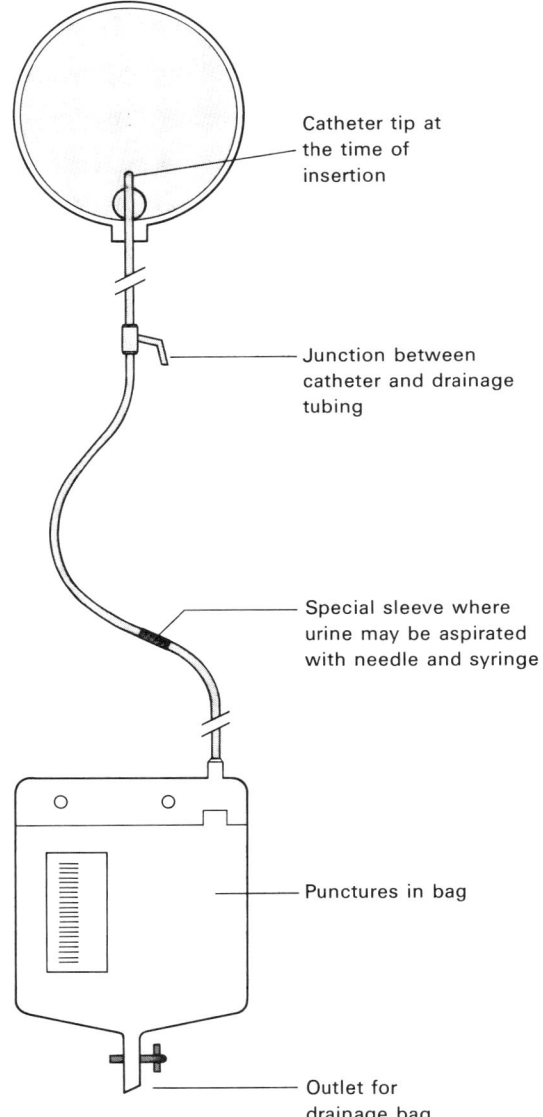

Fig. 8.1 The indwelling urinary catheter: points at which microorganisms can enter the system.

inner surfaces of the drainage system. They are given numerous opportunities to gain access:

(1) When the drainage bag is changed.
(2) When the catheter and drainage system are disconnected for traditional bladder irrigation.
(3) If disconnection takes place for specimen collection.
(4) If the drainage system becomes disconnected

by accident, which might occur, for example, if a disoriented patient pulled his catheter.
(5) If fluids used for bladder irrigation become contaminated.
(6) If the outlet of the drainage bag becomes contaminated when it is emptied, or is allowed to touch the floor. The drainage bag may become colonised by bacteria and behave as a reservoir from which they can be released if the bag is inverted or allowed to become kinked beneath the patient. A backflow of urine will travel up the tubing towards the bladder. Many bags are now fitted with non-return valves, but laboratory experiments have shown that these are not infallible. Infections may still result, possibly because bacteria travel through the valves with ascending air bubbles. Urimeters are still not generally fitted with non-return valves. In a small study conducted among 20 patients who had had an indwelling urinary catheter for more than 1 day, 17 patients developed urinary tract infections because the drainage bag had become colonised (Stamm, 1978)

BACTERIAL VIRULENCE AND URINARY TRACT INFECTION

Although *E. coli* is the most common urinary pathogen, the majority of nosocomial urinary tract infections for which it is responsible are caused by only a few of its serotypes (see Chapter 10), mainly those which form part of the normal bowel flora. Some bacteria are more virulent than others because they have developed particular morphological or physiological attributes which appear to contribute to their ability to attack the cells of the host (see Chapter 1). The cell surfaces of virulent *E. coli* serotypes are particularly rich in a polysaccharide called antigen K, which seems to protect the bacteria from attack by white blood cells, so that they escape destruction by phagocytosis. Serotypes with antigen K seem to be particularly successful when they ascend the ureters, because they are able to attack renal tissue. Strains which lack antigen K are more likely to remain in the bladder.

Before bacteria can invade cells they must attach themselves to the cell surface. Pili (hairs) which cover some strains of *Proteus* enable these bacteria to attach themselves successfully. Under experimental conditions they have been found to induce pyelonephritis more readily than those strains that lack pili. Various other species, including *Proteus*, appear to be successful urinary pathogens through their ability to secrete urease, an enzyme that digests urea to carbon dioxide and ammonium ions. Urea is a breakdown product of protein metabolism that is excreted in the urine. Large quantities of ammonium ions cause urine to become alkaline. A history of *Proteus* urinary tract infection and alkaline urine is associated with a high incidence of renal calculi and catheter encrustation.

The urinary tract seems to be particularly defenceless against invading bacteria. Urine is made by a process of filtration and selective reabsorption in the nephrons which make up the kidney. Proteins and other large molecules with a molecular weight of greater than 68 000 daltons are unable to pass through the pores of the glomerulus. Immunoglobulins are very large protein molecules, so they never enter the glomerular filtrate, and are not added to it at any stage as the filtrate travels along the nephron.

Urinary tract infections are particularly common in female patients because of the shortness of the urethra.

THE PATIENT'S PERSPECTIVE IN CATHETERISATION

Most of the research findings discussed above have been the work of microbiologists or doctors with a particular interest in urology. Others, including nurses, are now beginning to investigate the more 'patient-oriented' problems associated with catheterisation. As highlighted by Ferrie *et al.* (1979) these include: leakage, blockage, encrustation, bladder spasm, and genital oedema. All these problems are either related to infection or exacerbated by it.

Bladder Irrigation

Bladder irrigation may be performed to reduce or prevent catheter obstruction or urinary tract infection. It may be inevitable when the catheter lumen becomes blocked with debris, but conventional bladder washouts involve disconnection of the catheter and drainage bag. Opinions regarding their value vary: some researchers have reported a reduction in the amount of blockage and leakage following the introduction of routine bladder irrigation; whereas others recommend bladder washouts to be reserved exclusively for occasions when obstruction has actually occurred. A new bladder washout system called the Uro-Tainer (marketed by Clini-Med) has become available in the last few years. This removes the need to break the 'closed' system of drainage because fluid from the Uro-Tainer can be directed into the drainage bag through its outlet. The bag is then inverted so that the fluid comes into contact with the internal surfaces of the drainage bag while a clamp prevents it entering the urethra. Preliminary, though very small-scale trials (Kennedy, 1984) suggest that this new system is superior to conventional bladder irrigation. In the small study reported, the Uro-Tainer appeared to reduce the incidence of urinary tract infection and was commented upon favourably by patients, relatives and staff. However, 13 subjects entered the trial and nine completed it; these numbers are too small for statistical analysis and larger trials are needed to verify the results. Bladder washouts are not easy to perform in an aseptic manner and they are costly in terms of equipment and time. Common sense would suggest that the new system is an improvement on the old.

Opinions regarding the value of prophylactic antibiotic irrigation (and oral medication) during short-term catheterisation are mixed, but most authorities agree that they are inappropriate for long-term use. Some believe that disinfectants have a place in long-term catheter management, but others disagree on the grounds that they too can promote the development of multiresistant bacterial strains. Stickler *et al.* (1981) found that noxythiolin (Noxyflex) exerted no bactericidal effect unless it was allowed to remain in contact with infected urine for 2 hours; this is clearly impractical during clinical use.

Perineal Care

It is commonly believed that urinary tract infections can be prevented, at least to some extent, by cleaning the perineum and urethral meatus with a disinfectant at regular intervals. However, there is no clear evidence to date in support of this. Rates of infection were reduced in one group of patients whose daily programme included baths, cleaning the perineum afterwards with antibacterial spray (Brehmer and Madsen, 1972). Uncontrolled clinical trials have indicated that antibacterial lubricants and urethral disinfectants may be beneficial (McLeod *et al.*, 1963; Mulla, 1961). Later, prospective controlled studies, however, suggest that twice-daily cleaning with povidone-iodine has no effect upon infection rates (Britt *et al.*, 1976). This has led many microbiologists and nurses alike to believe that soap and water is the best method of cleansing the perineum. A team of British nurses is currently undertaking an exploratory study of methods of catheter toilet used throughout the country, to be followed by multicentre, controlled clinical trials. Until the results of these become available, there is little evidence in support of any one particular regime. It is always possible that handling the catheter to clean it may propel bacteria into the bladder along the periurethral space. Taping the catheter to the thigh may help to reduce the effect of this piston action when the patient moves; it will certainly help reduce trauma to the urethra.

Choice of Catheter

Catheters are manufactured mainly from four types of material: plastic, latex, teflon-coated, and silicone-coated latex. The range of designs is enormous and the materials may be used in combination to produce catheters which have different properties (Table 8.2).

Where no suitable alternative to long-term catheterisation is possible, individual assessment of the patient is of major importance, since tolerance to different kinds of catheter material is very variable. There have been relatively few trials to compare the effectiveness of these, except for one study conducted by Kennedy (1983) among 18 elderly female patients, which lasted for 9 months. Silicone catheters were removed after a mean period of 35 days. Only 19% remained *in situ* for 3 months, although throughout the trial they were removed only when problems were encountered,

Table 8.2 Foley Catheters: Materials and Types Available

(1) *Plastic*
   Advantages
      Good drainage. Suitable for use when the urine may contain clots or debris. Two and three-way drainage systems are available, allowing bladder irrigation
   Disadvantages
      Prone to encrustation. Not suitable for long-term use. Manufacturers recommend that they should not remain *in situ* for more than 14 days. Patients may complain of discomfort
(2) *Latex*
   Advantages
      Soft, comfortable, inexpensive
   Disadvantages
      Encrustation, urethritis. Manufacturers recommend use for 14 days only
(3) *Latex – teflon-coated*
   Advantages
      Manufacturers recommend use for up to 4 weeks
   Disadvantages
      Encrustation; discomfort (see text)
(4) *Latex – silicone-coated*
   Advantages
      Use recommended up to 3 months. Manufacturers claim that they are non-irritant and that good tolerance can be expected
   Disadvantages
      Relatively expensive compared to other types. In some products, the internal diameter is reduced, promoting blockage. Tolerance may not always be good (see text)

not routinely. Latex catheters remained *in situ* for a mean of 30 days, but very few for 3 months. Teflon-coated catheters fared least well; scarcely any of the patients were able to tolerate them for more than a few days.

The experience (not research-based evidence) of Blannin (1982) suggested that catheters with a small lumen should be used whenever possible and that small-capacity balloon catheters are to be preferred. This author observed that large lumens and balloons tended to irritate the bladder, causing spasm of the detrusor muscle, so that urine bypassed the catheter. There is now more conclusive evidence that large catheters aggravate this bypassing (Kennedy et al., 1983). Drugs given to reduce muscle spasm may help overcome this problem.

Frequency of Recatheterisation

Belief has grown among nurses that recatheterisation should not take place unless there are specific problems, because of the risk of introducing infection. Research conducted many years ago (Helmholtz, 1950), however, suggested that although the insertion of a catheter may transport bacteria up the urethra, the inoculum is so small that under normal circumstances problems are unlikely to result. If the catheter is removed soon afterwards, normal voiding of urine will wash these bacteria out again. There are other probably more important portals of entry, and the most influential factor is the length of time that the catheter is allowed to remain *in situ*.

Microbiological Monitoring of the Urine

McCormack (1977) advocated that when patients are catheterised long term their urine should be monitored at regular intervals for bacteria, to draw attention to the emergence of multiresistant strains; steps can then be taken to prevent cross-infection (see case study 10.1, p. 164).

PREVENTING NOSOCOMIAL URINARY TRACT INFECTIONS

Most of the methods currently available to help nurses prevent urinary tract infections focus upon reducing the entry of bacteria into a 'closed', initially sterile system of drainage, while persuading the patient to take adequate fluids, at least 2 litres daily. From the previous discussion, it should be apparent that these may not be very effective for a patient whose catheter is allowed to remain *in situ* for long. It is also important to emphasise that although drainage bags should not become overfull, the system should not otherwise be handled more than necessary. Some guidelines for catheter care are presented in Table 8.3. These are not intended to be prescriptive, since the circumstances of every patient will vary. They have been formulated from the research evidence currently available, with all the limitations of this work previously discussed.

Table 8.3 Guidelines for Catheter Care

(1) Avoid the use of long-term indwelling urinary catheters wherever suitable alternatives can be found
(2) *Never* leave the catheter *in situ* longer than necessary, and insert using full aseptic technique
(3) Assess and monitor every patient according to individual need
(4) Maintain adequate nursing records, including:
  - original date and reason for catheterisation
  - recatheterisation if necessary
  - type and size of catheter
  - capacity of the balloon
  - monitor the urine for evidence of infection
(5) Avoid disconnection of the catheter and drainage bag by
  - never using spigots
  - using bladder irrigation only when strictly necessary
  - withdrawing specimens from the special sleeve
(6) Ensure good drainage by
  - never allowing the tubing to become twisted
  - keeping the drainage bag below the level of the bladder
(7) Avoid ascending infection by ensuring that
  - the drainage bag hangs clear of the floor
  - the tubing and drainage bag do not become inverted
  - the drainage bag is emptied frequently
(8) Keep the risks of cross-infection to a minimum, reducing the number of people who handle the catheter by
  - careful patient allocation
  - teaching the patient to take care of his/her own catheter wherever possible
(9) Promote the patient's comfort and dignity by
  - providing information
  - good standards of hygiene
  - perineal and catheter toilet
  - choosing unobtrusive, bodily worn systems wherever appropriate
  - using small-size catheters, with small balloons

Precautions with Catheter Usage

It is fair to say that in order to prevent urinary tract infections, the use of indwelling urinary catheters should be avoided wherever a suitable alternative can be found. In cases of necessity (critical monitoring of urinary output in intensive care units) the catheter should never remain *in situ* for longer than absolutely necessary. Before first-time catheterisation every patient should be assessed individually and monitored carefully afterwards to determine how well the system chosen is tolerated.

Since silicone catheters are expensive, but not always the best possible choice, it is logical to start with an inexpensive variety (latex or plastic). Adequate nursing records should always be maintained. They should include the original date and reason for catheterisation, recatheterisation, type and size of catheter and the capacity of the balloon. Disconnection of the catheter and drainage bag should be avoided. Spigots should never be used and bladder irrigation only when it is really necessary (obstruction, clot retention). Uro-Tainer systems seem preferable to traditional methods of irrigation. Specimens should be withdrawn from the special resealing sleeve provided, using needle, syringe and full aseptic technique. Tubing should never be allowed to kink, twist or coil beneath the patient and the drainage bag should remain below the level of the bladder so that it will drain properly. It should never become inverted, or backflow of the urine to the bladder will result. The outlet should hang clear of the floor. Drainage bags should be emptied frequently so that any colonising bacteria receive as little opportunity as possible to migrate up the tubing. A bag that is too full drags uncomfortably on the genitals and looks unsightly. A sterile jug should, if at all possible, be used to catch the urine and the outlet should be cleaned before and after emptying with a suitable disinfectant (70% alcohol as an impregnated swab or spray). Opinions vary as to whether emptying should be regarded as a clean or aseptic procedure, but sterile disposable gloves should be worn whenever catheters or drainage bags are handled. Specimens should be sent routinely to the microbiology laboratory. Catheterised patients should not, if at all possible, be nursed in adjacent beds, as this increases the likelihood of cross-infection (Stamm, 1975). It is best for each nurse to be allocated no more than one patient with a catheter per span of duty so that risks of cross-infection are minimised. It is difficult to balance the risks associated with recatheterisation against the risk of infection that may occur if a catheter, allowed to remain *in situ* over an extended period, becomes heavily colonised. However, every fresh catheterisation will result in additional trauma to the urethra, and except in the event of problems, is probably best avoided. Indiscriminate recatheterisation is expensive and wastes time.

In the event of bypassing, water should never be added to the balloon and the catheter should not be replaced by one of a larger size. Instead, a smaller catheter with a smaller capacity balloon may be advisable, because it will irritate the bladder less.

Whenever possible, patients should be taught how to look after their own catheters. If the system is handled chiefly by the patient, the risk of cross-infection is reduced and the patient will further benefit from independence and being involved with his own care (see Chapter 11). This is especially important if long-term catheterisation is envisaged and he is expected to carry on using the catheter when he goes home. In this case, the system chosen will depend on factors related to acceptability and convenience as well as to infection control. At home the possibility of cross-infection will be a great deal smaller. Various discreet, bodily worn systems are now marketed, some with garments specially designed to hold and conceal the drainage bag. Nurses who look after patients likely to go home with a catheter must be informed about the different products available, their relative merits and cost.

Whether the patient is in hospital or the community, nurses must know how to recognise the signs and symptoms of urinary tract infections (discussed in greater detail in Chapter 10). Case study 8.1 below describes how a patient was assessed before a suitable regime of care was chosen, and the care plan in Table 8.4 explains how a urinary tract infection can be prevented from spreading to other patients.

Even if catheters are sometimes poorly managed, their use does appear to be declining. Nordquist (1984) improved matters on a geriatric ward by discontinuing the use of indwelling catheters in favour of a regime of careful observation, habit training and drugs to reduce the incidence of nocturia. Overall nursing requirements did not increase and antibiotic prescriptions declined by 90% compared to a control ward where urinary incontinence was managed in the traditional way. The incidence of septicaemia, bronchopneumonia and wound infections also declined in comparison to the control ward. Laundry costs, and expenditure on items such as incontinence pads fell by 46%. In this study 124 patients admitted to the innovative ward were followed up for a period of 4 years; 65% died during this time, but the great majority (78%) remained free of catheters and infection until their demise.

Table 8.4 Outline Care Plan for Antibiotic-resistant *Pseudomonas* Urinary Tract Infection

(1) Causative organism: *Pseudomonas aeruginosa*, resistant to gentamicin
(2) Reason for precautions: to prevent contamination of the environment and possible cross-infection to other patients
(3) Transmission
    nurses' hands
    contact spread on any damp objects: washbowls, flannels
(4) Items contaminated
    bedpans, catheters, jugs (urinals for men)
    soiled bedclothes (urine)
    patient's hands
(5) Need for a single room desirable, but not absolutely essential, depending on availability and circumstances
(6) Protective clothing: aprons and gloves

Case study 8.1

Mrs Jones, aged 65, had always leaked a few drops of urine when she laughed or coughed, dating back to when her children were born. They had always been good, big babies. With the passage of time her problem became slightly worse. Putting on weight and carrying heavy bags of shopping up the hill to her cottage did not help. Although she had had the same general practitioner for years, she somehow felt that her problem was not sufficient to bother him, and in any case she did not somehow fancy talking about it to a man. Some days the problem was worse than others, but she could generally contain the urine by wearing a sanitary pad.

Matters came to a head when Mrs Jones became unwell. For the first time the housework seemed to defeat her, and her 'problem' got so bad that she dared not leave the house. Her husband decided to take her straight to the doctor.

The doctor gave Mrs Jones a full physical examination, and tested her urine. It was full of sugar. The doctor explained that grown up people can develop 'adult-onset' diabetes and arranged for Mrs Jones to have an appointment at the diabetic clinic at the local hospital, where she was seen by both a doctor and a nurse. Mrs Jones did indeed appear to have diabetes mellitus, but it could successfully be controlled by diet. When Mrs Jones felt able to mention her incontinence the diabetic nurse did not seem surprised, and explained that this is a common problem among diabetics, especially when the disease is first diagnosed and symptoms have not yet been controlled. A sample of urine had already been sent to the laboratory to screen for infection, which can make the problem worse.

Mrs Jones felt better than she had for a long time. She was especially reassured when the nurse promised to visit her at home, but was a bit daunted when told that she must try to lose weight. In the meantime she was provided with a supply of larger, more absorbent pads.

The diabetic nurse visited Mrs Jones at home regularly. Her urine remained free of infection, although not always of glucose, and it was apparent that despite continued encouragement, Mrs Jones found a certain amount of difficulty keeping to her diet. Her stress incontinence never really improved to any great extent, and she was eventually persuaded to attend a clinic. A cystocele was diagnosed; the wall of the bladder had been damaged years ago, when Mrs Jones's children were born, and the problem was exacerbated now by obesity. Mrs Jones felt that she was too old to have surgery, and in the end she was visited by the district nurse, whose assessment revealed the following problems:

- Obesity: height 1.57 m (5ft 2in) weight 70 kg (154 lb).
- Urinary incontinence, now severe, occurring day and night, preventing Mrs Jones venturing out alone and significantly reducing her quality of life; her clothes were continually damp and she was concerned about odour.
- Mild, but rather poorly controlled diabetes; the urine generally contained at least a trace amount of glucose, but never ketones.

The district nurse explained the options open to Mrs Jones in the privacy of her own home, and included her husband in the discussion since he was so concerned. She pointed out the restrictions imposed by catheterisation, but Mrs Jones remained adamant that she did not want an operation, and Mr Jones agreed that since his wife had always been 'strongwilled', catheterisation would probably be best, as she was unlikely to change her mind.

Initially Mrs Jones was catheterised with a short-term indwelling Foley catheter, but this was later changed to a silicone one, with a small balloon. A leg bag was worn during the day, which could be concealed quite well beneath Mrs Jones's voluminous skirts, and she was now prepared to venture out as far as the nearby shops.

Reassessment of Mrs Jones's problems at this stage showed obesity and mild diabetes, both poorly controlled. But, on the positive side, Mrs Jones seemed quite happy. She was coping well with the catheter, was reasonably active and her quality of life had improved. Infection remained a potential problem in view of Mrs Jones's elevated blood sugar levels, but she emptied the catheter herself and she had at least been persuaded to drink 2 litres of fluid every day, and to observe her urine for colour and odour; this she did diligently.

Mrs Jones's catheter was size 14, with a small balloon. She checked the tubing every day for signs of blockage, and some weeks after it had been inserted she noticed that debris was collecting in the tube. She had been told that catheters could become encrusted, but wishing to be independent she did not mention this on the district nurse's weekly visit.

One night Mrs Jones woke suddenly with a colicky pain in her abdomen; the bedclothes were damp, as the catheter had leaked a little round the outside the previous day. Mrs Jones was taken to the accident and emergency department for the catheter to be replaced. Unfortunately she developed symptoms of urinary tract infection soon afterwards and had to be admitted to hospital when her husband became unable to cope. A specimen sent to the laboratory showed that the infection was due to *Pseudomonas*, and that the bacteria were resistant to gentamicin (see Chapter 4).

The nurses on the ward adopted the guidelines shown in Table 8.4 to prevent the spread of infection to other patients on the ward.

When she was admitted to the ward, Mrs Jones was frightened and rather disoriented. She was accompanied by her husband, who was extremely anxious. They were greeted by a nurse, who made an initial assessment of Mrs Jones's condition, identifying her main problems in relation to infection. These included:

- *Disorientation.* Mrs Jones did not really know where she was, or what was happening to her. Mental confusion is often associated with infection in older people, and may give a clue to the underlying problem. She was not pyrexial, but her pulse was accelerated.
- *Agitation.* Mrs Jones was not able to tell the nurse that she was in pain, but her discomfort was apparent from her restless behaviour, tugging at the catheter. Her clothes were damp with urine and perspiration.

The immediate aims of care were to obtain a specimen of urine for bacteriological examination, then remove the catheter and make Mrs Jones as comfortable as possible, while providing reassurance for her husband. Urinary tract infection was strongly suspected, but it was not known at this stage that multiresistant bacteria were responsible. In view of her disorientation, Mrs Jones was given a bed in the main ward, where she could be observed easily. Initially a catheter was not reinserted, but when, 24 hours later, it became evident that Mrs Jones was heavily incontinent, a decision was taken to recatheterise her for her own dignity, and because she was neither mobile nor mentally alert and was therefore at great risk of developing pressure sores. Plastic gloves were worn when handling the bedclothes, and the catheter and drainage apparatus.

When the laboratory results became available, the junior doctor asked the sister to move Mrs Jones to a single room. The sister was reluctant to comply, explaining to the doctor that Mrs Jones had been nursed on the main ward for more than 2 days, and that so far her infection had been contained by sensible infection control precautions. The ward specialised in the care of general medical patients, and although many of them were elderly, nobody but Mrs Jones had a catheter; there were no immunosuppressed or acutely ill patients. Moreover, the only single room available was occupied by a patient who was in considerable pain, and who had been in distress on the main ward.

The antibiotics prescribed for Mrs Jones were changed, so that she received intravenous carbenicillin, which is effective against *Pseudomonas*. The infection control nurse visited the ward, and emphasised the importance of good handwashing techniques and gloves to prevent contact spread. Mrs Jones was provided with her own washbowl. She was washed using soft disposable wipes and liquid soap. The nurses wore gloves and aprons whenever they touched her, and the need for these precautions were explained carefully to the patient and her husband.

Mr Jones, upset, could not understand why his wife had developed an infection because their home was very clean. He wondered how he could rid their house of all the 'germs'. It was gently pointed out that infection is a risk of having a catheter, and that the bacteria responsible normally live wherever there is dampness, only causing damage when they manage to enter a part of the body not usually accessible to them. In hospital the bacteria presented more of a problem than at home in view of other people whose bodily defences were similarly low. Mr Jones was comforted to learn that bacteria are not just associated with uncleanliness.

Mrs Jones responded well to antibiotic therapy. As she recovered, her needs were reassessed, and the nurses formulated the following aims; that before she left hospital Mrs Jones would be able to:

- Recognise and name the signs and symptoms of (a) incipient urinary tract infection, and (b) a blocked urinary catheter.
- Take action as soon as she noticed either problem, by contacting the district nursing service.

References

Ayliffe, G. A. J. 1971. Hospital acquired infection. In: *Proceedings of the International Conference on Nosocomial Infections*, Brachman, P. S. (ed.), p. 282. Waverley, Baltimore.

Blannin, J. (1982). The selection and management of catheters. *Geriatric Medicine*, 12: 57–60.

Brehmer, B. Madsen, X. O. (1972). Routine and prophylaxis of ascending bladder infection in male patients with indwelling catheters. *Journal of Urology*, 108: 719–721.

Britt, M. R. et al. (1976). The non-effectiveness of daily meatal care in the prevention of catheter-associated bacteriuria. Paper presented at the Sixteenth Interscience Conference on Antimicrobial Agents and Chemotheraphy, Chicago 1976.

Casewell, M., Phillips, I. (1977). Hands as a route of transmission of *Klebsiella* species. *British Medical Journal*, 2: 1315–1317.

Chin, P., Davies, D. G. (1976). Hand flora. *Journal of Hygiene*, 77: 93–96.

Clifford, C. M. (1982). Urinary tract infection. A brief selective review. *International Journal of Nursing Studies*, 19: 213–222.

Deegan, S. (1985). Intermittent catheterisation for children. *Nursing Times*, 81 (14): 72–74.

Dukes, C. (1928). Urinary infections after excision of the rectum; their cause and prevention. *Proceedings of the Royal Society of Medicine*, 22: 259–260 (International Congress and Symposium Series No. 23).

Dutton, A. A. C., Ralston, M. D. (1957). Urinary tract infection in a male urological ward. *Lancet*, 1: 115–117.

Ferrie, B. C. T. et al. (1979). Long term catheter drainage. *British Medical Journal*, 2: 1946–1947.

Garibaldi, R. A. et al. (1974). Factors predisposing to bacteriuria during indwelling urethral catheterisation. *New England Journal of Medicine*, 291: 215–219.

Gillespie, W. A. et al. (1960). The diagnosis, epidemiology and control of urinary tract infection in urology and gynaecology. *Journal of Clinical Pathology*, 13: 187–194.

Gould, D. J. (1985). Management of indwelling urethral catheters. *Nursing Mirror*, 161(10): 17–20.

Helmholtz, H. F. (1950). Determination of bacterial content of the urethra. *Journal of Urology*, 64: 158–162.

Johanson, W. G. et al. (1969). Changing pharyngeal bacteria of hospitalised patients. *New England Journal of Medicine*, 281: 1137–1140.

Kennedy, A. (1983). Long term catheterisation. *Nursing Times*, 79 (17): 41–45.

Kennedy, A. (1984). Trial of a new bladder washout system. *Nursing Times*, 80 (**46**): 48–51.

Kennedy, A. P., Brocklehurst, J. S. (1982). The nursing management of patients with long term indwelling catheters. *Journal of Advanced Nursing*, 7: 411–417.

Kennedy, A. P., Brocklehurst, J. C., Lye, M. D. W. (1983). Factors related to problems of long term catheterisation. *Journal of Advanced Nursing*, 8: 207–212.

Kunin, C. M. (1966). Prevention of catheter induced urinary tract infections by sterile closed drainage. *New England Journal of Medicine*, 274: 1155–1167.

McCormack, P. C. (1977). Nosocomial urinary tract infections. In: *Current Concepts of Infectious Diseases*, Hook, E. W. (ed.), pp. 233–241. Churchill Livingstone, London.

McLeod, R. W. *et al.* (1963). Prophylactic control of infection in the urinary tract as a consequence of catheterisation. *Lancet*, 1: 292–295.

Meers, P. D. *et al.* (1981). Report of the National Survey of Infection in Hospitals. *Journal of Hospital Infection*, 2: 23–28.

Mulla, N. (1961). Indwelling catheters in gynaecologic surgery. *Obstetrics and Gynaecology*, 17: 199–201.

Nordquist, P. (1984). Catheter-free geriatric care. Routines and consequences for clinical infection, care and economy. *Journal of Hospital Infection*, 5: 298–304.

Report of the Association of Incontinence Advisers (1984). Conference held in Bristol 1984. Reported in *Nursing Times Community Outlook Supplement*.

Sandford, J. P. (1964). Hospital acquired urinary tract infection. *Annals of Internal Medicine*, **60**: 903–914.

Stamm, W. E. (1975). Guidelines for prevention of catheter associated urinary tract infections. *Annals of Internal Medicine*, 82: 386–390.

Stamm, W. E. (1978). Infections related to medical devices. *Annals of Internal Medicine*, 84: 764–769.

Stickler, D. S. *et al.* (1981). Some observations of the activity of three antiseptics used as bladder irrigants in the treatment of urinary tract infection in patients with indwelling catheters. *Paraplegia*, 19: 325–333.

Turck, M. (1962). The urethral catheter and urinary tract infection. *Journal of Urology*, 88: 834–837.

Wastling, G. (1978). Long term indwelling urinary catheters. *Nursing Times*, **74**: 1176–1178.

Chapter 9

Wounds and Infection

INTRODUCTION

This chapter deals with wounds and the way that infection can disrupt wound healing. The factors which influence wound infection are described, followed by a discussion of the nursing management of patients with wounds. Since an appreciation of wound healing is central to the understanding of these topics, a section on tissue repair is also included.

EARLY DAYS OF WOUND HEALING

Early man observed that wounds bled less when they were covered, and that haemorrhages could be staunched by applying pressure. Materials available (water, herbs and clay) were probably applied on a trial-and-error basis. They *may* have influenced the rate of healing and the incidence of infection, but they were appreciated mostly for their soothing qualities. Evidence comes from murals painted on cave walls and from the papyri of the ancient Egyptians.

BC

The famous Edwin Smith papyrus which dates back to 1600 BC recommended that a penetrating wound to the head should be bound with fresh meat on the first day, then treated daily with honey, grease and lint! The Egyptians invented an adhesive bandage by applying gum to strips of lint and, like other early people, they had a range of primitive disinfectants at their disposal. These included a concoction made from willow leaves, mineral compounds and dung: minerals have antibacterial effects; dung introduced more bacteria into the wound.

Hippocrates (460–377 BC), the father of medicine, preferred nature to take its course. He advised washing wounds with tepid water, to which vinegar might be added and bringing the wound edges together to allow healing by first intention. Overzealous bandaging was known to promote gangrene. Greek medicine spread to Rome and became widely accepted. Fungating wounds were treated with fruits such as figs, which contain the enzyme papain, to break down slough. By the height of the Roman Empire surgery had become relatively sophisticated. A vast range of surgical instruments were found at Pompeii, indicating that cataracts, breast cancers and tonsils could be removed.

Early AD

Over the years, misconceptions about wound healing developed too. From the second century AD until Lister's time the appearance of pus ('laudable pus') was believed to form a necessary part of tissue repair. Physicians went to great lengths to *promote* infection in the wounds they treated, and a vast array of topical preparations were developed, their sole aim being to cause suppuration. In the 16th century air was considered to endanger the healing wound, so every effort was made to keep the wound warm, dark and moist. Infection was undoubtedly rife.

The approach to wound care was changed by accident, and like many surgical advances, it happened during a time of war. On the battlefield, Ambrose Paré ran out of eggs, which he required to promote pus formation, and was forced to treat wounds with oil. His patients experienced less pain and inflammation, and many more of them survived.

The 18th Century

Advances in chemistry during the 18th century led to the isolation of elements like chlorine and iodine, which have important disinfectant properties. The discovery of anaesthesia allowed the length of operating times to increase, and the rate of sepsis with it. Fortunately, Joseph Lister's work had resulted in the development of the antiseptic carbolic spray.

The 19th Century

By the 19th century various different dressing fabrics were in common use, lint, old clothes and rags being among the most popular. They were washed and reused; the older they became, the better, because they became softer! Cotton was introduced to Europe over 2000 years ago, but was not used as a dressing material until the 19th century, when the practice was introduced by a Birmingham surgeon called Joseph Gamgee.

The 20th Century

During the late 19th and early 20th centuries, medical advances proceeded at an ever-increasing pace (see Chapter 2), but surprisingly little attention was paid to the development of dressing materials and topical wound treatments until comparatively recently. The purpose of a dressing is to protect the wound, encourage healing and to prevent the environment becoming contaminated. One of the most significant advances was the development of disposable items and the introduction of hospital CSSD departments, both of which occurred in the early 1960s. Until this time, the average ward nurse could spend up to 3 hours every day preparing and sterilising dressings and instruments. The introduction of disposable items and the CSSD service were valued chiefly because they saved time, but they have almost certainly reduced the incidence of infection as well.

Numerous problems are associated with disposable items (cost, misuse, storage), but from the point of view of infection control, the most significant is the disposal procedure itself. Incineration is the answer, but this is a good deal more difficult to achieve in the community, especially in modern homes.

WOUND HEALING

The ability of tissues to undergo repair, like their ability to withstand infection, will depend on the general physiological condition of the patient and the condition of the wound itself (its specific microenvironment). Age, nutritional status, metabolic disturbance and genetically predetermined factors (for example haemophilia), all influence ability to heal. Healing takes place more readily when the individual enjoys good general health and when the tissues are in otherwise good condition. Repair proceeds more smoothly if cells can divide actively and if enzyme function is optimal. In the case of chronic wounds such as pressure sores and varicose ulcers, the patient's general condition must be improved before satisfactory healing will take place. A holistic approach seems most appropriate; the wound may be regarded as only one of many problems, and an outward reflection of underlying poor health, the cause which must be investigated and treated before tissue repair will occur.

The Inflammatory Response and Collagen Synthesis

The inflammatory response which follows tissue damage lasts for about 3 days (see Chapter 7). Heavy contamination due to microorganisms or any other cellular debris prolongs inflammation, and may require surgical debridement.

Towards the end of the inflammatory response macrophages in the wounded area attract fibroblast cells. These synthesise a meshwork of collagen (Fig. 9.1), which provides a scaffolding for the connective tissue that will ultimately fill the wound. Collagen is a tough, fibrous protein that forms the chief constituent of skin, fascia, tendons and ligaments as well as scar tissue.

In a surgical wound, collagen synthesis reaches a peak between the fifth and seventh postoperative day. Infection disrupts healing because pathogenic bacteria release an enzyme called collagenase, which digests the collagen fibres. Since it is these which provide tensile strength in repairing tissues, infection decreases the overall strength of the wound. Collagen formation depends on an adequate blood supply to provide oxygen and nutrients. Aerobic bacteria infecting a wound divide rapidly, competing for these.

Fibroblasts are stimulated to synthesise collagen in an environment where lactate ions and vitamin C are present in high concentrations. Both these substances are acidic; pH is low deep in the tissues, because the viable cells are metabolising and releasing lactic acid. Oxygen tensions are relatively low under these circumstances, so collagen tends to be generated deep down in the tissues. Tissue repair begins deep within the damaged areas and works outward.

Angiogenesis

New blood vessels also begin to develop at this stage in the healing process. New capillaries are stimulated by low oxygen tensions to grow from the healthy margins of the wound and to invade the area of regeneration. The formation of new blood vessels is called angiogenesis, and it commences outside the area of damage, working inwards.

Skin, Cells and Epithelialisation

Because it provides a continuous covering over the external surfaces of the body and is subject to a great deal of wear and tear, skin is the tissue most frequently subjected to trauma, and its relatively undifferentiated cells have retained considerable powers of regeneration. The same property is shared by endothelial cells lining other bodily surfaces, such as the gut. Less than 24 hours after a clean incision has been made, healthy epidermal cells from the margins of the wound begin to multiply, then to move in a sheet across its surface. Cells lining the sebaceous glands and hair follicles also divide and contribute to epithelialisation of the wound surface (Fig. 9.2). The wound is completely covered in an intact layer, several cells thick.

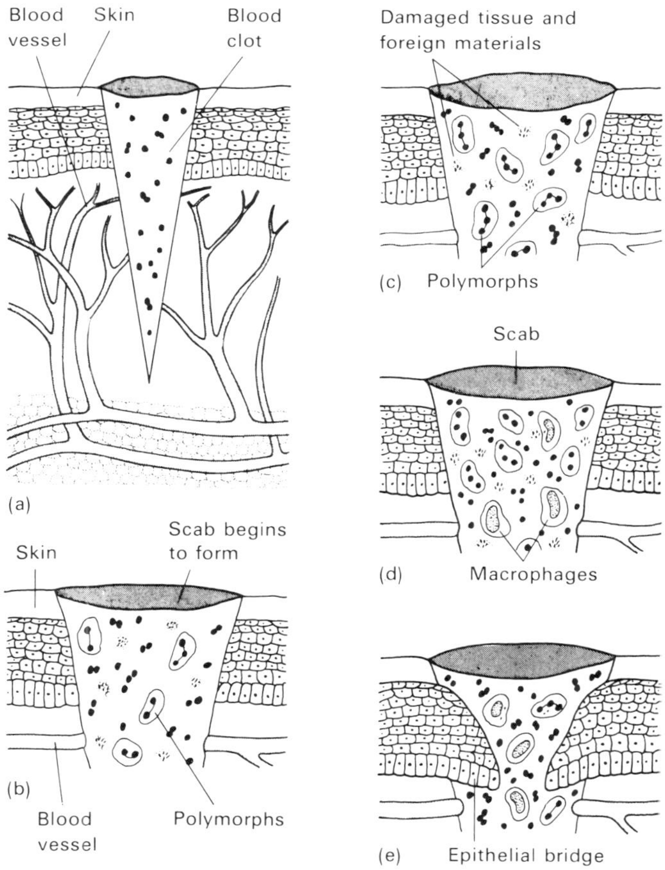

Fig. 9.1 Hour-by-hour view of the wound healing process (primary intention). (a) Immediately following surgery; (b) 2 hours postsurgery; (c) 6 hours postsurgery; (d) 12 hours postsurgery; (e) 24 hours postsurgery (reproduced with permission from Westaby, 1985).

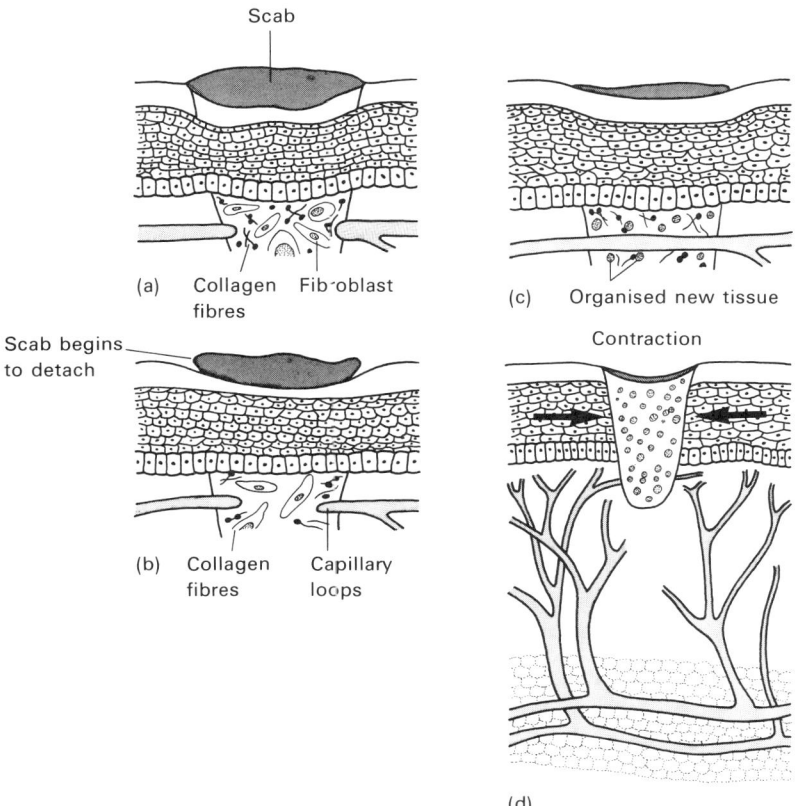

Fig. 9.2 Hour-by-hour view of the wound healing process (primary intention). (a) 48 hours postsurgery; (b) 6 days postsurgery; (c) 2 weeks postsurgery; (d) at 3–4 days contraction reduces the area of a wound with tissue loss (reproduced with permission from Westaby, 1985).

Where the cells meet at the middle of the damaged area, further movement is inhibited. Once epithelialisation is complete, a tough water-soluble protein called keratin is deposited in the cells, making them waterproof. Severely damaged tissues such as full thickness burns take longer to become epithelialised, because the hair follicles and sebaceous glands are destroyed.

The wound is now sealed from bacterial invasion by a delicate layer of cells. Epithelialisation of a clean surgical wound is generally complete by the third postoperative day – this is why dressings applied in the operating theatre are often removed at this time. The protective scab from the blood clot that formed over the damaged tissue is now able to slough away. A scab visible over a wound is indicative of underlying repair.

Formation of New Tissue

Collagen synthesis, angiogenesis and epithelial migration together constitute the proliferative phase of healing. Collectively they result in the formation of new granulation tissue made of fragile new capillary loops, suspended in a meshwork of collagen fibres and covered by a thin epithelial layer. Nurses will be aware that chronic lesions heal much more slowly than clean, surgical incisions. Regeneration is repeatedly interrupted with episodes of further inflammation, fibroblast activity, excess collagen deposition and further damage. Scarring is therefore more pronounced, due to the formation of excess granulation tissue. However, scarring from exuberant granulation can occur in poorly managed surgical wounds, and there may be hypertrophy in chronic or surgical wounds that have become infected, because the inflammatory response will continue over a longer period of time. Retention of necrotic tissue, foreign bodies or the use of excess suture material can result in hypertrophic scarring.

Tensile Strength

The tensile strength of the wound increases during the proliferative phase of healing, due to the collagen deposited by the fibroblasts. The rate at which tensile strength increases will vary from one site to another. Intestinal anastomoses may regain the original strength of the tissue within 7 days. Skin and fascia regain their strength more slowly. Wounds in which healing is delayed require prolonged support by sutures. Nurses must therefore explain to patients that they cannot compare their progress to that of others on the same ward.

Maturation of the Wound

The signs of inflammation are gradually lost during the proliferative phase of healing, but the wound retains its red, raised appearance and the patient will often complain that it is itching. At this point, examination under the high power of the microscope would reveal that the collagen fibres had become arranged haphazardly. During a phase of maturation, which may last for up to a year, they become realigned, so that they ultimately lie at right angles to the wound, lacing it together in a three-dimensional weave. Maturation of the wound is accompanied by decreasing vascularity, shrinkage of the fibroblasts and a gradual increase in tensile strength. The scar becomes stronger, but looks less pronounced. Patients need to be given this information *before* they leave hospital; once in the community they may have limited contact with health care staff, especially if minor surgery has been performed, and they may be concerned about changes in the scar.

CLEAN AND CONTAMINATED WOUNDS

There have been few nursing studies exclusively about the healing process. However David *et al.* (1983) in their multicentre study of the treatment of established pressure sores, observed that only a very small proportion of those falling into the infected category gave any indication of healing. The degree of contamination of a wound will influence the rate of healing.

Classifying Wounds

The National Research Council developed a method of classifying wounds in 1964, which has since been adopted by other research teams investigating problems associated with wound infection. In research studies, acceptance of a universal system of classification or series of definitions is always of great value, because it allows direct comparison of findings made by different people working within the same field. According to the 1964 definitions, wounds may be categorised as clean, clean-contaminated, contaminated and dirty. These are shown in Table 9.1.

The National Research Council suggested that any wound discharging pus should be regarded as 'infected'. Signs of inflammation and leakage of serous fluid were taken to signify 'possible infection'.

One of the main aims of the surgeon is to prevent wound infection wherever possible. 'Clean-contaminated' and 'contaminated' wounds are fre-

Table 9.1 Wound Classifications

Clean wounds: no evidence of inflammation, no lapse in aseptic technique during surgery and no entry into the respiratory and gastrointestinal tracts. Cholecystectomy, hysterectomy and appendicectomy without evidence of inflammation may be placed in the clean category.

Clean contaminated wounds: those generated by surgical procedures which involve entry into the respiratory or gastrointestinal tracts, but in which no significant spillage has occurred.

Contaminated wounds: those in which there is evidence of acute inflammation without the formation of pus, or where gross spillage has occurred from a hollow internal organ ('viscus'). An otherwise clean operation in which there has been a major breach of aseptic technique and recent traumatic wounds are considered to be contaminated.

Dirty wounds: those in which pus or a perforated internal organ are encountered. Traumatic wounds not of recent origin are also placed in this category.

quently encountered during abdominal surgery, and for most endogenous pathogens the number of bacteria necessary to result in an established infection is 10^6 microorganisms for every gram of tissue. Local cellular and humoral defence mechanisms can usually cope successfully with smaller doses, so that many bacteria present in contaminated wounds are destroyed. However, the local defence mechanisms may become overwhelmed when large amounts of necrotic tissue are present, providing a medium for bacterial growth. Under these circumstances the number of organisms constituting the infective dose rapidly increases. Foreign bodies in the wound or the action of anti-inflammatory drugs depress cellular and humoral defence mechanisms.

Surgical Intervention

Minor wounds heal spontaneously, but when the damage is more extensive surgical intervention is required to help speed repair and return to normal functioning, to avoid infection and help to minimise deformity. The method chosen by the surgeon to close the wound will depend on the amount of tissue lost. Directly suturing together the opposing edges of the incision is appropriate only for a clean wound where there has been no tissue loss, such as surgical wounds and lacerations caused by sharp, clean instruments like knives. When tissue has been lost, plastic surgery will be required. Flaps or skin grafts may be used. Three different methods of wound closure are illustrated in Fig. 9.3: primary closure, delayed primary closure and healing by secondary intention. They were evolved by surgeons with years of military experience, in which it was repeatedly demonstrated that immediate closure of infected or heavily contaminated wounds would promote the dissemination of microorganisms throughout the entire body. Septicaemia, abscess formation, wound dehiscence and death could follow. Although the surgeon will decide which method to use, nurses need to know the rationale behind their choice, as they spend more time with individual patients than do doctors, and must provide support to patients, and answer questions about treatment and likely progress when they arise.

Primary Closure

The method of closure finally chosen will depend to a large extent upon the estimated risk of infection. Primary closure is appropriate for clean and clean-contaminated wounds, and for those traumatic wounds for which debridement and mechanical cleansing have successfully removed all bacteria and contaminated matter. Delayed primary closure is the method of choice for heavily contaminated and dirty wounds. Damaged tissues succeed in developing resistance within 4 or 5 days of the injury. The wound can then be closed by sutures or grafting. Body cavities such as the pleura or peritoneal cavity must be sealed immediately if an injury exposes them, in order to prevent evisceration, but drains are inserted and the superficial layers of the wound are either left open or packed loosely. The mechanism enabling damaged tissues to develop resistance is not fully understood, but it is thought to coincide with the time at which the inflammatory response achieves its optimal level. Phagocytosis is then at its height.

The presence of a foreign body greatly decreases the threshold for infection; one silk suture can reduce the threshold for clinical infection by a factor of 10 000. Resistance to invading pathogens develops much more rapidly in wounds that have been held together by adhesive tapes than in those where sutures have been used.

Delayed Primary Closure

Where a policy of delayed primary closure has been agreed, the wound is covered with a sterile non-adherent dressing, then left undisturbed for 4 or 5 days. When closure takes place, the minimal amount of suture material is used. The patient will require a great deal of nursing support and encouragement: he may be disturbed about the eventual appearance of the wound and be anxious that any movement will either damage it or cause pain; a comfortable position may be difficult to achieve, especially when the wound involves the chest or abdomen; chest infection may result because the lungs cannot be fully expanded, and the patient is afraid to cough.

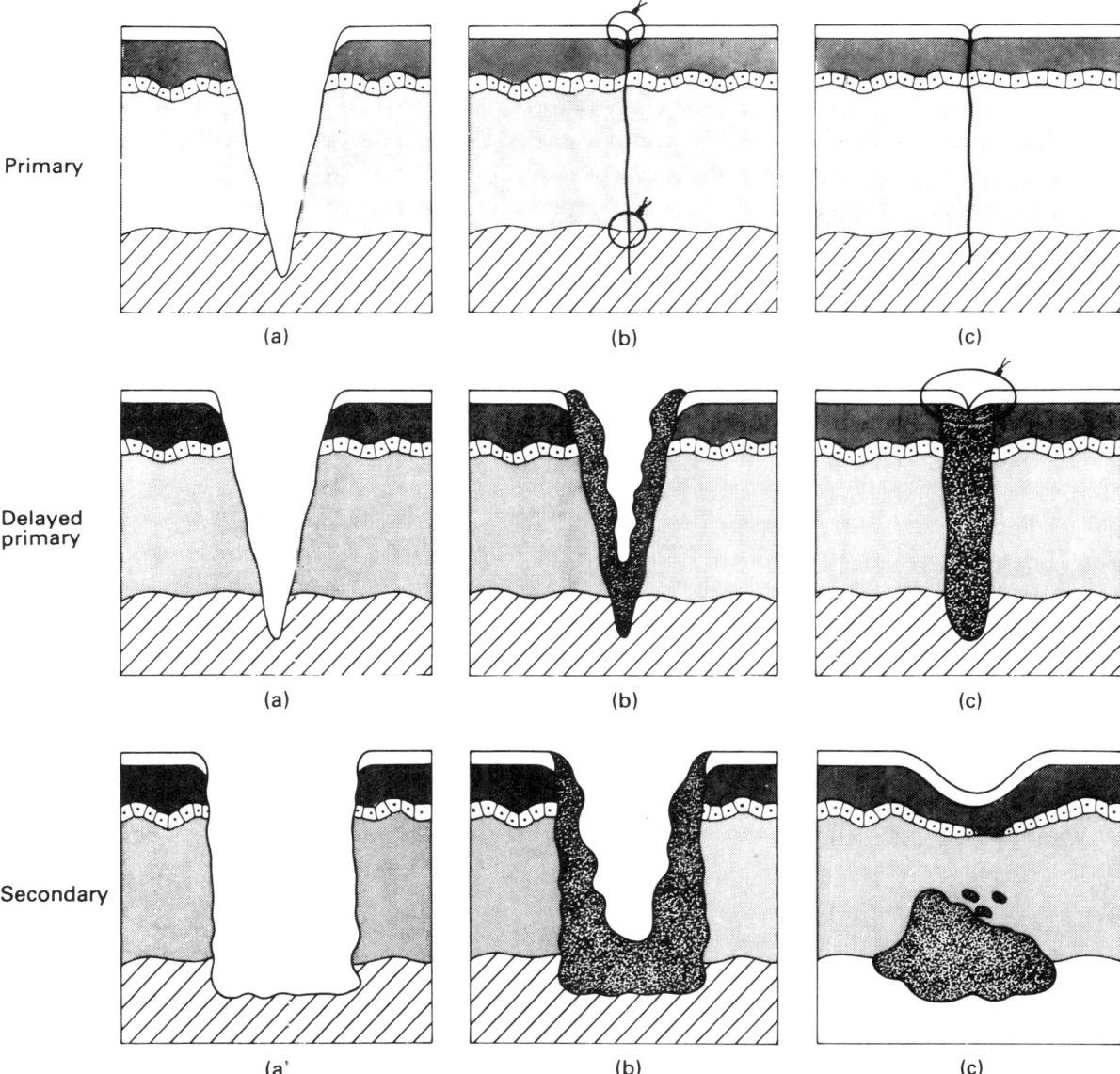

Fig. 9.3 The top row illustrates healing by primary closure; the middle row healing by delayed primary closure and the bottom row healing by secondary intention. Least scarring appears in healing by first intention (reproduced with permission from Westaby, 1985).

Secondary Intention

When healing by secondary intention takes place, the wound is allowed to close itself through a gradual process of contraction and epithelialisation. Healing by secondary intention is generally permitted for wounds that are very heavily contaminated, or for superficial burns and donor sites, where loss of tissue has been extensive, but the wound is not deep. Disadvantages include scarring, contracture and distortion, effects that are much less marked on the trunk than on skin covering bones or joints; this is because there are more areas of loose, overlapping tissue on the trunk.

It is important for nurses to appreciate the different methods of wound closure so that they have insight into the techniques used by different surgeons.

Eventually all unattended wounds would heal by secondary intention, provided that the patient's general health was originally good.

WOUND INFECTION

Prevalence studies have shown that nosocomial infections develop among 10% of inpatients (Meers *et al.*, 1981). In the National Prevalence Survey, wound infections were found to be the second most commonly occurring hospital acquired infections. Some wound infections are exogenous, others form part of the normal flora of the patient's gut or skin. The bacteria most commonly implicated in wound infection are shown in Table 9.2.

Table 9.2 Bacteria Frequently Associated with Surgical Wound Infection

Bacteria	Postoperative day of onset
Staphylococcus	3–5 days
Gram-negative rods	5 days
Streptococcus	2–3 days
Clostridium welchii (gas gangrene)	1–3 days

Cruse and Foord's Study

Cruse and Foord (1973) are responsible for a major study of wound infection rates in which 23 649 surgical wounds were examined over a period of 5 years. A 10 year follow-up study has now been completed. The first study took place in a Canadian hospital with 830 beds and ten operating theatres. All the wounds were examined by the same researcher (the nurse member of the team), every day until the 28th postoperative day (patients who had had burns, oral, rectal or vaginal procedures and circumcisions were excluded from the study); 1124 wounds became infected, giving an overall rate of 4.8%. The rates of infection for the different categories of wounds are shown in Table 9.3. The infection rate of dirty wounds was 20 times greater than that for clean wounds.

Table 9.3 Infection Rates for the Different Categories of Surgical Wounds

	Per cent
Clean	1.8
Clean-contaminated	8.9
Contaminated	21.5
Dirty	28.3

The findings of Cruse and Foord suggest that the wound infection rate associated with a particular hospital or with a particular surgeon is largely dependent upon the type of operation most commonly undertaken. Standards are best judged by the infection rates of clean wounds. Most hospital infection control committees would consider a clean wound infection rate of 1% as exemplary, a 1–2% rate as acceptable, and levels higher than this to merit special investigation and perhaps recommendations for future practice. Much depends, however, upon the kinds of patient who are routinely operated on. A consultant who performs radical surgery on elderly people in the advanced stages of malignancy can expect a higher rate of sepsis than his colleague who works exclusively with a younger age group undergoing mostly minor procedures.

The study by Cruse and Foord is considered to be methodologically sound not only because of its size, but also because of its design. It was a *prospective* study: wounds were examined and details about them were recorded soon after each operation had taken place. The alternative would be a *retrospective* study, in which details of surgery and its outcome would be obtained by perusal of the casenotes some time after the operations had been performed. A prospective study is ongoing, and allows for individuals to be examined over a predetermined length of time, which in this study was 28 days. In a retrospective study, the records are examined once, and there is little provision for follow-up of cases. Some retrospective studies in hospitals have taken place long after the patients have been discharged. Casenotes are notoriously unreliable because they may be mislaid, or illegible, and because the significance of the information that they contain may be difficult to interpret after the event. In terms of research, prospective studies are always considered to be a superior source of information, although they are more time-consuming and more expensive. Examination of casenotes is a poor substitute for direct observation.

The findings of the National Prevalence Survey (Meers et al., 1981) described in Chapter 3 are not directly comparable with the findings of Cruse and Foord. A prevalence study gives a 'snapshot' view of the situation examined at one particular point in time: the team led by Meers looked at hospital patients on the same day and judged whether they were infected on that day only. Cruse and Foord undertook an incidence study, examining the number of new cases of infection developing in a hospital population over a predetermined span of time.

From their findings, Cruse and Foord concluded that those parameters which influence the development of surgical wound infection could be divided into two categories:

(1) the dose of contaminating bacteria,
(2) the resistance of the patient.

These will be considered in turn.

The Dose of Contaminating Bacteria

Filtered Air Systems

Evidence suggests that clean wounds become infected when the internal tissues are exposed in theatre (Whyte et al., 1982). Exogenous infection in theatre may occur by the airborne route or by contact spread. Staphylococci are usually present in the air of a conventionally ventilated theatre, but the numbers that fall into the wound are generally small. However, a single skin scale from a staphylococcus carrier may transport up to 100 individual bacterial cells. The chances of this happening are increased by the duration of the operation, a long incision, large numbers of people present in the theatre, and considerable movement while the operation is in progress.

Staphylococcus aureus has been identified as the causative agent in many episodes of postoperative sepsis. *Staphylococcus epidermidis* was for many years considered to be non-pathogenic, but in recent years it has been implicated in wound infections, especially orthopaedic implant operations. This can have devastating consequences for the patient. The presence of the infection may not become apparent for months or even years, but ultimately result in a sequence of chronic ill-health, return to theatre and removal of the prosthesis.

Laminar Air Flow

Laminar air flow and the body exhaust system developed by Charnley (1964) reduce the number of airborne particles in the theatre (see Chapter 5). They have been widely used during orthopaedic procedures, and in 1974 the Medical Research Council and DHSS jointly funded a large-scale retrospective study to compare the sepsis rates when ventilation systems were used, compared to traditionally ventilated theatres (Lowbury et al., 1978). Records were obtained for 8500 orthopaedic operations conducted in 19 different hospitals: 75% of the patients had had total hip replacements; the remainder had had prosthetic surgery to the knee. Sepsis was confirmed among 86 (1.7%), diagnosis being made on the findings of a second operation. Infection rates were significantly lower among patients whose operations had been conducted under laminar air flow.

Inevitably the results of this study prompted health care workers to suggest that laminar air flow should be available for all surgical cases. It is, however, very expensive, and cost benefit analysis has emphasised the impracticality of installing laminar flow in all operating suites. Instead, the rate of sepsis may be reduced by keeping the number of people in the theatre to a minimum and restricting unnecessary activity among those who are present. Non-woven materials should be chosen for theatre garments (bacteria and small skin scales can move through spaces in traditional weave) and the ventilation system should be checked regularly by the hospital engineers. Filters in the system should be renewed at regular intervals. If the number of postoperative infections for clean surgery rises to unacceptably high levels (more than 1 or 2%), the number of airborne particles in the theatre should be checked using slit sampling equipment, as the filtering system may be faulty. If there have been a number of infections due to *Staphylococcus aureus*, a carrier may be implicated. Screening of all theatre staff will be necessary to identify the carrier, who will need treatment (see Chapter 10).

Duration of the Operation

The risk of infection increases according to the length of time that the tissues are exposed. After the first hour, the infection rate will double for each additional hour that the operation is prolonged. Complicated and lengthy surgery has been associated with relatively high rates of sepsis, even when the wounds have all been clean.

Preoperative Showering with Antiseptics

The study by Cruse and Foord showed that preoperative showering with an antiseptic containing hexachlorophane on the evening before surgery would significantly decrease the rate of wound infection. The same reduction was not observed when hexachlorophane was replaced with ordinary soap. These findings have been widely publicised by pharmaceutical manufacturers, but in a more recent survey, also conducted on a large scale, antiseptics did *not* appear to influence the wound infection rate (Ayliffe *et al.*, 1977).

Shaving

Shaving the operation site the day before surgery with a razor is known to influence risks of wound infection. The epithelium is damaged, increasing the growth and multiplication of bacteria already present. Shaving is obviously necessary when hair is growing over the site of the incision, but it should take place as early as possible using an electric razor. In other cases it may be possible to clip the hair. A study by Seropian and Reynolds (1971) has shown that the postoperative wound infection rate is lowest when shaving is avoided altogether. Depilatory creams were no more effective than shaving in this study.

Skin Preparations

Numerous independent research teams have reported that the handscrub used by the surgeon, the nature of the patient's skin preparation, and the use of plastic skin drapes do not appear to influence the incidence of wound infection (Alexander-Williams *et al.*, 1972; Psiala *et al.*, 1977).

Wound Site

The site of the wound appears to be a major determinant in the development of postoperative sepsis. For example, incisions in the inguinal region associated with radical vulvectomy and removal of the inguinal lymph nodes are notoriously difficult to heal. Wells (1983) reported a high incidence of infection in the external wounds of patients who had undergone coronary artery bypass grafting when the veins for the grafts had been obtained from the legs. The bacteria responsible were nearly always of faecal origin. The author suggested that the legs should be regarded as a contaminated site, and that the surgeon responsible for harvesting the veins should put on a clean gown and gloves before rejoining the operating team.

Mechanical Cleansing

The purpose of mechanical cleansing is to remove noxious substances from the wound and to protect the healing mechanism by improving local conditions within it. In theatre wounds can be irrigated before they are closed. Alternatively, the surface of a heavily contaminated or infected wound may be irrigated on the ward. A stream of sterile, antiseptic fluid is driven across the wound by hydrostatic pressure, but solution does not remain in contact with the tissues for long. Its main effect is to dislodge contaminants, reducing bacterial colonisation. There is some risk that the high pressure necessary may damage the tissue defences, so a compromise is offered by intermittent episodes of irrigation from a conventional syringe. Although this method is probably less damaging, it removes fewer bacteria.

Length of Preoperative and Postoperative Stay

The longer the period spent in hospital before surgery, the higher the risk of sepsis. This is mainly because the patient stands a greater chance of becoming colonised with hospital-acquired multiresistant bacteria. Cruse and Foord (1973) reported an overall infection rate of 1.1% among people who had been in hospital for just 1 day prior to surgery. This rate rose to 2% for those who had been in hospital for 1 week before undergoing surgery, and

4.3% for a stay lasting more than 2 weeks. Clearly there are very good reasons for keeping people out of hospital for as long as possible before the day on which planned surgery has been scheduled.

In the 1950s large outbreaks of staphylococcal cross-infection led to the closure of many hospital wards. On the positive side, these outbreaks were carefully investigated and research led to the development of hospital policies designed to reduce the risks of spread. Gram-negative sepsis is now undoubtedly a scourge in hospitals, and this has led to a shift of attention away from the problems associated with staphylococcal cross-infection. However, an editorial published in the *Journal of Hospital Infection* in 1983 cited sufficient evidence to suggest that the problem may be returning, and that it is largely due to preoperative colonisation by multiresistant staphylococcal strains.

Antibiotic Therapy

Antibiotic prophylaxis given systemically to surgical patients has reduced the incidence of surgical wound infection dramatically. However, its aim should always be to protect a *particular* patient from bacteria known to represent a *specific* threat. Antibiotics should not be employed as part of a blanket policy to destroy 'all known germs' (Easmon, 1984).

Although the decision to give prophylactic antibiotics will depend very much upon the judgement of the individual surgeon, in accordance with the policies developed by the infection control team working within the hospital, it should be apparent from Chapter 1 that no nurse can afford to remain ignorant of the dangers associated with indiscriminate antibiotic use.

Topical Antiseptics

Gilmore and Martin (1974) showed that the incidence of wound infection fell sharply when abdominal incisions were sprayed with povidone-iodine. This broad-spectrum antiseptic destroys not only a wide range of viable bacteria, but their spores as well (see Chapter 5). It is used widely by nurses as a topical treatment for established pressure sores (David *et al.*, 1983; Gould, 1985), possibly because it is commercially available in the form of a spray. Bacteria can never be eradicated completely from the skin and povidone-iodine has no healing properties other than those of antisepsis, so the continual and unselective use of the spray is of questionable value. Spraying a spirit-based solution onto a raw area causes the patient considerable discomfort.

Vasculation

The beneficial effects of inflammation depend upon a good blood supply. If vasculation is impaired, the rate of tissue repair will be reduced and bacteria will multiply causing extensive damage. This sequence may be inevitable in traumatic wounds, but in other cases the problem may be inherent in faulty surgical technique. In the past there have been suggestions that wound infections may to a large extent be the consequence of poor surgical technique, and that sepsis may be avoided despite contamination, provided that the surgeon has been meticulous (Dunphy and Jackson, 1962). Tissue necrosis may result from rough handling, excessive use of diathermy or by knotting ligatures so tightly that the tissue held between them becomes 'strangled'. Where skin sutures are placed too closely to the margins of a wound, they may cut through the flesh, causing it to gape open again. Dehiscence, which occurs most often following abdominal surgery, is a frightening experience for the patient and is associated with a high rate of mortality. When dehiscence occurs, the wound has often been infected.

Foreign Bodies

Foreign bodies and haematoma formation both promote infection. It has been demonstrated within the field of plastic surgery that haematomas exert toxic effects independently of any damage caused by bacterial multiplication within them.

Sutures

The foreign bodies most frequently associated with sepsis are sutures. Bulky, braided materials are more often implicated with episodes of sepsis than monofilamentous ones because they provide interstices in which bacteria can be concealed from the host defence mechanisms. Over the past 30 years there has been a dramatic increase in the varieties of commercially available suture materials, but there have been relatively few evaluative studies of their performance. The surgeon's choice is generally based upon established tradition and personal preference.

Wound Drainage

Drains are inserted after surgery or trauma when fluid is expected to collect. The secretion may be serous exudate, blood, pus or body fluids such as bile, which form part of the normal physiological secretions of the body. Table 9.4 summarises most of the drains in common usage. If fluid is unable to drain it will accumulate in the tissues, providing a focus for infection, forming abscesses. An abscess that is too large to be resolved by the bodily defence mechanisms (see Chapter 7) will release toxic substances into the neighbouring tissues. The patient will feel very unwell, with fever, rigors, profuse sweating, dehydration and anorexia. Progressive enlargement of an abscess may damage vital structures. For example, a collection of pus in the brain will soon exert pressure on neighbouring tissues because the rigid cranial cavity will limit expansion. Purulent pericarditis causes cardiac tamponade. Antibiotics are insufficient to resolve infection because the drugs cannot penetrate to the centre of the large mass of pus. Drainage is *essential* – without it, the patient may die.

Cruse and Foord (1973) found that closed suction drainage offered a significant reduction in the incidence of postoperative sepsis. When a drain was not inserted into a clean-contaminated wound, the rate of infection was 2.2%. Penrose drains (of soft latex) were associated with a sepsis rate of 1.8% when they were inserted through a separate stab wound. This rate rose to 8.8% when drainage was allowed to track through the wound itself. When closed suction (Redivac) drains were used, the rate fell to 0.6%. There is a certain amount of evidence, however, to suggest that drains may occasionally contribute to the development of a wound infection rather than help prevent it. Bacteria which normally live on the skin surface have been recovered from the inside of abdominal drains (Nora *et al.*, 1972); it appears that they can move in either direction along the drain, from inside the wound to the exterior, or from outside into the tissues. Infection will be set up if sufficiently large numbers are able to gain access. Wound drains should therefore be handled with full aseptic precautions.

Anaesthetic Equipment

Anaesthetic equipment may be a source of bacteria, particularly Gram-negative species which flourish in its warm, moist tubing, and may contribute to the risks of cross-infection and postoperative sepsis. To minimise this hazard, anaesthetic equipment should be thoroughly cleaned each time that it is used, and care taken to avoid recontamination when it is reassembled.

Bowel Preparation

Bowel operations are often followed by sepsis, especially after emergency operations. The bacteria responsible are usually Gram-negative bacilli and anaerobes which form part of the normal bowel flora. Infection is therefore endogenous. Bucknall (1982) examined over 1000 subjects who had had a laparotomy. He found that infections were more common after bowel surgery than procedures in which the gut was not involved.

Bowel preparation can help prevent these infections (Irvin and Goligher, 1973). Mechanical bowel preparation has been recommended for all patients scheduled to undergo elective bowel surgery, because it reduces the number of bacteria in the colon. Traditional purgatives and enemas have now been replaced by whole gut irrigation in some centres. A nasogastric tube is passed and fluid allowed to flow into the gut in large quantities. Prophylactic antibiotic therapy is usual whichever method is chosen by the surgeon. Nurses may have

Table 9.4 Wound Drainage

Corrugated drains	generally used to drain the subcutaneous tissues of contaminated wounds
Tubes/catheters	for pus, and fluids, for example, chest drainage
Penrose drains	soft latex filled with gauze that acts like a wick to draw up fluid
Closed suction drains	for example, Redivac drains.

little influence about the regime of treatment prescribed, but they have a vital role in helping to support the patient during the stressful preoperative period. Whatever the method chosen, it will add discomfort. The nurse has a key part to play in explaining the need for treatment, to ensure compliance and dispel unnecessary fears.

The factors discussed above have been included because, on the basis of critical examination, logic suggests that each might have some influence on wound sepsis. In some cases, research has either demonstrated or failed to demonstrate a relationship, and conclusive evidence is still wanting. Despite this, many such procedures form an established routine in hospitals. Patients are still shaved the night before surgery and made to add antiseptic solutions to the bath. Sometimes the routine is established at the surgeon's request, but in others decisions may be shared between nursing and medical staff. The work of the infection control committee in developing these policies is described in Chapter 10.

Westaby (1985) summarises the following as particularly valuable in reducing the dose of infecting bacteria during surgery:

(1) strict aseptic technique,
(2) removal of all debris, extraneous materials and necrotic tissue,
(3) gentle handling,
(4) using the minimal amount of suture material,
(5) keeping the time of operation as short as possible,
(6) irrigating the wound with an antiseptic solution *before* closure.

The Resistance of the Patient

Factors which influence general susceptibility to infection have been discussed in Chapter 4. This section is addressed more specifically to the aetiology of wound infection.

Bucknall (1985), writing from the surgeon's point of view, argues that the patient's resistance should be enhanced in order to reduce the possibility of multiplication by contaminating bacteria. The doctor's contribution will include assessment and correction of electrolyte balance, haemoglobin levels and diabetes. A nursing assessment should assess risk factors such as predisposition to chest infection, the possibility of anorexia or malnutrition, anxiety and the need for information. Telling the patient what to expect when he wakes up, and providing chest and leg exercises have been found in at least one study to allay stress and postoperative infection (Boore, 1978). The various factors that may influence the patient's resistance are outlined below.

Age

Ayliffe *et al.* (1977) surveying 38 hospitals between 1967 and 1973 found that postoperative sepsis was lowest among people between the ages of 20 and 40. This undoubtedly reflects the state of development of the immunological system. Infections were reported quite frequently among children, but the incidence declined towards adulthood, presumably because the immune defence mechanism matured. Among older people, degeneration of immunodefence mechanisms probably explains the increasing risk of infection. This has clear implications for nursing, since the average age of patients undergoing general surgery today is over 60 years.

Sex

In the same study Ayliffe's team compared postoperative sepsis between male and female patients undergoing surgery of the gastrointestinal tract, hernia repair (herniorrhaphy), nephrectomy and stripping of the varicose veins. Males developed significantly more infections; they are more often carriers of *Staphylococcus aureus* and tend to disseminate the bacteria to a greater extent than female carriers.

Nutritional Status

Cruse and Foord (1973) noticed a significant association between obesity and infection. For clean wounds overweight people had a 13.0% rate of sepsis, compared to 1.8% for those whose weight remained within desirable limits. Adipose tissue is present mainly in the subcutaneous tissues, where it may impede haemostasis. The resulting haematoma will provide an excellent medium for bacterial growth. Obese patients encounter further problems postoperatively, as bacteria, especially Gram-negative bacilli, thrive in moist skin folds. A good standard of hygiene is therefore more difficult to achieve, and greater ingenuity may be required to hold a dressing in position. The wound will be more easily contaminated, and more likely to contaminate the environment. Increased difficulty in mobilisation, and positioning may lead to chest infections. Coughing will then add to the stress placed on the wound.

Malnourished patients are also at a greater risk of postoperative sepsis. Cruse and Foord (1973) reported a wound infection rate of 16.6% among malnourished subjects.

Ascorbic acid deficiency increases the risk of developing a wound infection by damaging phagocytosis, and the attraction of white blood cells to the site of injury. Several independent research teams have recommended vitamin C supplements for postoperative patients who are at particular risk of developing infection (Davidson et al., 1971), especially elderly patients, whose ascorbic acid levels are sometimes very low. Nurses can help by ensuring that patients eat a well-balanced diet rich in vitamin C both preoperatively and postoperatively; however, the body cannot store vitamin C, unlike other vitamins, and has no reserves to draw upon after a period of shortage. Medication may sometimes be necessary when patients have had to fast for several days.

The inflammatory response, immunological processes and tissue repair also depend upon a good supply of protein. A negative nitrogen balance will impede healing, increasing the opportunity for bacteria to invade the wound.

Metabolic Disorders

Metabolic disorders alter the ability of the tissues to withstand contamination. The disease most often mentioned in this context is diabetes mellitus, probably because it is so common. Cruse and Foord (1973) quote a 10.7% rate of sepsis for clean wounds in diabetic patients. Polymorphs appear to be less readily attracted to the infected area compared to migration in healthy people. Treatment with vitamin A may help prevent this happening. Work on this is still in the experimental stages.

Steroids

Steroids depress the immune response by suppressing the activities of the white blood cells and inflammation. However, there is some evidence to suggest that these effects constitute a problem only in heavily contaminated wounds. Lindstrom (1977) found that sepsis does not usually complicate recovery from clean operations such as transplants, even though the patients are given steroids specifically to reduce transplant rejection.

Hypovolaemia

Low circulating blood volume and a reduced oxygen supply to the tissues increase susceptibility to infection, so haemorrhage therefore increases the risk of wound infection. The effect may be reduced by giving the patient a large dose of vitamin C, because this enhances phagocytosis.

Malignancy

Malignant diseases of all kinds are associated with increased susceptibility to infection and delayed healing. In Bucknall's (1982) study, conducted with more than 1000 patients undergoing laparotomy in a London teaching hospital, malignancy and its associated problems of anaemia and malnutrition resulted in a significantly higher infection rate.

WOUND MANAGEMENT: THE NURSING CONTRIBUTION

The remainder of this chapter is concerned with the nursing aspects of wound management. Most surgical wound infections are initiated in theatre. The bacteria responsible originate from the skin, gastrointestinal tract or upper respiratory tract of either the patient or the operating team. Transfer may be via the airborne route or by direct contact. Theatre nurses can help minimise the risks of infection by ensuring that the policies and procedures planned for their department by the infection control team are strictly adhered to.

Evidence from older studies suggests that outbreaks of wound infection due to multiresistant staphylococci have occurred through cross-infection on the wards. But there is little evidence to suggest that this is so today. Clean, undrained wounds seal within 1 or 2 days; in most hospitals the theatre dressing is not removed until the third postoperative day.

Many of the most problematic wounds, from the nurses' point of view, are chronic rather than the result of deliberate trauma. They include pressure sores, varicose ulcers and fungating wounds which develop in cases of advanced malignancy. Traditionally these have failed to secure medical interest, but their numbers exceed that of problematic surgical wounds. Over 10 years ago, Fernie (1973) estimated that the treatment of established pressure sores cost the NHS over £60 000 per annum. Dale (1984) calculated that in a population of 100 000, 1690 people suffer from leg ulcers. Most are managed in the community and form a major part of the district nursing workload.

Wound Dressing Materials

Until fairly recent years, the materials available for wound care had undergone little change for several decades. Research by commercial manufacturers and the advance of technology have rapidly brought a wide variety of products within the reach of the average nurse. These are revolutionising wound management, but many of the products are expensive and 'functionally specific', designed for the care of a particular type of wound. It is no longer possible to prescribe the same dressing regime for every lesion or every patient. Individual assessment is necessary, taking into account the patient's overall condition and the reason for the development of a chronic lesion with its associated reluctance to heal. Nurses must therefore be properly informed about the dressing materials currently available and their likely performance for a given kind of wound. Products must be chosen so that healing is maximised and the risk of spreading or acquiring secondary infection is reduced. Knowledge must be used to develop specific goals and nursing care plans should be realistic. Vague aims such as: 'Mr Brown's varicose ulcer will heal' are of very limited usefulness because they fail to explain how this will be promoted, to define the endpoint at which healing can be considered to be complete, or to suggest how progress may be evaluated. More realistic aims are shown in case study 9.1.

Nurses' skills of observation and their ability to monitor their patients' progress need refinement, and records must be kept accurately.

Choice of Dressing Materials

Although the healing process may not be speeded significantly by medical or nursing intervention, choice of a suitable wound treatment can optimise local conditions within the wound and may improve the natural result. The particular preferences of ward sisters or consultants and their bias towards certain products may lead to repeated use of the same materials, often because of a spectacular and isolated 'success' in the past. David et al. (1983) in their multicentre trial found that 98 different products were used to dress established pressure sores. Many were the favourite remedy of one particular ward or unit and not found outside it (see Chapter 3).

Factors Influencing Healing

Healing will depend upon the general condition of the patient and on factors operating within the local environment of the wound, including: humidity, gaseous exchange, pH, a supply of nutrients, and temperature.

Humidity

There is a critical balance between wound humidity and the absorption of excess exudate. A wound that is allowed to become too dry will form a hard scab over its surface, impermeable to gaseous exchange. The migration of epidermal cells across the surface of a wound will take place only in a moist environment. All physiological processes require oxygen and this will diffuse into living cells only when it is in solution. The presence of a hard, dry scab will therefore impede healing. Occlusion beneath a dressing designed to retain moisture (polyurethane dressings such as OpSite or hydrocolloid dressings such as Granuflex) promotes epithelialisation, angiogenesis and granulation, as well as reducing discomfort. Winter (1978) reported that in experimental animals epithelial

Case study 9.1

Mr Brown was admitted to hospital with a varicose ulcer which resisted healing. He had suffered from bronchitis for years and it was felt that the ulcer should be treated by conservative methods if possible, because of the risks of anaesthesia. As soon as Mr Brown arrived on the ward a wound swab was taken. The result indicated secondary colonisation of the damaged tissues with a mixture of *E.coli* and *Streptococcus faecalis*.

Mr Brown's condition was assessed by the nurse who would be responsible for most of his care. He was a frail gentleman of 70 who lived alone, although he was visited every day by his daughter, and twice weekly by a home help.

The following problems were identified:

- Poor nutrition. Mr Brown's daughter did all his shopping and much of his cooking, but his appetite was reduced because of the pain and offensive odour from the ulcer.
- Reluctance to go out of the house, because of embarrassment due to the ulcer. Mr Brown was becoming a recluse; he would no longer visit his daughter, even when transport was provided.
- Reduced mobility around the house, because of leg pain.
- Depression due to self-imposed loneliness and worry about his condition.
- Shortness of breath on exertion as a result of bronchitis. Oxygen perfusion of his tissues, especially the extremities, could be assumed to be poor. He had been a smoker for many years, but had stopped on the advice of his general practitioner.

The ulcer involved an extensive area of skin over the toes, heel and lateral aspect of the left leg, with some destruction of underlying tissues. The pain was worse on walking and at night. The lesion had developed quite rapidly after Mr Brown had knocked his leg, and he had been persuaded by the home help to see his general practitioner.

It is important not only for the nurse to examine the ulcer, but to take some time obtaining a careful history from the patient, because successful management depends on understanding the aetiology of the ulcer. In Mr Brown's case, the ulcer seemed to be ischaemic in origin. These lesions are due to malnutrition of the skin resulting from poor arterial blood supply. Although often spontaneous, they may follow trauma or pressure from ill-fitting footwear. Venous ulcers are generally shallower lesions, less destructive and painful, with insidious onset, and their management is different.

The aim of Mr Brown's care was to improve his overall condition by relieving his pain, improving his nutritional status and trying to alleviate his feelings of depression, as well as providing more localised care at the site of the wound.

The aims of the specific wound care were to:

- Resolve infection.
- Arrest further chronic inflammation.
- Remove slough.
- Promote healing.

Initially, the outline of the wound was traced onto a piece of sterile cellophane and the diameter measured at its widest point to give a baseline for measurement following increases or decreases in size. The daily dressing regime involved:

- Cleansing the wound with 1% cetrimide solution to destroy the mixed, superficial bacterial colonisation. Analgesics were given before handling the wound. Strict asepsis was maintained, because the ulcer had already eroded some underlying tissue, and invasive bacterial infection could lead to cellulitis and further deterioration in Mr Brown's general condition, as well as locally, with a need for systemic antibiotics.
- Before the cleansing agent was applied, a topical desloughing agent (Varidase) was used to remove necrotic debris. The solution was reconstituted immediately before use, drawn up into a syringe and gently poured onto the affected areas.
- A non-adherent dressing was chosen to cover the surface of the wound. There was little discharge, and therefore no need for bulky, absorbent dressings.
- A bandage was applied loosely over the affected area, as tight bandages would further obstruct blood supply and cause pain. The purpose of the bandage was to hold the dressing in position, avoiding the need to attach adherent tape to the delicate tissue at the margins of the wound, to retain heat and to protect the tissues. This was necessary in Mr Brown's case because long periods of sitting can further reduce impaired blood supply to the legs. In order to walk about the ward he needed to feel confident that the damaged area would not be subject to further trauma and, because he felt sensitive about its appearance, that it would be covered.
- The toes of the affected foot were parted with gauze to prevent further friction, pressure and ulceration.

After 1 week, the plan of care was reviewed by:

- Repeated bacterial monitoring
- Measuring the size of the lesion, although during the stage of debridement it was recognised that decrease in size could not really be expected.

- Mr Brown's general condition was also reassessed at this stage.

At the end of the first week of treatment, slough had been removed from the wound, so that it now appeared deeper than before. This assessment was based on the nurses's impression at this stage of the treatment. No further bacteria were isolated from the wound.

The aims of care were now reformulated:

- promotion of granulation,
- further resolution of inflammation,
- to continue to encourage Mr Brown to eat a nutritious diet and to be mobile.

The wound care regime now involved the use of an elastomer foam (silastic foam) to fill the deeper parts of the wound. A stent of foam was made by pouring the newly prepared, still liquid foam into the cavity, then holding the solidified stent loosely in position with a bandage.

Mr Brown's general condition had improved considerably. His pain was controlled and he felt more cheerful now that progress was being made. Consequently, the care plan was adjusted so that the wound would be re-examined and evaluated again in only 3 days' time, when the same methods of assessment showed that the wound was:

- still not infected,
- smaller across its diameter by 2 cm.

The depth of the wound could now be assessed using objective measurements for the first time; the new stent was 0.5 cm shallower than the first one.

One of the main aims of care was now to teach Mr Brown how to manage his own dressing with supervision, so that he could go home.

Two weeks after admission Mr Brown was discharged into the care of the district nurse, who, after her initial visit to assess the patient's condition, visited twice weekly. Mr Brown was able to inspect the skin around his wound for inflammation and apply bandages himself.

The endpoint of healing was defined as the time when the damaged area was completely epithelialised and intact, with no further pain, or swelling and only slight pinkish discoloration of the newly replaced tissues. In the meantime Mr Brown was educated about the need for:

- good general nutrition,
- mobilisation,
- choosing comfortable, well-fitting footwear,
- inspecting his legs and feet for further signs of damage, so that prompt action could be taken.

---

migration proceeded about three times faster after wound occlusion compared to lesions in which a thick scab has been allowed to form, and the cosmetic effect was improved. The white blood cells become trapped in scab material and cannot function (Rovee, 1972).

The differences between a wound that has been covered and one that has been exposed are summarised in Fig. 9.4.

The main objection to occlusive dressings seems to be the fear that bacteria will multiply in the exudate that collects beneath. However, exudate is known to contain large numbers of active white blood cells which help to combat any bacteria present on the skin before the dressing was placed over it (Randolph May, 1983). Provided that the dressing is properly fixed over the wound, no new bacteria can reach the damaged tissues. Excess exudate can be aspirated from the wound with a needle and syringe. A scab may promote the multiplication of anaerobic bacteria in the slough which collects beneath. Both hard crust and scab may need removal manually, a procedure that is usually uncomfortable for the patient.

Gaseous Exchange

The importance of adequate oxygen supply to a healing wound was emphasised by Winter (1971). The rate of metabolism in healing tissues is very high. Epithelialisation and phagocytosis place heavy demands on the oxygen supply. There is, however, little evidence to suggest that skin cells are able to obtain oxygen directly from the atmosphere, although this is a popular belief among nurses and may be the rationale behind applying oxygen directly to the surface of a wound (Gould, 1985). Winter and Perrins (1970) found that hyperbaric oxygen would increase the rate of epithelial migration in surgically induced porcine wounds that had been covered with occlusive dressings. The hyperbaric oxygen, however, succeeds by increasing the oxygen tension of the blood supplying the wound. Another important differ-

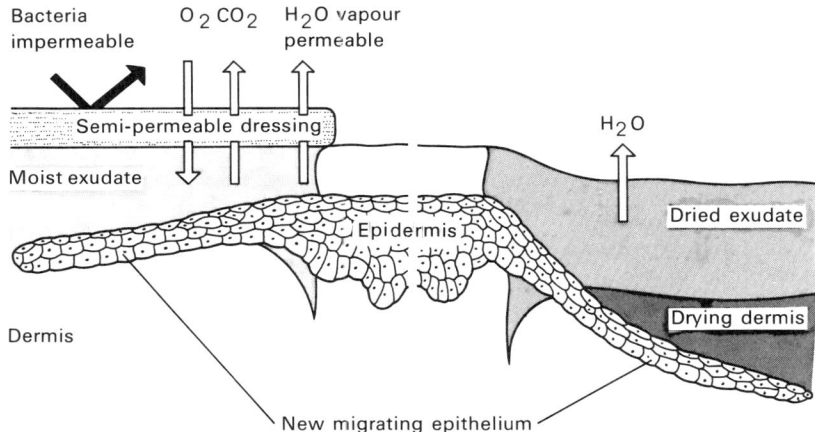

Fig. 9.4 Difference between covered and exposed wound.

ence is that the healing process is slower and more complex in chronic wounds than those resulting from surgical trauma, and that they often contain large areas of necrosis. Dead cells do not metabolise. Hyperbaric oxygen, if it is of any value when externally supplied, will benefit only living cells.

pH

Gaseous exchange has a critical influence on the pH of the regenerating tissues. Cells die outside a very narrow pH range, because their enzymes, particularly those necessary for cellular respiration, become inactive. Alterations in pH halt epithelialisation and phagocytosis. This is significant when applying cleansing and debriding agents which do not have a physiological pH. Eusol, for instance, is an alkaline solution; hydrogen peroxide is acidic.

Supply of Nutrients

Rapidly dividing cells depend on the blood supply for nutrients and the prompt removal of toxic metabolic wastes. The local application of albumin in the form of egg white, an old treatment for established pressure sores, is potentially harmful. The skin cells cannot absorb it in any appreciable quantity, but egg white provides an excellent culture medium for bacteria.

Temperature

Wounds require thermal insulation to body core temperature (Locke, 1979). The rate of cell division doubles in wounds maintained at a steady temperature of 37 °C compared to skin surface temperature. A decrease in temperature delays cell division, which may take 3 hours to recover (Turner, 1982). White blood cell activity may fall to zero (Lawrence, 1982). Long dressing changes and the application of cold antiseptics reduce wound temperature. Locke showed that a newly cleaned wound took 40 minutes to return to its former temperature.

Protective Functions of the Dressing

The protective function of the dressing includes its capacity to absorb excess exudate and its properties of non-adherence.

Although a dressing must keep the wound surface moist, it must also absorb excess exudate, or sloughing may occur. One of the chief priorities in the management of a high exudate wound is the choice of a product that will permit free drainage of fluid yet prevent contamination. The dressing must be highly absorbent, but not allow soaking to occur to the outer layer. Once 'strike through' occurs, a pathway is established allowing bacteria to travel down into the dressing, or in the opposite direction, up from the wound (Colebrook and Hood, 1948).

Adherence to the wound is a major problem with many products, and generally occurs because serous exudate has dried onto the dressing. When the dressing is changed, the scab and dermis attach to it and are torn away (Winter, 1971), adding to the discomfort experienced by the patient and delaying healing by provoking a fresh inflammatory response. More rarely, capillary loops may grow up onto the weave of a traditional dressing material like gauze. Wood (1976) found that cotton fibres from gauze could become incorporated into the healing tissues. This may result in granuloma formation, reducing the strength of the wound and its cosmetic appearance, and causing keloid scarring. Instead of incorporating gauze squares into the standard dressing pack, hospital CSSD departments should perhaps move towards greater use of non-adherent dressings.

Clinical evaluation of the new, 'functionally specific' wound care products is an essential part of their performance. A great deal of work is done by commercial manufacturers, often in conjunction with clinicians. Nurses who participate in work of this kind should draw attention to the need to care for the patient as a whole person. A patient may, for example, remain in hospital after the initial phase of recovery because his wound needs redressing at frequent intervals. If he can be taught how to apply an elastomer dressing such as silastic foam and feels confident to do so, he may be discharged earlier, with regular supervision and encouragement from the district nurse. Table 9.5 compares some of the more commonly used wound care products.

The Aseptic Dressing Technique

Ayliffe et al. (1982) point out that the need for aseptic handling of the wound is commonly believed to have grown out of increasing recognition of the dangers associated with bacterial contamination, although the evidence for this is scanty (see Chapter 3). Ability to perform this technique has been so central to nursing skills that it was used for years as a standard assessment during general nurse training. However, a study by Hunt in 1974 showed that nurses working in three general hospitals failed to perform dressing techniques according to the policies set by their respective hospitals, and frequently with little regard for the principles of asepsis. The aseptic dressing technique varies between one hospital and another. In some centres masks are still worn, and nurses are not encouraged to talk to the patient when wounds are dressed. In others, masks, originally discarded to reduce expenditure, have been found to offer no added protection, and the dressing procedure is regarded as a good opportunity to talk to the patient.

The content of dressing packs, preferred wound disinfectants and the method of cleaning the dressing trolley are all subject to considerable local variation. Ayliffe et al. (1982) describe the aseptic dressing technique as 'surrounded by mystery and ritual'. They discuss the problems of combining the patient-centred approach with pre-existing routines, for example ensuring that all beds are made before wounds are exposed. In most hospitals at the present time, ward sisters carry limited influence with domestic staff and may not be able to organise wound dressing and cleaning sessions so that they take place at mutually exclusive times. There is, however, little evidence that this failure has contributed to any increase in ward-acquired infection. Ayliffe et al. (1982, p. 47) found that even when bedclothes were vigorously shaken, the particles which became airborne seldom rose as high as the tops of traditional bedside curtains.

The aim of the non-touch technique advocated for dressings is to avoid contact with fingers that might be contaminated. It is generally achieved with forceps, but bacteria may be heavily dispersed when a large, soiled dressing is removed with a forceps inadequate for manipulation. Now that plastic disposable forceps are often incorporated into CSSD packs, this is a common occurrence. Sterile plastic gloves may be better than forceps. In the case of a large dressing, the hand may be protected with a plastic bag, which can then be inverted so that it contains the entire dressing. Commercial packs (Hampshire dressing) are available for this purpose, and are of particular value to nurses who work in the community.

In many hospitals nurses are taught to perform dressings working in pairs, one acting as the 'clean', and the other as the 'dirty' partner. This

Table 9.5 Commonly Used Wound Care Preparations (adapted with permission from J. Draper, *Nursing Times*, Oct 9 1985)

Agent	Action	Composition	Relative cost*	Advantages	Limitations	Comments
Eusol	Chemical debriding agent	Chlorinated lime (0.25%) Boric acid (1.25%) Water	+	Cheap Easily obtainable	Cold pH 8 Non-specific in action – may destroy healthy skin	Use has never really been evaluated Said to lead to an increase in blood urea and prompt renal failure Often diluted beyond effectiveness
Eusol and paraffin	Chemical debriding agent with lubricant properties	As above plus liquid paraffin	+	Cheap Easily obtainable	As above	As above, but even more dilute
Malatex cream	Chemical debriding agent	Benzoic acid (0.02%) Malic acid (0.36%) Salicylic acid (0.006%) Propylene glycol (1.7%)	++	Good debriding agent Effervescent, helps to separate tissues	pH acidic Non-specific action Dries rapidly – dressings needed twice daily Some reports of delayed healing	May damage healthy epithelial tissue Aserbine is a solution of Malatex, but six times stronger
Varidase	Enzymatic debriding agent	Streptokinase (105 μ) Streptodornase (23 μ) Thiomersal (2%)	+++	Specific action on necrotic tissue Physiological pH	Cost Slow action Does not destroy bacteria Enzyme molecules are easily destroyed by prolonged storage of reconstituted solution, storage above or below 4°C or by shaking vigorously during preparation	Good results are achieved only with skilled use and correct reconstitution
Hydrogen peroxide	Mechanical debriding agent and cleanser	Used as 5–7% solution	+	Cheap pH 7 Destroys odour Relatively non-toxic Destroys anaerobic bacteria	Cold Brief action	
Bactigras	Medicated wound dressing	Cotton gauze impregnated with yellow paraffin and 0.5% chlorhexidine	+	Retains moisture Permeable to O_2 Permits drainage Range of sizes available Cheap	Not absorbent Does not thermoinsulate May not be as non-adherent as manufacturers claim Permeable to bacteria	Paranet – lacks chlorhexidine Sofra-Tulle impregnated with antibiotics, thus promoting antibiotic-resistant bacterial strains
Gauze	Wound dressing	Cotton cloth, available as swabs or pads in different sizes	+	Cheap Insulating Permeable to oxygen	Adherent Permeable to bacteria Permits wound leakage Dehydrates	

Wounds and infection

Product	Type	Description	Rating	Advantages	Disadvantages	Notes
Melolin	Non-adherent wound dressing	Acrylic viscose pad with perforated polymer film in contact with the wound and non-woven fabric backing	+++	Permeable to O_2 Thermal insulation Range of sizes	Often becomes adherent Permits exudate to escape – 'strike through' Permeable to bacteria Dehydrating	An advance on gauze, suitable for sutured wounds that are not discharging
Lyofoam	Wound dressing	Polyurethane foam in a 'cellular' structure with hydrophilic contact surface	++	Absorbent Non-adherent Permeable to O_2 Retains moisture Thermoinsulating Comfortable	Lateral 'strike through'	Valuable on exudating wounds and around tracheostomies
OpSite	Occlusive wound dressing	Transparent polyurethane dressing with adhesive strips at each side, made of polyvinyl	+++	Permeable to O_2 H_2O vapour, but not bacteria or H_2O Retains wound exudate with bactericidal effect Comfortable Wound easily observed Soothing for burns Reduces the need for frequent dressing changes	Lateral leakage of exudate Skill in application Requires margin of dry, undamaged skin Exudate may build up, so aspiration is required O_2 permeability decreases if the number of dead cells build up	
Cetrimide	Wound disinfectant	Tetradecyl trimethyl ammonium bromide (0.1–1%)	+	Cheap	Limited disinfectant properties Cold Readily inactivated by organic matter	Savlon – solution of cetrimide and chlorhexidine with detergent properties
Noxyflex	Wound disinfectant	Reconstituted from powder consisting of: noxythiolin (2.5 g) amethocaine (10 mg)	+++	Fair antibacterial and antifungal spectrum Can be used to irrigate wounds	Pain on application	
Chlorhexidine	Wound disinfectant	5% Solution chlorhexidine gluconide	++++	Low toxicity	Restricted antibacterial activity Expensive Cold Rapidly inactivated by organic matter	
Povidone-iodine (Betadine, Disadine)	Wound disinfectant	Povidone-iodine – various dilutions are used	+	Broad spectrum – destroys spores Not readily inactivated by organic matter Rapid action Cheap	Stains skin and clothes	

Table 9.5 (continued)

Agent	Action	Composition	Relative cost*	Advantages	Limitations	Comments
Debrisan	Wound dressing	Dextran polymer in the form of granules	++++	Prevents dehydration Absorbent pH unchanged Impermeable to environmental bacterial Permeable to O_2, CO_2, H_2O vapour Promotes granulation	Expensive Skill needed to use Not a debriding agent	Wounds must be debrided *before* Debrisan can be successfully applied. Old Debrisan must be carefully cleaned away – it can look like pus, so the wound may be mistakenly thought to be infected
Silastic foam	Wound dressing	Dextran polymer in the form of granules	+++++	Non-adherent Permeable to oxygen Thermal insulator Comfortable Fits wound contour Saves time – dressing changes seldom need be undertaken	Can be used only in wounds that are not infected Can become hard *Very* expensive Accurate reconstitution needed	Patients can be taught to do their own dressings with supervision, leading to earlier hospital discharge and reducing risks of cross-infection

* Relative cost on scale of +–++++

may be impractical on busy wards, and some infection control teams have modified the recommended procedure, so that only one nurse is necessary, but does not have to leave the bedside. Older procedures demanded the dressing pack to be opened, the wound exposed and the nurse to wash her hands at the nearest sink. Any delay would result in prolonged exposure of the wound and the contents of the pack, while the patient would remain anxiously waiting behind drawn curtains. A good non-touch technique should ensure that the hands never come into contact with the wound or the dressing. Even if they do, any contaminating bacteria would probably form part of the patient's flora, and be present in numbers too small to constitute an infective dose. The need for a final handwash after taking down the dressing is therefore debatable, and it is redundant if the hands are rinsed with 70% alcoholic rub at the bedside.

The Purpose of Aseptic Techniques

The time-consuming and ritualistic aseptic technique demands critical examination in several other respects. The *purpose* of applying a fresh dressing should be questioned on every occasion. Sometimes a clean rather than a strictly aseptic procedure would appear more logical. If the dressing is applied purely to prevent clothing irritating the surface of a healed wound, because a patient dislikes the appearance of the scar, or so that a confused patient is unable to interfere with it, then a clean technique appears sufficient. Many chronic wounds are heavily contaminated, and the purpose of the dressing is to protect the environment rather than the tissues. If a patient has just emerged from a bath, then there is little rationale behind the slavish application of the complex aseptic procedure, and little justification for applying disinfectant solutions to a wound that is already clean and dry. Contact with the skin is momentary. Bacteria are removed mainly by the mechanical action of swabbing. Poor technique and extra handling merely increase the risk of contamination. Gram-negative bacteria thrive in antiseptic solutions, but this risk has been eliminated by the introduction of individual, prepacked sachets, the outer surfaces of which are sometimes wiped with an alcoholic

solution before use. If the surface of the pack is clean and dry, bacteria are unlikely to be present in numbers large enough to constitute an infective dose. The procedure is therefore of little value.

The purpose of this discussion is not to encourage a slipshod attitude, but to promote a more critical approach, and to encourage nurses to apply the basic principles of microbiology. The amount of effort invested in a particular procedure ought logically to be reflected in the amount of infection prevented. The NHS is becoming more cost-consious and all resources, time as well as money, are becoming increasingly scarce.

References

Alexander Williams, *et al.* (1972). Abdominal wound infections and plastic wound guards. *British Journal of Surgery*, **59**: 142–146.

Ayliffe, G. A. J. *et al.* (1977). Surveys of hospital infection in the Birmingham region. *Journal of Hygiene*, **79**: 299–313.

Ayliffe, G. A. J. *et al.* (1982). *Hospital-acquired Infection: Principles and Prevention.* Wright PSG, Bristol and London.

Boore, J. (1978). *Prescription for Recovery.* Royal College of Nursing, London.

Bucknall, T. E. (1982). Burst abdomen and the incisional hernia – a prospective study of 1,129 major laparotomies. *British Medical Journal*, **284**: 931–933.

Bucknall, T. E. (1985). Factors affecting the development of surgical wound infections: a surgeon's view. *Journal of Hospital Infection*, **6**: 1–8.

Charnley, J. (1964). A clean air operating enclosure. *British Journal of Surgery*, **51**: 202–205.

Colebrook, L., Hood, A. M. (1948). Infection through soaked dressings. *Lancet*, **2**: 682.

Cruse, P. J. E., Foord, R. (1973). A five year prospective study of 23,649 surgical wounds. *Archives of Surgery*, **107**: 206–210.

Davidson, J. *et al.* (1971). A bacteriological study of the immediate environment of a surgical wound. *British Journal of Surgery*, **58**: 326–333.

Dale, J. J. (1984). The Lothian and Forth Valley Leg Ulcer Study. *Proceedings of the Royal College of Nursing Research Society 1984*, 38. Imperial College, London.

David, J. *et al.* (1983). An investigation of the care of patients with established pressure sores. *Report of the Northwick Park Nursing Practice Research Unit.*

Dunphy, J. E., Jackson, D. S. (1962). Practical applications of experimental studies in the care of the primarily closed wound. *American Journal of Surgery*, **104**: 273–282.

Easmon, C. S. F. (1984). Prevention is not always the best antibiotic cure. *Hospital Doctor*, **15**: 10.

Editorial (1983). Methicillin-resistant *Staphylococcus aureus*. *Journal of Hospital Infection*, 4: 327–329.

Fernie, G. R. (1973). Biomechanical aspects of the aetiology of decubitus ulcers in human patients. *PhD thesis*, University of Strathclyde.

Gilmore, O. J. A., Martin, T. D. M. (1974). Aetiology and prevention of wound infection in appendicectomy. *British Journal of Surgery*, 61: 281–287.

Gould, D. J. (1985). Pressure for change. *Nursing Mirror*, 161 (16): 28–30.

Hunt, J. (1974). *A Study of Dressing Techniques in Three Hospitals*. Royal College of Nursing, London.

Irvin, T. T., Goligher, J. C. (1973). Aetiology of disruption of intestinal anastomoses. *British Journal of Surgery*, 60: 461–463.

Lawrence, J. C. (1982). What materials for dressing? *Injury*, 13: 500–512.

Lindstrom, B. L. (1977). Surgical complications of 500 kidney transplantations. In *Dialysis, Transplantation and Nephrology*, Robinson, B. H. B. (ed.). Pitman Medical, London.

Locke, P. M. (1979). Paper given at the Symposium of Wound Healing, Helsinki.

Lowbury, E. J. L. *et al*. (1978). Multi-hospital trial on the use of ultraclean air systems. *Journal of the Royal Society of Medicine*, 77: 800.

Meers, P. D. *et al*. (1981). Report of the National Survey of Infection in Hospitals 1980. *Journal of Hospital Infection*, 2: 23–28.

National Research Council (1964). Postoperative wound infection. *Annals of Surgery*, 160, Supplement 2: 1–192.

Nora, P. F. *et al*. (1972). Prophylactic abdominal drains. *Archives of Surgery*, 105: 173–179.

Psiala, J. *et al*. (1977). The role of wound drapes in the prevention of wound infection following abdominal surgery. *British Journal of Surgery*, 64: 729–732.

Randolph May, S. (1983). Physiological activity from an occlusive wound dressing. *Wound Healing Symposium*, pp. 35–51. Medical Education Services, Oxford.

Rovee, D. (1972). Effect of local wound environment on epidermal healing, pp. 152–81. In *Epidermal Wound Healing*, Maibach, H. I. and Rovee, D. (eds.). Year Book Medical Publishers Incorporated, Chicago.

Seropian, R., Reynolds, B. M. (1971). Wound infections after preoperative depilatory versus razor preparation. *American Journal of Surgery*, 121: 251.

Turner, T. D. (1982). Synthaderm – an environmental dressing. *Pharmaceutical Journal*, 3: 49–50.

Wells, F. C. (1983). Wound infection in cardiothoracic surgery. *Lancet*, 1: 1209–1210.

Westaby, S. (1985). *Wound Care*. Heinemann, London.

Whyte, W. *et al*. (1982). The importance of airborne bacterial contamination in wounds. *Journal of Hospital Infection*, 3: 123–136.

Winter, G. D. (1971). *Healing of Skin Wounds and the Influence of Dressings on the Repair Process*. Bradford University Press, Bradford.

Winter, G. D. (1978). Wound healing. *Nursing Mirror*, 146: 10.

Winter, G. D., Perrins, B. J. (1970). Paper given at the Fourth International Conference on Hyperbaric Medicine, Lgkushoia, Tokyo.

Wood, R. A. B. (1976). Disintegration of cellulose dressings in open granulating wounds. *British Medical Journal*, 1: 1444–1445.

Further Reading

Ayton, M. (1985). Wounds that won't heal. *Community Outlook*, 16–19. (*Community Outlook* is a supplement in the *Nursing Times*; this one accompanied the issue: (1985) 81 (41)).

Bishop, W. J. A. (1959). *A History of Surgical Dressings*. Robinson, Chesterfield.

David, J. (1982). Pressure sore treatment: a literature review. *International Journal of Nursing Studies*, 19: 183–191.

Verhonick, P. J. (1961). Decubitus ulcer observations measured objectively. *Nursing Research*, 10: 211–214.

Chapter 10

Using the Infection Control Service Effectively

INTRODUCTION

Nurses, as well as doctors, need to know about the services provided by the infection control team so that they can use it effectively. Sometimes difficulties arise through failure to appreciate the extent or limitations of the hospital microbiology department or the way in which its work is organised. The purpose of this chapter is to describe the role of the infection control team and the people who contribute to its effective functioning within both the hospital and community. In the second part of the chapter, laboratory procedures are explained, pointing out how nurses can contribute to the success of microbiological investigations.

THE INFECTION CONTROL TEAM

The department of diagnostic microbiology is staffed by laboratory technicians (medical laboratory scientific officers) and the service is coordinated by a chief technician. Each health district employs at least one consultant microbiologist who provides specialist advice about all matters relating to infection.

In England and Wales, provision of hospital infection control services is left to the discretion of each health district. In consequence, it has become dependent upon the influence and enthusiasm of individual members of staff. However, all hospitals are required by statute to have an infection control committee and to employ an infection control officer. The key person is generally the microbiologist, although others, often surgeons or paediatricians, have set up infection control services. The sporadic way in which the service has been allowed to develop has tended to hamper the communication of findings. Generally the work has not been well coordinated between one health district and the next.

Suggestions were made in the 1950s that a member of the medical staff should be appointed as an infection control officer. The Ministry of Health (1959) agreed that this should be a part-time post held by a senior member of the existing medical staff. A good deal of research into the mechanism of hospital-acquired infection was then taking place and many infection control committees date from this time, although their work is subject to considerable variation. The main aims of a typical hospital infection control committee are outlined below.

The Infection Control Committee

The overall function of the committee is to provide advice about the prevention of infection within the hospital and the community. The chairman has direct access to the hospital management team and liaises with other members of the medical staff, but the committee usually functions in an advisory capacity. Medical staff retain a high degree of clinical freedom, so that clinical practice remains relatively free of administrative direction, including that of the infection control committee. The impact made by the committee therefore depends very much upon the cooperation of all the medical staff employed within the hospital.

The structure of a typical infection control service, also subject to variation, is shown in Table 10.1. The infection control officer and nurse are shown as key members of the team, but since the committee is concerned with infection problems in all hospital departments, including pharmacy, domestic services, catering, engineering, laundry and CSSD, representatives from all these will be included (Table 10.2). The clinical areas are represented by a surgeon, and if there is an occupational health department within the hospital, this will probably be represented as well. Sometimes a community health specialist will sit on the committee. Normally there will be a senior nurse representative and an administrator to advise the committee on the administrative viability of its

Table 10.1 Structure of the Infection Control Service (⇌ denotes flow of information in both directions)

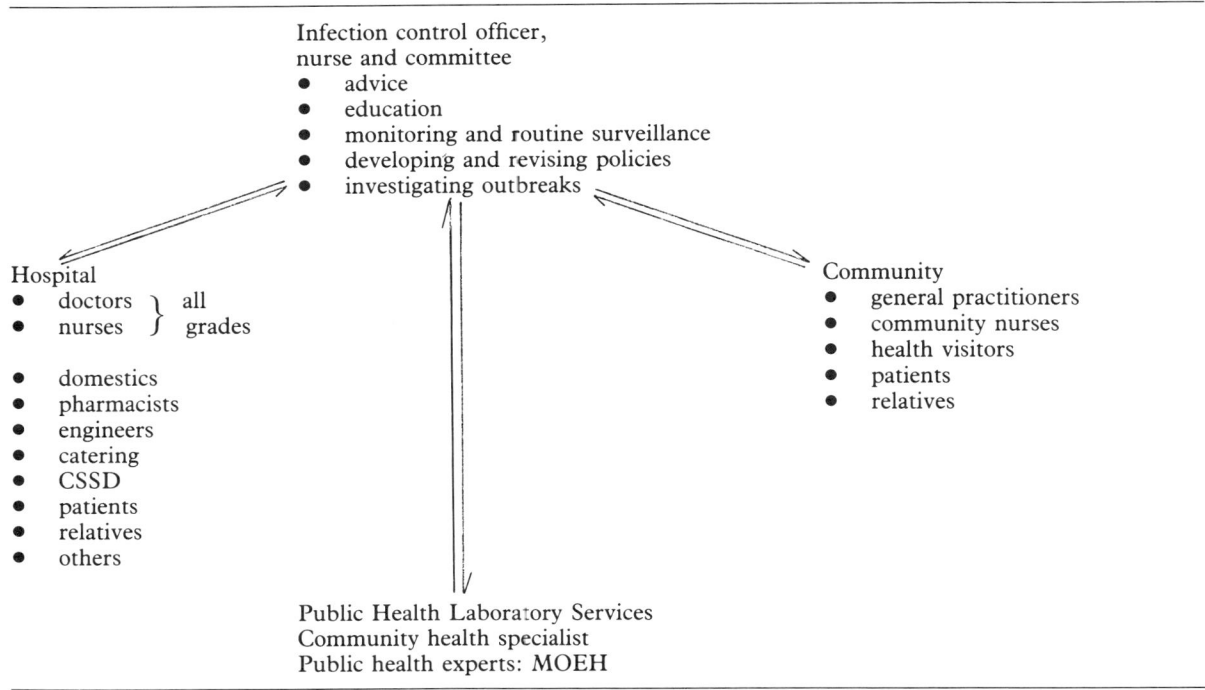

Table 10.2 Members of a Typical Hospital Control of Infection Team

- Infection control officer
- Infection control nurse
- Surgeon and/or paediatrician
- Specialist in community medicine*
- Nurse manager
- Domestic services manager
- CSSD manager*
- Pharmacist
- Hospital engineer*
- Catering manager*
- Administrator
- Laundry manager*

*May be coopted when necessary

recommendations and the cost that they will incur. He will take suggestions made by the committee to the management team. Members of the committee are preferably senior members of their respective departments, to ensure that they can speak with authority when representing their colleagues and disseminating information.

The committee members are jointly responsible for establishing the standards necessary to prevent infection and to provide advice about tackling outbreaks when they occur. The hazards of nosocomial infection are reduced as far as possible through adequate preventive measures including policies for the use of:

- disinfectants,
- antibiotics,
- sterilisation,
- isolation procedures for infectious patients.

Some committees also take an interest in the purchase and use of materials or equipment which involve a possible risk of infection to patients or staff – for example, bedpan washers, 'sharps' disposal boxes, ventilators and wound dressing materials.

When new policies are developed, perhaps during the commissioning of a new hospital building, or when wards are upgraded, members of the committee meet often. Frequent meetings may also become necessary when existing policies are re-examined. Once infection control programmes have become established, meetings may be reduced to only a few times each year, or only in the event of problems. Reports on the incidence of infection are often provided by the infection control nurse, and these may be discussed during routine meetings or circulated to members. Additionally, the committee may evaluate reports involving infections risks, such as in hospital kitchens.

The Infection Control Officer

Throughout England and Wales 75% of all officers are consultant microbiologists. The officer heads the infection control team and is usually the chairperson of the committee. However, either of these appointments may be held by another clinician with a special interest in infection control. Responsibility involves identifying problems associated with infection and providing advice about necessary control measures. Members of the committee will jointly prescribe the policies, but these may have to be modified to meet the everyday demands of the service. A policy may state, for example, that all victims of food poisoning must be isolated in single rooms. If the number of patients affected in an outbreak exceeds the number of single rooms available, the help of the infection control officer will be sought. The chief factors to be considered include the severity and communicability of the infection and the possibility of effective treatment. Extensive outbreaks may involve the closure of a ward, or even an entire hospital, so the officer must have immediate access to the hospital authority responsible for making those decisions – usually the senior manager.

The Infection Control Nurse

The infection control nurse is generally the only full-time member of the infection control team, and she has the responsibility of dealing with day-to-day infection control problems, which she reports back to the officer. Her task is to help other hospital staff to prevent infection wherever possible and to identify and minimise the effects of any infection that occurs. She is usually accountable to the microbiologist, with whom she liaises, and also to a senior nurse manager. The work also demands liaison with a wide variety of hospital service employees from doctors and nurses of all grades to administrators, domestics, catering staff and the hospital occupational health service. The work of the infection control nurse will vary according to the hospital or district in which she is employed, but some of the key functions are detailed below.

(1) Helping the microbiologist and experts from other departments to draw up policies designed to reduce the incidence of infection and to look after infected patients safely.

(2) Ensuring that the infection control policies are readily available to all members of staff, and that they are implemented correctly.

(3) Monitoring infection rates. This task may be too great to undertake for the entire hospital. Instead, continuous records may be maintained for high-risk areas such as the intensive care and special care baby units, with occasional checks made on other areas, or in response to particular need. Records may be kept manually or computerised. In many microbiology departments a chart is kept of the patients who have developed a particular infection. Shaeffner (1984) believes that the introduction of computers will permit better documentation and greater opportunities for infection control in the future.

(4) Helping to investigate and control outbreaks when they occur.

(5) Educating all grades of staff about the importance of infection control. Teaching may take place informally in the work place; formal lectures and demonstrations may be arranged during inservice education programmes and in the school of nursing.

(6) Researching into infection. Some infection control nurses participate in research studies, others may undertake research projects of their own.

Infection control nurses were first employed in the 1960s. News of the beneficial effects of their employment spread, and posts were subsequently created in many hospitals. However, there is no existing legislation to enforce any hospital or hospital district to employ an infection control nurse and some do not. A few districts employ more than one nurse in this capacity, encouraging teamwork.

The scope of the work undertaken varies considerably between hospitals in, for example, a rural health district, where much travelling may be involved, to a compact inner city area, with a high population turnover, poverty and crowded substandard living conditions, according to local needs and priorities. Infection control nurses do not work shifts, but they may be required to work outside normal office hours and must be contactable in an emergency.

The role of the infection control nurse is sometimes misunderstood by her colleagues. Like the infection control officer and the committee to which she reports, her main function is to provide specialised advice. The extent to which her recommendations are heeded and implemented will depend on the degree to which other members of staff are prepared to draw upon her expertise. Cooperation is vital to the effective performance of infection control, since good advice will be redundant unless it can be introduced into clinical practice. To function effectively, the infection control nurse therefore requires not only a fund of specialist knowledge, but the ability to communicate it both verbally and in reports. Case study 10.1 illustrates the need for good interpersonal skills, the educational role of the infection control nurse and her autonomy.

Infection control nurses have more autonomy than their ward-based colleagues, and must be able to work alone, often with little supervision, knowing when it is necessary to take initiative. It is not always possible to share immediate problems with colleagues, so most infection control nurses appreciate the opportunity to discuss their concerns with their counterparts from other hospitals. They receive a great deal of help and support from their professional body, the Infection Control Nurses' Association, which arranges local meetings and an annual conference. The Infection Control Nurses' Association was formed in 1970 and has over 150 full members as well as associate members, mainly microbiologists, CSSD managers and commercial members. The conferences, regular

---

Case study 10.1

A fireman aged 27 years was involved as a pedestrian in a serious road traffic accident. He sustained head injuries resulting in gross brain damage and was artificially ventilated. His condition stabilised, but he remained deeply unconscious. After much discussion, ventilation was discontinued with the agreement of his relatives, but the patient maintained his own respirations and was transferred from the intensive care unit to a general surgical ward. He was physically robust and it was evident that his twilight existence might continue for months or years.

Attempts to transfer the patient to a hospital for the chronically sick were defeated. He remained permanently on an acute surgical ward where the nurses grew very fond of both the patient and his family. At the time of the accident he had been married for only 6 weeks and his very young wife lived nearby. He was an only child and his parents travelled over 100 miles to visit him each weekend. His condition was discussed with them and everyone agreed that he should be spared aggressive treatment, and that he would not receive antibiotics if he developed an infection. He continued to receive excellent nursing care.

The infection control nurse had received bacteriology reports while the patient was in the intensive care unit, but observed that the laboratory had ceased to receive specimens after his transfer to the surgical ward. She knew that he had a long-term indwelling catheter which could easily become colonised or infected with Gram-negative bacteria. These would represent a serious threat of cross-infection to the other gravely ill patients nursed on the same ward (see Chapter 8). When the infection control nurse visited the ward, the sister explained that the nurses would prefer to remain ignorant of any infection that the patient might develop, because they knew that he would not be actively treated.

The infection control nurse discussed the hazards of catheter-associated infection and the risk of cross-infection. She explained that urine from the unconscious patient could be monitored by the microbiology department at regular intervals and bacteria tested for antibiotic sensitivity, so that early precautions could be taken to prevent spread to others. She emphasised that the patient would not be treated against the wishes of his family or the clinicians despite these measures. The ward sister agreed to send a catheter specimen to the laboratory every week and to ensure that the urinary drainage system was handled only by nurses wearing gloves.

Ultimately the patient's condition deteriorated and he died of a chest infection. He received no antibiotics. Before he died Gram-negative bacteria had been isolated from his urine, but sufficient precautions had been taken to ensure that they had no chance to spread to other patients on the ward.

publication of the journal of the Association, and the introduction of training courses (organised by the English National Board) provide members with valuable opportunities to update their specialist knowledge. It is only fair, however, to point out that the work of infection control nurses has never been formally evaluated in Britain or comparisons made between health districts in which they are and are not employed. This would present a formidable task because the appointment of the nurse may bring to light problems and reveal infections which had previously not been acknowledged. Many of the policies developed by the infection control team are planned to operate over a long period. Criticism of their effectiveness soon after they have been implemented would not be valid.

The situation in the United States contrasts sharply against that in Britain. The Americans, who have always had a more cost-effective approach to medical care, took the lead from Britain, first appointing infection control nurses in the 1960s. Whereas Britain has only a few hundred infection control nurses, the United States now has over 3000. Hospitals cannot be licensed (and therefore cannot admit patients) unless they have infection control policies that are shown to be implemented and effective, and a person responsible for surveillance of these policies. Regular infection control statistics form part of the quality control programme in a country where patients, who generally expect to pay for their health care, are on the whole better informed about health matters. People are not prepared to accept morbidity from nosocomial infection as a normal risk and suing for malpractice due to nosocomial infection accounts for 5% of all claims.

The Occupational Health Department

The occupational health department has a major role to play in the control of infection, and the nurse who works in it will probably liaise closely with the infection control nurse. Screening for possible infection will form part of the regular medical examination of all newly appointed staff. New employees will all require a chest X-ray to exclude tuberculosis and will be asked to provide evidence of immunisation. A history of exposure to infectious illness must be taken and those who have never had rubella may be offered the vaccine. Stool specimens must be obtained for microbiological examination from all new members of the catering department.

One of the most important functions of the service is to provide health education and, where necessary, counselling and reassurance concerning health-associated topics, particularly infection. The nurse may teach staff about the hazards of hepatitis B, explaining the precautions necessary when handling blood products and the importance of avoiding needlestick injuries. Members of staff placed at risk can be given passive immunisation in the form of immunoglobulin (see Chapter 4). Those who work in high-risk areas, for example with the mentally handicapped, can be offered the hepatitis B vaccine. The success of a vaccination programme depends very much upon publicity and the quality of information provided to employees. The infection control and occupational health nurses may work together when a major screening or vaccination programme is planned (Tyman, 1986).

Records kept in the department should be strictly confidential, and not available to managers, otherwise uptake of the services available may be hesitant.

Infection Control Policies

The policies agreed by the members of the committee may be presented in a manual or looseleaf folder, so that additions and amendments are possible. Every ward and department should have a copy of the policies pertinent to their work. Information can never be of practical value unless staff know that it exists, can find and readily understand it. Gould (1985a) found that in a typical sample of nurses drawn from one health district, a high proportion claimed that they had never seen the infection control policy on their current ward, although the document had been distributed to every ward in all the hospitals concerned.

Periodic checks must be made to ensure that the policies are correctly implemented, are achieving their aims, and that they are acceptable to staff.

The most carefully designed policy is unlikely to be effective if practical difficulties prevent it becoming operational. The excellence of any policy will depend as much upon those who use it as on those who were responsible for its planning. Any problems should be reported to representatives of the infection control committee and put on the agenda for discussion. All newly appointed employees must be given the opportunity to familiarise themselves with policies and to receive inservice training at regular intervals in order for them to remain safe as practitioners. Many health districts ensure that recently appointed staff attend an induction day, followed, if possible, by regular study days. Infection control nurses may contribute to the organisation of these programmes and participate in teaching.

Concepts about microorganisms and their behaviour change with the progression of research and with new developments in technology. Consequently, infection control policies must be reviewed at intervals and updated as necessary. The legal implications attached to this are illustrated in case study 10.2 below.

The Public Health Laboratory Service (PHLS)

This service includes twelve regional laboratories, and a series of specialist reference and research units, the two main centres being Colindale in London and Porton in Wiltshire. These provide an extensive microbiological service, including much advice about infection control. Teams of microbiologists and epidemiologists monitor the trends of infectious disease reported throughout the country, providing specialist advice for its management. In the case of particularly large or problematic outbreaks, the PHLS may also provide help with investigations. Following the outbreak of legionnaire's disease in the Midlands in 1985, the PHLS became involved with investigations and the followup of those who became infected. In a later survey undertaken among 40 British hospitals, 28 showed evidence of the causative organism, *Legionella pneumophila*, in their water supplies. Cooling systems existed in twelve of the hospitals included in the survey, and five of these were infected despite chemical treatment to destroy the bacteria. In the survey 104 hotels were also investigated; 55 showed signs of contamination.

Case study 10.2

A patient was admitted to a regional burns unit, having sustained extensive injuries over a large area of his body. He developed staphylococcal wound infections during the course of his stay but recovered and was discharged. He decided to sue the hospital authorities for negligence resulting in infection, and the infection control officer was asked in court to give evidence to show that he had provided reasonable precautions against cross-infection in the burns unit.

The officer demonstrated that the infection control policies were reviewed by the committee every 2 years and that they took into account the most recent developments. He pointed out that the infection control nurse had personally distributed a copy of the most recently updated infection control manual to every ward and department in the hospital, including the burns unit, obtaining a signature on receipt from every senior nurse. Induction days were arranged for all newly appointed nurses. The infection control nurse always contributed to these, spoke for an hour about the practical importance of infection control, and showed the manual containing all the policies. The school of nursing where these sessions took place had kept records of attendance for several years. These demonstrated that all the nurses employed in the burns unit throughout the patient's admission had been present at an induction day. Records kept by the infection control nurse showed that she visited the burns unit every week, including the period when the patient was there.

The evidence given satisfied all who were present that reasonable precautions had been taken to prevent the spread of infection on the unit.

Water was tested from 17 business establishments, and twelve were found to be contaminated.

Many of the outbreaks followed up by the PHLS are in connection with food poisoning, which has already been described in some detail in Chapter 1. Most outbreaks involve meat, eggs or shellfish, but occasionally other kinds of food are implicated. Several years ago a number of people became ill after they had eaten chocolate, a food product not normally associated with gastrointestinal upset. *Salmonella napoli* was isolated and the chocolate was traced to a market stall in the south of England. Investigations revealed it to be an inexpensive variety exported from Italy where in the factory the source of the infection was traced to the cocoa beans. Previously the manufacturing process had involved heating these to a high temperature, but this had recently been superseded by a newer process which involved more moderate temperatures, so that the bacteria were not destroyed.

The PHLS also collects weekly information on a range of infectious diseases, published in the *Communicable Diseases Surveillance Report*, which is sent to all hospital microbiology departments. However, the contribution of information is voluntary, except for those diseases which are notifiable (Table 10.3), so the service depends to a large extent upon the goodwill of those in a position to contribute.

Table 10.3 Diseases Notifiable to the Medical Officer of Environmental Health (MOEH) in England and Wales*

Acute encephalitis	Ophthalmia neonatorum
Acute meningitis	Paratyphoid fever
Acute poliomyelitis	Plague
Anthrax	Rabies
Cholera	Relapsing fever
Diphtheria	Scarlet fever
Dysentery	Smallpox
Food poisoning	Tetanus
Infective jaundice	Tuberculosis
Lassa fever	Typhoid fever
Leprosy	Typhus fever
Leptospirosis	Viral haemorrhagic fever (VHF)
Malaria	Whooping cough
Marburg disease	Yellow fever
Measles	

*The list differs slightly in Northern Ireland and Scotland

Other Organisations Concerned with Infection Control

Hospitals can obtain advice from several outside agencies besides the PHLS, including the Medical Research Council (MRC), university departments and industry. Research funds and sponsorship for courses of study are often provided by commercial enterprise. The DHSS advises hospitals on planning and the development of equipment. Many of its departments have an interest in infection control, but their input is not always well coordinated. However, the DHSS has in the past organised educational programmes with an infection control content and set up committees and working parties for special purposes, such as investigating staphylococcal outbreaks in hospital and providing guidelines for laboratory safety. In 1985 a working party was set up to explore safety guidelines for hospital staff, particularly laboratory technicians dealing with AIDS.

Manufacturers have contributed to the prevention of infection by endeavouring to meet increasingly rigorous standards of safety, particularly those demanded by disinfection and sterilisation processes, and there is consultation with infection control specialists during the design and development of new products.

The Medical Officer of Environmental Health (MOEH)

The MOEH has a considerable role to play in the prevention of infection within the community. Certain infectious diseases are notifiable to the MOEH and the attending doctor, whether in hospital or the community, must ensure that he has been informed (see Table 10.3). The MOEH and his team of community health physicians try to find the origin of the infection and to prevent its spread within the community. The work may include taking specimens from contacts and obtaining negative specimens before the patient leaves hospital or returns to work. A specialist in community infection may be represented on the infection control committee.

Coordinated Functioning of the Infection Control Team

From the discussion above it should be apparent that members of the infection control team do not operate in isolation from the rest of the hospital. On the contrary, their work may involve liaison with colleagues in the community and agencies outside their own hospital. Two case studies (10.3 and 10.4) illustrate the integral functioning of the infection control team.

The group A haemolytic streptococcus is responsible for a wide range of infectious illnesses, including tonsillitis, acute glomerular nephritis, scarlet fever, puerperal sepsis, erysipelas and rheumatic fever. Some are local infections, others are generalised. An outbreak on any hospital ward will therefore always be regarded with concern.

Case study 10.3

In July 1979 bacteriology results from a paediatric ward showed that several children had become infected with beta (β)-haemolytic streptococcus Lancefield group A. The same bacteria were isolated from the throats and nasal passages of several members of staff who had become ill. An emergency meeting was convened between the consultant paediatrician, the infection control officer and nurse, the senior nursing officer for the unit and the hospital administrator. As a result, admissions to the ward were cancelled unless they were emergencies and environmental sampling of the ward took place. The infection control nurse compiled records of all the patients who had been admitted to the ward during the same month. Names were checked against laboratory records for previous streptococcal infection and nose and throat swabs were taken from all the remaining children on the ward. The occupational health nurse made records of all the staff who had worked on the ward since the beginning of July, including nurses, doctors, ancillary staff and volunteers, and obtained nose and throat swabs from them all. The infection control team hoped that they would be able to identify a carrier as the source of the infection. However, everybody who yielded positive laboratory findings had also been clinically ill. All were asked to remain away from work until a course of appropriate antibiotics had been completed and further nose and throat swabs were shown to be negative.

A temporary children's ward was opened for emergencies in a geographically separate part of the hospital and all staff were screened before they were allowed to work on it. Altogether 121 swabs were taken (excluding repeat swabs) and 15 were positive for group A streptococcus. A culture of each was sent to the Streptococcus Reference Laboratory at the PHLS. Investigations showed that eight were of the same strain (they all had the same type of antibodies on their cell surfaces), and this particular strain was also represented in dust from environmental sampling. (Data from Ayton, 1981.)

Beta-haemolytic streptococci are classified according to the presence of a specific antigen on the cell wall. There are fourteen Lancefield groups, numbered from A to O. Group A is responsible for 95% of all human streptococcal infections, and within this group about 57 different strains can be differentiated, according to further antigenic testing. This allows the successful tracing of an outbreak.

Between 6% and 8% of the general population are either nose or throat carriers of group A streptococcus, the rate of carriage tending to be higher among children. In view of this, paediatric wards merit careful surveillance by the infection control team.

Carriers disperse the bacteria by coughing, sneezing or spluttered conversation. Dust can become contaminated by the streptococci when the moisture in the droplets has evaporated, but the bacteria themselves are then much less virulent than if moist. Recognising that this was a possible mode of transmission, the infection control team recommended that the paediatric ward illustrated in case study 10.3 should be thoroughly cleaned to remove all traces of contamination. A phenolic disinfectant (Clearasol, see Chapter 5) was chosen because it is effective against group A streptococcus and not inactivated by the presence of organic matter. All linen, even fresh items from the ward cupboard, were returned to the laundry. The ward curtains were changed. All items that could be autoclaved were sent to the CSSD. Boxes of disposables that had been opened were incinerated. Toys which could not withstand washing in disinfectant were destroyed. Wherever possible, soft furnishings (armchairs, mattresses) were put out into the sun to air, as ultraviolet light destroys bacteria.

When cleaning was complete, repeated environmental sampling demonstrated that the streptococci had successfully been eradicated and the ward could open again. However, the venture had been expensive and the waiting list for elective admissions delayed.

For practical purposes, an outbreak of infection is regarded as two or more cases, related in space or time. Case study 10.3 illustrates the difficulties in tracing the source of an outbreak. Ayton (1981) and her colleagues were able to uncover a certain amount of circumstantial evidence to suggest the source of the epidemic strain of streptococci. Not long before the outbreak occurred, a child was admitted to the paediatric ward directly from the accident department. He had eczema, and swabs were taken from the lesions as soon as he arrived on the ward, but as it was a Friday evening they did not reach the laboratory until after the weekend. After this child arrived, three more patients, two nursery nurses, the ward clerk and a visiting parent became clinically ill, and investigations revealed that all these infections were due to the epidemic streptococcus. One of the patients had also been admitted with eczema, but his skin swabs had been negative at the time of admission. Streptococci were isolated only *after* the admission of the 'carrier' patient. Group A haemolytic streptococcus has a short period of incubation 2 or 3 days at maximum, and the child with infectious eczema had been admitted only a few days before the other epidemic cases began to appear. However, he had been admitted directly into an isolation cubicle, and had had no contact with any of the other people who subsequently became infected. However, it is quite possible that a member of staff became heavily contaminated following contact with this child. Inadequate handwashing may have resulted in contact spread, and contamination of the ward environment.

From Ayton's report it is apparent that hospital visitors are placed at risk of infection, for the epidemic streptococcus was isolated from the throat of a mother whose child was also in isolation. This child had leukaemia, but fortunately did not become infected, as the consequences of streptococcal infection in an immunocompromised child may be serious, even fatal.

Outbreaks of food poisoning are often reported in the national press and they sometimes occur in hospital, especially where elderly people are nursed. Case study 10.4, documented in a medical journal (Horan, 1984), describes an outbreak of food poisoning.

In cases where patients have become infected by food poisoning from staff, it is often the most incapacitated who become victims, because they require the most handling. Case study 10.4 is unusual in this respect, since the infected patients were mobile and fully continent. However, all three were taking either cimetidine or a drug with antacid properties. Both depress the secretion of hydrochloric acid in the stomach, so bacteria that have been swallowed may not be destroyed (see Chapter 1). The patients also shared the same WC. There is now evidence that bacteria responsible for food poisoning may also be able to contaminate the environment, resulting in contact spread. A report from the PHLS has implicated *Salmonella* in hospital outbreaks of this nature (Abbott *et al.*,

Case study 10.4

Two patients on a geriatric rehabilitation ward developed diarrhoea and were found to be infected with *Shigella sonnei*, the causative agent of dysentery. There were 36 beds on the ward and the patients occupied them according to their degree of dependency; they did not all share the same toilet facilities. The infected patients were transferred to cubicles on the same ward and isolation procedures were instigated, but soon afterwards a third patient who had died of pneumonia was found at post mortem to be colonised with *Shigella sonnei*. Stool cultures revealed that bacteria of the same strain were infecting two nurses, both of whom had profuse diarrhoea for approximately a week before the first symptoms appeared among the patients. Neither had stayed away from work, but each was instructed to stay away until she had produced three consecutively negative stool specimens. One nurse was away from work for 4 weeks. Screening the remaining staff failed to reveal an asymptomatic carrier and the source of the outbreak was never uncovered.

1980). Members of a specially convened subcommittee reviewed 552 hospital outbreaks of *Salmonella* that had occurred between 1968 and 1977. The source of the outbreak was successfully traced in only 76 cases, and of these, food was implicated in 24 outbreaks. In the remaining 52 outbreaks, environmental contamination may well have led to contact spread, especially as many of the outbreaks occurred on units where faecal contamination is particularly common: geriatric, paediatric, psychiatric and maternity units.

Cruikshank (1984) discusses the importance of environmental sampling when this type of outbreak is traced. To be successful, swabbing must be planned and systematic. The considerable cost in terms of time and finance cannot otherwise be justified. Clinical and epidemiological data are required, and vital information will include:

- the exact dates and time of onset of symptoms (obtained where necessary from ward records),
- dates of special investigations such as endoscopy, in which instruments may have acted as fomites,
- dates on which patients were admitted and discharged,

- data about all food eaten by all members of staff (doctors, nurses, ancillary staff and volunteers) as well as patients, remembering that relatives may bring food to the ward,
- a plan of the ward, pointing out the beds of all the affected patients, their WC facilities and the positions usually occupied in the day room,
- a histogram to relate the number of cases of the infection to the dates of onset.

If food was the source of the outbreak, the cases will cluster together over a clearly defined period of time (Fig. 10.1). In the case of *Salmonella*, clustering will be within a period of 72 hours, its incubation period. The incubation period of *Shigella* is similar, but staphylococcal food poisoning, due to toxins in contaminated food and not to the bacteria themselves, may be distinguished by its much more rapid onset (about 6 hours after ingestion). In the event of contact spread, the time of onset of the symptoms will be spread over a much longer period (Fig. 10.2). Staphylococcus toxin does not, of course, set up cross-infection in this way.

The infection control and occupational health nurse have a major role to play in persuading staff to comply with stool screening. Many people feel embarrassed, secretly dread being discovered as the 'guilty' carrier and worry about being absent from work in the event of positive findings. When staff are away from work because they are found to be carriers, they receive their normal basic salaries, but in a hospital where it is usual to receive remuneration for working shifts and unsociable hours, financial loss may be incurred.

Outbreaks of antibiotic-resistant bacteria often occur in hospital. Coleman (1984) describes how isolates of *Serratia marcescens* obtained from 30 different patients admitted to the same general hospital were all resistant to the antibiotic cephalosporin. No common source was found, but there was some evidence that antibiotic resistance was actively transmitted between the bacteria by con-

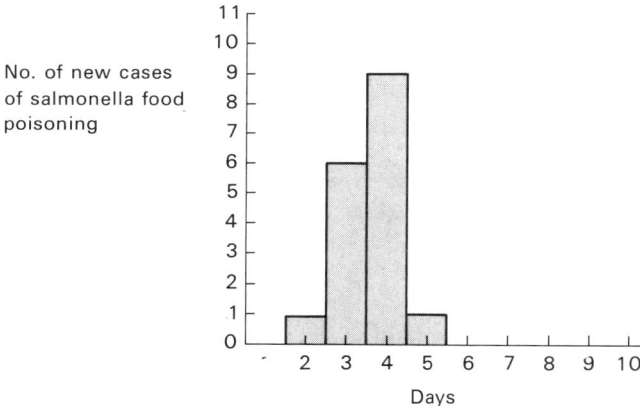

Fig. 10.1 Histogram constructed to show relationship of salmonella food poisoning developing in relation to time.

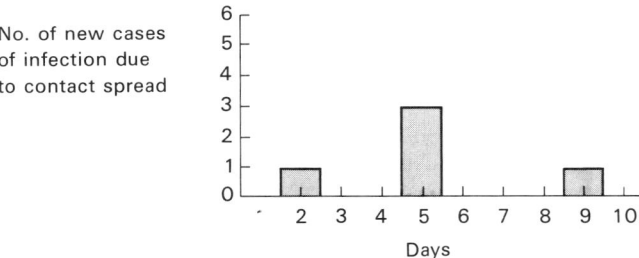

Fig. 10.2 Histogram to show cases of infection due to contact spread in relation to time.

jugation (see Chapter 1). Hill and Ferguson (1984) reported carriage of multiresistant *Staphylococcus aureus* among 35 neonates in a special care baby unit over one calendar year. Only two babies became clinically ill, but one of them died. The unit was then closed for several weeks in an attempt to eradicate the bacteria, but this was not effective. In this case the route of transmission was impossible to determine.

The difficulty of controlling an outbreak even when the source has been determined is illustrated by a report from another neonatal unit, this time in the Netherlands (Gerards, 1984) where 16 infants (66%) developed gastroenteritis caused by *E.coli*. One of the babies died; four nurses on the unit were found to carry the same strain, but their stools became negative after they had been treated with the antibiotic colistin for 2 weeks. However, it proved more difficult to treat the babies effectively and the epidemic was terminated only by instituting strict isolation precautions and improving the standards of hygiene on the unit.

The identification of pathogenic microorganisms and testing their sensitivity to antibiotics is the work of the diagnostic microbiology department. Every nurse needs at least some insight into this work because the successful operation of the department depends so heavily upon cooperation between nurses. Developments in technology have had a major impact on virtually every aspect of hospital life, and in the haematology department, for example, the use of sophisticated equipment now means that testing of blood samples is almost fully automated. In the microbiology department, however, this is not the case. The identification of bacteria is still an art. If an inadequate or poorly taken specimen is received, then no bacteria may grow at all. Dixon and Kolyvas (1984) designed a study to illustrate the trends of hospital staff in ordering and collecting microbiology specimens. In 77% of the episodes examined, it was impossible to determine who had ordered that a specimen should be taken. Only 20% could be medically justified either because they were needed to confirm a diagnosis or to monitor the effectiveness of therapy. The majority were obtained for inappropriate reasons, suggesting considerable misunderstanding of the correct use of the laboratory.

In view of these findings, the second part of this chapter is concerned with the effective use of the laboratory services. Of course the doctor is ultimately responsible for the patient and in theory the medical staff should sanction all microbiological investigations. In practice, it is often the nurse who notices that a patient has developed an infection and valuable time may be lost if she waits for a doctor to visit the ward before obtaining a specimen. It is, after all, the nurse who will first observe any inflammation and pus when she dresses a wound, foul urine when she empties a catheter, and it is to the nurse that the patient will generally complain about wound soreness or dysuria. In the community the nurse attending the patient must always take the initiative if she has reason to believe that infection has developed.

USING THE LABORATORY SERVICE EFFECTIVELY

Broadly speaking, microbiological investigations are undertaken for one of the reasons below:

(1) To identify the pathogen responsible for an obvious infection.
(2) To monitor the progress of recovery following an infection.
(3) To confirm or eliminate a specific site of the body as a focus of infection or colonisation.
(4) To determine whether a convalescent who has had an infectious condition is still harbouring the pathogen responsible.

Factors Affecting Microbiological Findings

Several factors influence the success of these investigations.

(1) The time at which the specimen was obtained, *before* receiving attention in the laboratory.
(2) The method used to obtain the specimen.
(3) The transport medium (if any).
(4) Appropriateness of the specimen.
(5) The quantity of material available to be examined.
(6) The provision of adequate clinical details, including correct labelling of the specimen and its accompanying form.

Under optimal conditions, many bacteria, including most pathogens and opportunists, will divide approximately once every half an hour. Pus, urine and many other body fluids provide ideal media in which very rapid multiplication may take place. Suppose, for example, that a specimen of urine was taken from a patient who did not in fact have bacteriuria, but that a few bacteria were transferred to the urine as it was poured into the specimen container. If the specimen reached the laboratory soon after the event, the presence of a few contaminating bacteria could be dismissed, especially in the absence of any clinical symptoms indicative of infection. If, however, the urine was allowed to remain in a warm room for several hours, the number of contaminants would increase dramatically, and the presence of a clinical infection would at least be considered.

In contrast, certain very delicate microorganisms will not survive for long once they have been removed from the tissues and there is a danger of false-negative results. *Neisseria meningitidis*, for example, causing meningitis, will not live for long outside the body, so cerebrospinal fluid should be sent to the laboratory as soon as possible. Patients with a provisional diagnosis of meningitis are generally very ill and nobody should be subjected to the discomfort of lumbar puncture unless it is absolutely necessary.

Specimens (with a few exceptions) must always be collected with aseptic technique and placed in uncontaminated containers to avoid false-positive results.

Types of Specimen

Urine Specimens

It is particularly important that urine should be obtained in an uncontaminated receptacle, to exclude any of the bacteria which normally inhabit the tip of the urethra in the specimen. To obtain a midstream specimen male patients can be instructed or helped to withdraw the foreskin, cleanse the urethral meatus and collect the middle part of the stream directly into a sterile container. A disinfectant should *not* be used for cleansing, because it may damage the bacteria and irritate the delicate urethral mucosa. Sterile water or normal saline are both inexpensive and suitable cleansing agents.

Collecting an uncontaminated urine specimen from a female patient is never easy and presents a particular problem when the patient is bedbound or too disoriented to cooperate. The external genitalia and the urethral meatus should be cleansed, and the patient asked to micturate with the labia separated, catching the middle part of the specimen in a sterile container.

Fewer difficulties are encountered when obtaining catheter specimens because a needle and syringe can be used to aspirate freshly passed urine from the special sleeve on the catheter tubing. The tubing and drainage bag should never be disconnected to obtain a catheter specimen because of the risk of introducing infection. Urine from the drainage bag will not yield satisfactory microbiological results because it is likely to be contaminated and may have been passed some time ago (see Chapter 8).

Wound Swabs

As much pus as possible should be collected on the swab, to increase the possibility of growing the pathogen responsible for the infection once it has reached the laboratory. The likelihood of successful identification and culture is enhanced if pus can be scraped from the wound with a clean disposable spatula and poured into a specimen container. Liquid pus may be aspirated with a needle and syringe.

Stool Specimens

Stool culture may be necessary to identify bacteria, viruses or parasites, such as worms. Entamoeba is microscopic, but parasites, particularly worms, may be clearly visible to the naked eye, although their ova and cysts are only revealed by microscopic examination.

When diarrhoea or suspected food poisoning are investigated, a series of specimens (generally at least three) are sent to the laboratory from consecutive bowel movements. Rectal swabs are unsatisfactory for stool culture because insufficient material is collected.

Parasitic cysts and ova are adapted to withstand

unfavourable environmental conditions, and can still be detected after a specimen has been stored. However, many freeliving parasites die very soon after leaving the host because they are unable to tolerate the external body temperature. Identification is difficult once protozoa and microscopic worms have ceased to move, so if their presence is suspected the laboratory must receive the stool *immediately* it has been passed. These 'hot stools' can only be processed by the laboratory during normal working hours.

Sputum

Pathogens responsible for bronchitis and pneumonia grow in the lower, normally sterile parts of the respiratory tract. Sputum may be gathered from the patient directly into the specimen container, but often saliva is sent to the laboratory instead, either because the patient is genuinely unable to expectorate, or because he has not been given sufficient explanation about providing a sample. The physiotherapist may help to collect sputum for microbiological examination.

Nasopharyngeal Secretion (Trap Sputum)

Very sick patients who have been intubated or who require regular suction often succumb to Gram-negative opportunist infections. The sputum withdrawn from the nasopharynx should therefore be sent to the laboratory for monitoring at regular intervals.

Nose and Throat Swabs

To obtain a specimen of secretion from the nose, the tip of the swab is gently wiped around the inside of the anterior nares. Throat swabs are best obtained if the tongue is depressed with a spatula before the tip of the swab is passed over both tonsil areas and the posterior pharyngeal wall, collecting any exudate present. Patients generally find these procedures unpleasant and should be warned in advance about the gag reflex when the swab contacts the back of the throat. A high proportion of those requiring nose and throat swabs are children, so parents can help by holding the child firmly while the specimens are obtained. Very young or nervous children may be wrapped in a blanket to restrict movement.

Pernasal Swabs

These are necessary to confirm a diagnosis of whooping cough. The causative organism, *Bordetella pertussis*, is most readily isolated from the posterior nasopharynx, especially if the specimen is obtained just after a bout of coughing. The tip of the swab is connected to a fine, flexible wire that can be introduced more readily into the posterior nasopharynx.

Blood Cultures

Blood should always be obtained from the patient with full aseptic technique. If it is to be sent for microbiological examination it must be placed immediately into specimen bottles containing the appropriate culture media. At least two bottles will be inoculated, one to be incubated aerobically, the other anaerobically. Transfer to the bottles, via their rubber stoppers, is also a strictly aseptic procedure to avoid contamination by environmental organisms. Patients who require blood cultures are often very ill and the specimens should be dispatched to the laboratory at once.

Nurses who work in the intensive care unit may take blood specimens, but on general wards obtaining blood cultures is more often the responsibility of junior medical staff. However, medical students receive little instruction about aseptic technique during their training, so it is generally prudent to supervise their activities when blood cultures are set up, particularly since the patient may be too ill or disoriented to cooperate.

Vaginal and Cervical Swabs

Vaginal and cervical pathogens are not easily confused with environmental contaminants, so the specimens may be stored for longer on the ward if necessary. Storage at room temperature may actually be helpful to the technicians since it permits pathogens like *Trichomonas vaginalis* to multiply; but the specimens must be sent to the laboratory in special transport media. The diplococcus which causes gonorrhoea is an exception because it cannot survive for long outside the host, and to be identified it is best for smears to be spread onto a microscope slide and examined as soon as Gram-staining has taken place. Cultures must be incubated immediately in an atmosphere enriched with carbon dioxide. This is why patients who require examination for sexually transmitted infection often stand a much better chance of rapid and accurate diagnosis if they attend a special clinic rather than their own general practitioner. Nurses working in the clinic receive inservice training so that they can identify the bacteria under the microscope and set up cultures to be sent to the laboratory. If microscopic examination indicates a positive finding, treatment can be given immediately in the clinic and preparations made for any necessary contact tracing. If a patient on the ward is thought to have a sexually transmitted infection, he will generally be taken to the clinic for investigation and treatment (which are, of course, confidential).

Vaginal swabs are no substitute for cervical swabs, or vice versa. The vagina is lined with a tough stratified epithelium, the cervix with more delicate, columnar cells, and the pathogens which invade these different types of cell are not the same. In an adult female, *Neisseria gonorrhoeae* will not be recovered from the vagina and positive results will be obtained only by inserting a Cusco's speculum and obtaining material from the cervix.

Collecting and Handling Specimens

Under ideal circumstances, no specimens, apart from those obtained from the female genital tract, should be received by the laboratory more than 2 hours after they have been obtained. In practice this can sometimes be difficult to ensure, because most are collected from wards and departments in batches at intervals throughout the day. Transport is provided by the portering staff. All wound and urine specimens not immediately dispatched must be stored in a ward specimen refrigerator at 4 °C to arrest any further multiplication. Urgent specimens are best sent to the laboratory at once, after an advance telephone call. The decision to refrigerate less urgent specimens will depend on the efficiency of the portering service and the speed with which the specimen is likely to receive attention once it arrives on the laboratory reception desk. At busy times of the day, particularly before the laboratory closes for the evening or weekend, an influx of specimens may cause delay. Nurses who work shifts to maintain a continuous 24 hour service for every day of the week may not realise that outside 'normal' working hours (9.00 to 5.00), the laboratory will employ only a skeleton staff to provide an emergency service. Often specimens have to be discarded, particularly following a weekend, either because they have been stored for too long on the ward, or because they have not received attention in the laboratory within a reasonable amount of time.

Some bacteria and a great many viruses will fail to survive unless they are sent to the laboratory in special transport media, which may often be obtained from the laboratories. Vaginal swabs are placed in charcoal medium. Wound swabs dry out easily and, if possible, should be transported in medium.

All laboratory specimens potentially contain pathogens and should be collected so that contamination of the environment and the people who will handle them is kept to a minimum. Specimen containers must be transported in individual plastic bags, which should always be sealed. Some hospitals have established 'specimen handling committees' where representatives from the laboratory and portering staff can develop policies to ensure that specimens arrive safely and promptly at the appropriate laboratory. Porters should always be advised against handling specimen containers that are leaking.

If leakage occurs during transit, it should be cleared away by a responsible person wearing the appropriate protective garments (disposable gloves and apron). Disposable wipes should be used, so that they may be incinerated. The contaminated area must be treated with the disinfectant recommended in the infection control policy (see Chapter 5). 'Danger of infection' or 'Biohazard' labels should always be attached to the specimens and request forms when the following are suspected:

- tuberculosis,
- syphilis,
- hepatitis B,
- AIDS.

Hospitals generally draw up a list of the particular infections which are felt to constitute a particular hazard.

Microbiology Request Forms

Specimens and their accompanying request forms must both be fully labelled, because they will be unsealed and separated on the laboratory bench. Confusion will result if the information disagrees, or if more than one patient has the same name. The necessary information is shown in Table 10.4 (see Fig. 10.6). When the clinical information provided is inadequate or insufficiently detailed, the conclusions drawn from microbiological investigations may be erroneous, and inappropriate treatment may be recommended when the completed report is received from the technician. For example, from Chapter 8 it will be apparent that when a patient has an indwelling urinary catheter information must be provided about the length of time that it has been *in situ*, the reason for catheterisation, the patient's diagnosis (since this will affect overall susceptibility to infection) and the colour and odour of the urine. Specimens from a patient who has developed puerperal sepsis will be processed quite differently in the laboratory to those obtained from a patient with vaginal discharge. When the clinical details provided are scanty, laboratory staff may have to contact the ward for additional information.

Table 10.4 Information Which Should Be Provided on a Microbiology Request Form

---

Name of the patient
Hospital number
Age
Ward or department
Site from which the specimen was obtained.
Nature of the specimen, for example, pus or urine
Date and time at which the specimen was obtained
Antibiotic therapy (type, route, dose, frequency of administration, length of course and if completed)

Clinical details: to include relevant points about the patient's symptoms: pain, pyrexia, dysuria or wound soreness, as well as the primary diagnosis, and anti-inflammatory drugs

---

Laboratory Procedures

The time at which the specimen reaches the laboratory reception desk is recorded with details of the patient's name, age, ward and the site from which the specimen was obtained. Specimens are sorted according to the laboratory bench at which they will receive immediate attention; the steps taken during diagnostic microbiological examination are outlined below:

(1) examination of a direct film of the material under the microscope and Gram-staining,
(2) inoculation onto suitable culture media and incubation overnight at 37 °C,
(3) examination of any microorganisms that have grown, counting, identification and, in the case of bacteria, testing for antibiotic sensitivity.

Results are recorded on the microbiology request form by the technician, but in many departments the microbiologist will look at the forms and sign them, perhaps adding comments about suitable treatment before they are returned to the ward. Urgent or unexpected findings may be telephoned before the results are sent. Each of the stages outlined above is examined in further detail, with descriptions of some of the more common microbiological tests.

Morphology and Staining

The morphological features of an animal, plant or microorganism refer to its size, shape and general appearance, and they will be described during the initial microscopic examination. Rays from the light source of an ordinary microscope shine through microorganisms, so in order to visualise them it is necessary to spread a thin film of material on to a glass slide and use stains or dyes to add colour, and help to classify the bacteria. The most frequently used staining method is the one developed in 1884 by the Danish bacteriologist, Hans Christian Gram. The significance of *Gram-staining* has already been indicated in Chapter 1. The stain differentiates bacteria into two broad groups according to the structure of their cell walls. Stages in Gram-staining are outlined below.

(1) A thin film of the specimen is spread over the

surface of a microscope slide and passed through the hot flame of a bunsen burner to kill ('fix') the bacteria.
(2) The film is then covered with a solution of gentian violet dye, which is washed away quickly with running water to prevent overcoloration.
(3) The slide is flooded with a solution of iodine. This acts as a mordant, helping the gentian violet to stain intensely, but it is not left in contact with the cells for more than a few seconds. Examination of the material at this stage would reveal all the bacteria to be stained dark purple, irrespective of their Gram-staining properties.
(4) The slide is next washed with ethanol, an alcohol that will decolourise some of the bacteria.
(5) The slide is rinsed with water and covered with a red dye called safranin.
(6) After a final rinse the specimen is blotted dry, covered with a coverslip and is ready to be placed under the microscope. Bacteria which have retained the purple colour of the gentian violet are said to be Gram-positive. In the remaining, Gram-negative bacteria, the alcohol washes away the gentian violet and the cell walls remain colourless but for the addition of safranin, which makes them red.

The *acid-fast staining* method is used specifically to identify *Mycobacterium*, a genus which includes the bacteria causing tuberculosis and leprosy.

(1) After the film has been fixed it is treated with a red dye called carbofuchsin.
(2) It is then dried in the flame of a bunsen burner.
(3) The film is rinsed with water, and if it were examined at this stage all the bacteria would appear red.
(4) Alcohol is applied to decolourise all but the 'acid-fast' *Mycobacterium tuberculosis* or *M.leprae*.
(5) Methylene blue is applied as a counterstain, which is taken up by the non-acid-fast bacteria.

A number of special stains are occasionally used to help identify particular morphological structures where confirmation of their presence would constitute a valuable diagnostic acid. Particular staining techniques are available to show whether flagella, capsules or spores are present.

Inoculation and Incubation

Inoculation is a laboratory procedure in which microorganisms are transferred to a suitable culture medium. The procedure is an aseptic one, to avoid the growth of unwanted contaminants. The medium is sterilised in batches ready for use and the microorganisms are transferred onto it via the tip of a wire loop that has been held in the flame of a bunsen burner for a few seconds, then allowed to cool.

The medium is incubated at 37 °C, the optimal temperature for the growth of most microorganisms of medical significance. The length of time before growth appears is variable, depending on the type of microorganisms present and the suitability of the culture medium. Many different kinds of media are available and they are very important in diagnostic microbiology. Basic culture medium is a nutrient broth, a clear infusion reminiscent of soup. It is kept in sterile bottles, into which bacteria may be inoculated.

However, solid culture media are also used very extensively in the laboratory. To make them, nutrient broth is mixed with molten agar, an inert polysaccharide substance obtained from seaweed. Agar melts rapidly at about the same temperature as boiling water and in the laboratory it is usually maintained in its molten state in warm water baths. It solidifies rapidly at 40 °C, a temperature that does not damage bacteria. Molten agar is generally mixed with medium and poured either into flat petri dishes with closefitting lids, or into test tubes that are stoppered and allowed to cool at an angle, to form 'slopes' (Fig. 10.3).

When an inoculating loop is swept over the surface of solid agar, the cells of the individual bacteria separate, and after they have been incubated each individual cell or small groups of cells will give rise to a colony. All the bacteria which make up a particular colony will, of course, be of the same type. Bacteria are unable to digest agar, only the nutrient broth, so the colonies remain separated from one another (Fig. 10.4).

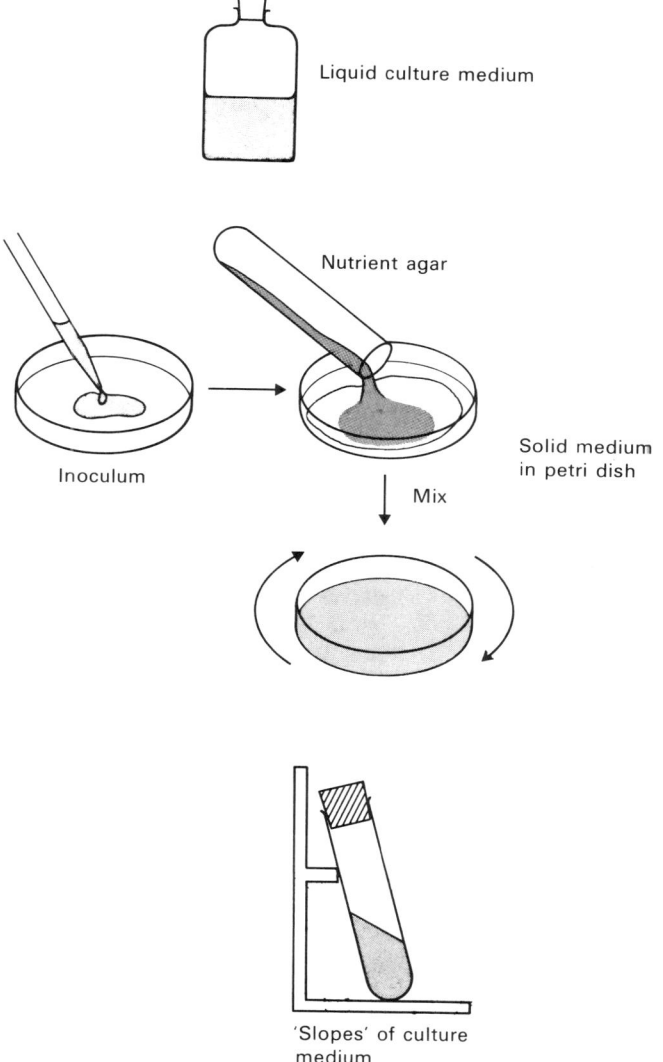

Fig. 10.3 Culture media.

The size of a colony will vary from 0.1 mm to 0.4 mm; most are easily visible to the naked eye, so the number present may be counted.

Their shape, colour, texture and adherence to the medium for a particular bacterial species remain constant, hence colony formation is a valuable diagnostic tool. Some bacteria, like *Proteus*, which are flagellated and highly motile, spread over the surface of the culture medium rather than remaining in discrete colonies. *Staphylococcus aureus* is identified by the golden colour of its colonies on solid agar, *Staphylococcus epidermidis* by its white colour.

In Chapter 1 it was pointed out that some bacteria are undemanding in their growth requirements, while others are exacting or 'fastidious'. Nutrient broth may therefore be an adequate culture medium for some bacteria, but not for others. A few, like *Treponema pallidum* and *Mycobacterium leprae*, will *never* grow outside the tissues of a living host and cannot, strictly, be regarded as having fulfilled Koch's postulates (see Chapter 2,

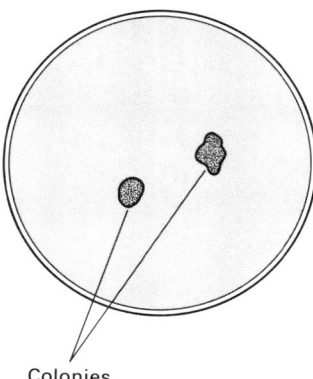

Fig. 10.4 Bacterial colonies growing separately on agar.

p. 37). Selective and differential media are of diagnostic importance and may be used to suppress the growth of particular bacteria, while encouraging the growth of more fastidious ones. *Salmonella typhi*, which causes typhoid, may be selected by culturing faeces on agar to which bismuth sulphate has been added. Sabouraud's glucose agar is used to isolate fungi while suppressing the growth of competitive bacteria; dyes like crystal violet and methylene blue inhibit Gram-positive bacteria. Blood agar is used to identify bacteria like the beta-haemolytic streptococcus, which can destroy red blood cells. If bacteria of this type are present, their colonies on the surface of the agar will be surrounded by a clear halo. MaConkey agar contains bile salts and crystal violet dye, to which lactose may be added; the bile salts promote the growth of intestinal pathogens such as *Salmonella* and *Shigella*, while the crystal violet inhibits the growth of Gram-positive bacteria. The addition of lactose allows differentiation of *Salmonella* and *Shigella*, since one can metabolise it while the other cannot.

A chemically defined medium is one in which the precise chemical composition is known. In practice, most bacteria and fungi are routinely cultured on complex media, where the exact chemical composition may vary a little between one batch and the next, depending on the range of nutrients (plasma, serum, polypeptides, whole blood) that have been added. Some culture media are made in the laboratory, others are purchased from commercial suppliers.

Moisture, pH and the presence or absence of oxygen are other critical factors that influence bacterial growth (see Chapter 1). Strict anaerobes will only grow in a medium from which oxygen has been excluded (Fig. 10.5). The inoculated petri dishes are stacked inside jars and the air is withdrawn and replaced with hydrogen. The jar must remain tightly sealed while it is incubated.

Specimens of urine, pus and other infected bodily fluids frequently contain more than one species or strain of microorganism. These are said to be 'mixed'. Inoculation onto a solid medium will produce several, visibly different colonies. To obtain pure cultures, a few cells from each colony must be inoculated onto a different culture plate and incubated again. Pure cultures may be examined in greater detail. Sometimes a strain that has not grown well in mixed culture may be transferred to an 'enrichment' culture, where its growth may be enhanced by the addition of further supplements.

Antibiotic Sensitivity

Ability to tolerate different antibiotics can vary within a particular bacterial species: for example, some strains of *Staphylococcus aureus* are able to grow in the presence of penicillin, while others are not. The explanation for this phenomenon was described in Chapter 1 (p. 12).

In the laboratory, bacteria which have been isolated and grown in pure culture are exposed to a range of different antibiotics in order to determine their sensitivity patterns, a very important point when deciding how to treat a particular infection. However, the drug of choice will always take into consideration the condition of the patient as well as bacterial sensitivity. For instance, gentamicin is not a suitable antibiotic for patients who have a history of renal impairment, because it is nephrotoxic, so the blood levels of this antibiotic must always be carefully monitored. Tetracyclines should not be given to pregnant women because of their teratogenic properties. Some patients are allergic to penicillin and alternative therapy must be found. Case study 10.1 showed that simply because antibiotic sensitivity patterns need to be monitored, antibiotic treatment is not necessarily desirable. Sensitivity patterns may be used to

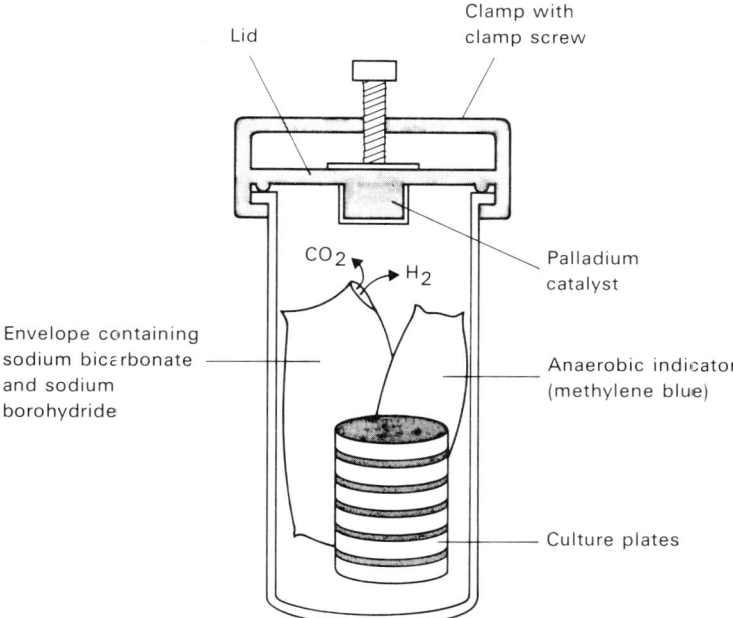

Fig. 10.5 Anaerobic culture technique.

identify strains of bacteria to exclude or demonstrate instances of cross-infection.

Serology

Antigen–antibody reactions and their role in defending the tissues of the host, were discussed in Chapter 7. These reactions can also take place outside the body (*in vitro*) and they are used extensively to diagnose disease. The branch of immunology concerned with *in vitro* antigen–antibody reactions is called serology. Serological tests can be performed quickly and offer a high degree of sensitivity and specificity, and several different tests are employed:

- agglutination reactions,
- precipitation reactions,
- complement fixation reactions,
- neutralisation reactions,
- immunofluorescence techniques.

Agglutination Reactions

Agglutination reactions occur between high molecular weight antigens bound to the cell surface of the bacteria and antibodies in solution. Combination of antigen and antibody results in cells becoming clumped together, hence the term agglutination. This forms the basis of the Widal test for typhoid; serum from a patient who has typhoid contains specific antibodies that will agglutinate with cells of *Salmonella typhi* if the two are allowed to mix.

Agglutination reactions can be used to estimate the concentration of antibody present in the serum taken from a patient. An increase in the titre of antibody to a particular microorganism during the course of disease strongly indicates that this microorganism is the causative agent.

Antibody titre is determined by adding a suspension of cells (carrying the antigens on their surfaces) to a series of test tubes, each containing a different solution of serum. The test tubes are incubated, then the greatest dilution of serum able to demonstrate an agglutination reaction is identified. The titre will be the reciprocal of this dilution; if, for example, there is a visible agglutination in a dilution of 1:160, but none in a dilution of 1:320, then the titre is taken as 160.

Haemagglutination reactions are those which involve red blood cells, and include blood grouping tests (ABO system, rhesus factor), as well as diagnosis of infectious agents.

The *Paul Bunnell test* for infectious mononucleosis (glandular fever) is a haemagglutination test. In humans this disease promotes the formation of an antibody that can agglutinate the red blood cells (erythrocytes) of sheep (a heterophilic antibody). The test is valuable because it is quite specific for infectious mononucleosis.

Precipitation Reactions

Precipitation reactions occur when low molecular weight antigens react with antibodies such as IgG or IgM. Unlike the antigens which can agglutinate, those which take part in precipitation reactions are soluble. Combination of these antigens and antibodies will result in the formation of large, interlocking aggregates that then precipitate from solution. The success of the test depends on mixing the antigen and antibody in the correct ratio; an excess of either will upset the balance and interfere with results.

In the precipitation ring test, serum containing specific antibody is added to a capillary tube and soluble antigen layered carefully on to its surface. A positive reaction is indicated by the appearance of a white ring of precipitation at the interface of the two solutions. This type of test has been used in the grouping of streptococci.

Precipitation reactions can also be performed on solid agar; they are then known as *immunodiffusion tests*. Exotoxin production by isolates of *Corynebacterium diphtheriae* has been examined in this way (Elek test).

Complement Fixation Tests

The function of 'complement' is to attack and destroy antigens (see Chapter 7). In the majority of antigen–antibody reactions, the complement is used up completely ('fixed'). Hence the process of complement fixation can be used to detect the presence of antibody.

The *Wasserman reaction*, formerly used in the diagnosis of syphilis, was a complement fixation reaction. It has now been replaced by the *VDRL test* (Venereal Disease Research Laboratory).

Complement fixation tests are performed in two stages. The serum from the patient is first heated to 56 °C for 30 minutes so that any complement which it contains is destroyed. The antibody to be tested can withstand this treatment. The serum is then mixed with a specific amount of known antigen and fresh complement from a laboratory animal. This mixture is incubated for 30 minutes, but the antigen–antibody reaction cannot immediately be visualised because only very dilute concentrates of both are used. An indicator system must be employed to determine whether the complement has remained free or become fixed. This forms the second part of the test. The indicator system consists of red blood cells obtained from a sheep (sheep erythrocyte cells) and specific antibodies to them. The combination of these with complement results in lysis of the red blood cells, and a visible colour change is therefore produced. If complement has been fixed during the first part of the test, it is not available to cause haemolysis, and a positive result with no colour change will follow. Unfixed complement will also provoke colour change. The test is quantitative, because the degree of haemolysis will indicate the amount of unfixed complement and therefore the amount of antibody present.

Neutralisation Reaction

In a neutralisation reaction the toxic effects of an exotoxin are eliminated by the action of a specific antibody. Neutralisation reactions were first observed in 1890, when two researchers, Emil von Behring and Shibasaburo Kitzato described an immune response that could neutralise the toxins produced by *Clostridium tetani*. They coined the term *antitoxin* for the neutralising substance present in the serum. Antitoxins are now defined as specific antibodies synthesised by host tissues in response to bacterial exotoxin. An antitoxin exerts its effects by combination with the toxin, so that the antigenic determinants on the toxin responsible for cell damage are inactivated.

Neutralisation reactions form the basis of the *Dick test* for scarlet fever and the *Schick test*, which determines the extent of an individual's immunity to diphtheria. A small quantity of diphtheria exotoxin is inoculated under the skin: if sufficient antitoxin is present, the exotoxin is neutralised and there is no reaction; if too little exotoxin is present to stimulate neutralisation, it will damage the skin at the point of entry, causing inflammation. Immunity to diphtheria is therefore unsatisfactory. These tests are seldom used today, but neutralisation tests have now been developed for the diagnosis of viral infections.

When a virus invades a cell, neutralising antibodies are produced by the host. They bind to sites on the surface of the virus and may prevent its successful attachment. The ability of a particular virus to damage the host cells, and detection of neutralising antibodies can be examined in tissue culture.

Immunofluorescence Techniques

Fluorescent antibody (FA) techniques are used to identify microorganisms present in clinical specimens, or to detect the presence of specific antibody in serum after it has been exposed to a pathogen. Fluorescent dyes are combined with the antibodies so that their presence can be detected by the reaction when they have been exposed to ultraviolet light.

The identity of a microorganism is determined by direct fluorescent antibody tests. The specimen that contains the antigen to be identified is put onto a glass slide and the fluorescent antibody is added. Incubation then takes place. The slide is washed to remove any excess unbound antibody and examined under the ultraviolet light microscope.

In indirect fluorescent antibody tests, used to detect the presence of specific antibody in serum, a known antigen must be placed on to the glass slide. The serum itself is then added, and if antibody specific to the antigen is present, they will react to form a complex. In order to visualise this reaction, fluorescent-labelled human gammaglobulin antibody is added to the slide. After incubation and washing away the excess antibody, the slide is ready for examination. If the known antigen is fluorescent, then its specific antibody must have been present. This is the basis of the *fluorescent treponemal antibody (FTA) test* for syphilis. *Neisseria*, *Haemophilus*, group A streptococcus and *Bacteroides fragilis* can all be identified by direct immunofluorescence. The Epstein-Barr (EB) virus, and those responsible for herpes and rubella can be identified by indirect immunofluorescence.

Phage Typing

The nature of bacteriophages was explained in Chapter 1. They are small viruses which attack bacteria and they usually destroy particular bacterial strains. A drop of medium containing phage particles on a plate seeded with sensitive bacteria will show colourless areas where the bacteria have been destroyed following a suitable period of incubation. This provides yet another method of identifying bacteria when outbreaks of cross-infection are traced.

Ordinary hospital laboratories do not have facilities for phage typing, and samples must be sent to a reference laboratory. Strains of *Staphylococcus* can be identified by phage typing, and outbreaks of cross-infection caused by *Staph. aureus* have been traced using this method.

The diagnostic microbiology tests described have followed one another in an increasing level of complexity and sophistication. Testing for sensitivity takes place routinely in the smallest department, but phage typing is the tool of only a very specialist laboratory. However, the range of diagnostic tests that can be performed in laboratories with limited conventional facilities and even in the surgery of a general practitioner are now expanding rapidly. Chemical engineers have developed miniature kits that contain all the materials necessary to perform a wide variety of standard tests. The success of these still depends on the technique of the person who performs the test. In a surgery, this may well be the practice nurse.

INTERPRETING THE RESULTS OF MICROBIOLOGICAL TESTS

Microbiology test results require interpretation. Technically, this is of course the duty of the doctor, but nurses are often puzzled because a particular course of action has been decided by the clinician or recommended by the microbiologist. Moreover, the choice of topical treatment for a chronic wound such as a pressure sore is generally left to the nursing staff (see David *et al.*, 1983). The type of specimen which a nurse most frequently has to collect is undoubtedly urine, but the interpretation of the findings seems to cause some of the greatest difficulty (Gould, 1985b).

Urine Tests

If a patient has developed a urinary tract infection, the urine will appear cloudy due to the presence of white blood cells, or it may even contain frank blood. However, the dark colour of extremely concentrated urine may obscure these signs. If the patient does not have an indwelling catheter he may complain of frequency and dysuria. A catheterised patient may be irritated by the catheter and continually feel the urge to micturate despite its presence. A patient who is confused may begin to pull the catheter and even succeed in disconnecting it. Urinary tract infections should always be suspected when a disoriented patient suddenly becomes restless, or when a previously continent patient has episodes of incontinence.

Infected urine has an offensive odour reminiscent of fish; *Pseudomonas* urinary tract infections are particularly troublesome in this respect. The patient often becomes pyrexial, although elderly people and neonates generally do not develop raised temperatures despite infection.

A genuine urinary tract infection will be accompanied by an inflammatory response, but unlike inflammation in the superficial tissues it is not directly visible, and can only be detected by microscopic examination of the urine.

Sometimes urine that has collected in a drainage bag will present the dark, concentrated appearance and malodour associated with infection, not because infection has actually become established, but because bacteria have colonised the drainage system. There is no actual infection because the bacteria have not yet invaded the bladder, and no inflammatory response, so no white blood cells will be seen. The bacteriologist may recommend irrigation with a disinfectant solution (chlorhexidine or noxythiolin), or changing the catheter and drainage system rather than antibiotic therapy (see Chapter 8). However, colonisation of the drainage bag may lead to the migration of bacteria up the catheter and into the bladder. Hence it is vital to monitor the urine of all catheterised patients for bacteriuria (see case study 10.1, p. 164, and to obtain specimens by aspirating freshly passed urine from the special sleeve positioned on the drainage tubing, not from the drainage bag.

Fortunately, it is possible from the findings in the laboratory to distinguish between the presence of bacteria due to genuine infection or colonisation and contamination. If the infection is genuine, then it is likely that a single kind of microorganism will be present in the urine in large numbers. Most laboratories consider that a bacterial count of 10^5 bacteria per ml of urine is indicative of active infection. If a mixed growth consisting of many different types of bacteria is found on the initial microscopic examination, contamination when the specimen was obtained, or colonisation is more likely to explain their presence, especially if the total number of each is very small.

The inflammatory response is characterised by the appearance of large numbers of white blood cells in the urine. The laboratory technician will quantify the number that he sees when he examines the specimen after Gram-staining (Fig. 10.6). Absence of white blood cells and mixed, low bacterial counts are highly indicative either of contamination or colonisation.

A midstream specimen is likely to be contaminated if the urethral meatus was not adequately cleansed before collection. This will be apparent since the number of epithelial cells in the specimen will then be much higher, a point that the technician will comment upon.

Misunderstandings about microbiology investigations can have serious consequences; this is illustrated by case study 10.5.

People often perceive what they would like to believe; in an emergency they may equally read into a situation what they would most *dislike* because it is uppermost in their mind. Case study 10.5, which took place in a small hospital only a few years ago, illustrates the need for specialist infection control advice.

SUMMARY

Nurses and doctors who work in particular specialities themselves (special baby care, dialysis or drug dependency units) may fully appreciate the *particular* infection control problems that they encounter every day. With the training that they receive as

SURNAME	FIRST NAME	~~MR~~.MRS.~~MISS~~	DATE COLLECTED	TIME COLLECTED
Mattews	Susan		20./02./1987	
DATE OF BIRTH	AGE IN YEARS	UNIT NO./HOSP.		A.M./~~P.M.~~
20. 6. 1912	75	XY 13407	DESTINATION OF REPORT	LAB. REF.
CONSULTANT		WARD		
Mr Jones		Gabriel Ward	Bacteriology	
INVESTIGATION REQUIRED	NATURE OF SPECIMEN		SIGNED	DATE
Microscopy, culture + sensitivity	CSU		H Jones	20/02/1987

RELEVANT CLINICAL & OTHER DETAILS

Cerebrovascular accident
1. 12. 86 catheterised for
intractable urinary
incontinence 10. 2. 87
Urine offensive and
dark, with debris

Is patient on anti-bacterial drugs? ~~Yes~~/No

During previous week? ~~Yes~~/No

If yes, give details of treatment below:

RESULT

WBC + + +
Epithelial cells +
E. coli 10⁵/ml.

CLINICAL MICROBIOLOGY J.B. Cook bacteriologist

Fig. 10.6 Specimen bacteriology form to show required information and typical result of a patient with urinary tract infection.

Case study 10.5

An elderly lady was admitted to a geriatric rehabilitation ward after falling at home. She was progressing well when, 7 days after admission, she developed profuse diarrhoea and abdominal pain. No other patients on the ward were affected. In view of this, the infection control team considered a diagnosis of food poisoning unlikely. They supported their argument by pointing out to the clinician that the patient had eaten nothing but food from the hospital kitchen for a week, that she had been in hospital for longer than the incubation period for most gastrointestinal pathogens (incubation for *Salmonella* is about 3 days), and that she was taking oral iron preparations, which are often associated with episodes of gastrointestinal upset. There was, therefore, insufficient evidence to merit isolating the patient, but anyway a stool specimen was sent to the laboratory.

The incident took place on the Friday evening before a bank holiday weekend. The infection control nurse visited the ward to explain the decisions reached between the infection control team and the consultant in charge of the case. She emphasised the lack of evidence in support of food poisoning, but reminded the staff about the importance of good hand hygiene. She noticed that the patient no longer had diarrhoea, and that although a little disoriented she was continent, and with a little reminding she was able to take care of her own hygiene needs adequately.

The microbiology report arrived on the ward the next morning. The busy staff nurse in charge glancing at it quickly saw the words '*Salmonella* isolated' and hastily informed the very junior house officer and the senior nurse in charge of the hospital. The news was particularly unwelcome to the senior nurse, who knew that too few staff had been allocated to the ward over the weekend to support the extra demands of isolation nursing. She was reluctant to contact an agency because of the added fee over the bank holiday, but had no other choice. She was also concerned that a period of confinement might be damaging to a patient who was already somewhat confused and only just beginning to settle down in her new environment.

In the ward, the nurses instituted isolation procedures as best they could in the only cubicle available. A very noisy patient had to be moved out into the main ward area, causing a certain amount of disruption. Further problems resulted when the family of the isolated patient arrived. They had been suspicious of the ward policy to mobilise patients and promote independence when their elderly mother had first been admitted, but within the last few days they had been favourably impressed with her improvement, and had hoped that as soon as the diarrhoea had settled she might be discharged into a private nursing home. Now they were disturbed to find her unhappily incarcerated in a tiny room complete with a commode in the corner, and all the regalia of isolation nursing to prevent contact spread. Their faith in the hospital suffered a dramatic decline when they were told that their mother had apparently developed food poisoning while in its care, and they were resentful that their plan to move her to a nursing home had been postponed indefinitely.

The agency nurse who arrived with the new shift at lunch time was allocated to the care of the isolated patient. She introduced herself, organised the room in a more suitable way, and then decided that since the patient was resting after her meal, she would familiarise herself with the casenotes. She decided to file the recent microbiology report and was mystified when she read 'Loose, dark brown stool received. No *Salmonella* isolated.'

part of their work, they usually learn to cope very well. However, when unusual problems develop they need advice. The national health service is now committed to a policy of improved patient care through increased efficiency. The services of the infection control team are vital if these objectives are to be achieved, and all nurses, both in hospital and in the community, should know when to ask for help and how to participate in the smooth running of the microbiology department, so that they get the best possible results for their patients out of that service.

References

Abbott, J. D. *et al.* (1980). *Salmonella* infections in hospital. A report from the Public Health Laboratory Salmonella Subcommittee. *Journal of Hospital Infection*, **1**: 307–314.

Ayton, M. (1981). An outbreak of streptococcal infection in a childrens' ward. *Nursing Times: Journal of Infection Control Nursing Supplement*, **77 (10)**: 13–15.

Coleman, D. (1984). Simultaneous outbreaks of infection due to *Serratia marcescans* in a general hospital. *Journal of Hospital Infection*, **5**: 270–282.

Cruikshank, J. G. (1984). Investigation of *Salmonella* outbreaks in hospital. *Journal of Hospital Infection*, **5**: 241–243.

David, J. *et al.* (1983). An investigation of the care of patients with established pressure sores. *Report of the Northwick Park Nursing Practice Unit*.

Dixon, C. M., Kolyvas, E. (1984). The generation and utilisation of bacteriology information by members of the health care team. *Journal of Hospital Infection*, **5**: 63–68.

Gerards, L. J. (1984). An outbreak of gastroenteritis due to *E.coli* 0146 H6 in a neonatal department. *Journal of Hygiene*, **5**: 283–288.

Gould, D. J. (1985a). Isolation procedures in one health district. *Nursing Times Occasional Paper*, **81 (7)**: 47–50.

Gould, D. J. (1985b). Management of indwelling urethral catheters. *Nursing Mirror*, **161 (10)**: 17–20.

Hill, S. F., Ferguson, D. (1984). Multiple resistant *Staphylococcus aureus* (bacteriophage type 90) in a special baby care unit. *Journal of Hospital Infection*, **5**: 56–62.

Horan, M. A. (1984). Outbreak of *Shigella sonnei* dysentry on a geriatric assessment ward. *Journal of Hospital Infection*, **5**: 210–212.

Ministry of Health (1959). *Staphylococcal Infections in Hospitals*. HMSO, London.

Schaeffner, W. (1984). Priorities in infection control: the impact of new technology. *Journal of Hospital Infection*, **5**: 1–5.

Tyman, S. (1986). Protecting the carers. *Nursing Times*, **82 (2)**: 41–42.

Chapter 11

Infection: Education and Counselling

INTRODUCTION

Infection is frightening. In modern western society it has become associated with uncleanliness. Emphasis is placed upon clean clothes, and clean homes; deodorised bodies are regarded as desirable and socially acceptable. Sales of deodorants have never been higher; manufacturers advertise detergents that wash whitest and household disinfectants guaranteed to destroy all known 'germs'. In supermarkets food products are inevitably labelled with expiry dates, assuring the consumer that they are fresh and wholesome. Very few homes lack a refrigerator.

Infection is regarded as dirty and dangerous. The practice of isolating people with infectious diseases described in Chapter 2 shows how, for centuries, the general public has feared infection. Its modern equivalent is illustrated by the treatment of AIDS in the media, and the way in which the hepatitis B carrier is too often treated in hospital.

Faced with the threat of infection, many people cease to behave rationally. They instinctively want the 'strongest' (most potent) disinfectant, to use it undiluted, irrespective of pharmaceutical instructions and the evidence discussed in Chapter 5 to show that the most concentrated form of a disinfectant may not be the most effective. Such behaviour is not just the prerogative of members of the general public. Hospital staff are not immune from fears associated with infection. Research by Gould (1985) (see Chapter 6) has indicated that qualified nurses and those in training preferred to confine their infected patients to single rooms, behind closed doors, irrespective of their condition or the way in which the causative agent was spread. Even when the irrational nature of their behaviour was discussed, they remained difficult to convince.

Fear of infection may be regarded as an instinctive, adaptive response, because it helps the individual avoid exposure to a source of potential danger. However, a great many of the infections encountered in ordinary hospitals today are of little danger to healthy people, and with intelligent precautions based on scientific principles rather than tradition, the risk attached to these and to most other infectious conditions is small. Anxiety is of little practical value to nurses who encounter infection as an everyday part of their working lives, because they need to provide skilled care and support for their patients.

Nurses need to have a sound understanding of basic microbiological principles in order to protect:

- patients,
- visitors,
- staff (including themselves),
- the hospital environment.

Knowledge is of no practical value unless it can be translated into practice, and to achieve this effective communication must take place. The nurse is in the best position to counsel and provide information for other people because she is the coordinator of patient care, and provides a 24 hour service on the ward.

The patient who has developed an infection has a right to know how this will affect his progress, and the sanctions that may be placed on him during his stay in hospital and when he goes home. His wife is entitled to learn about any precautions that will be needed before she visits and well before her husband is discharged. Dieticians, physiotherapists and other professionals need to know how restrictions placed upon the patient should alter his treatment and precautions for their safety. Domestic staff who clean the patient's room must feel confident not only that they are protected, but that their activities will not spread infection to other areas that they clean, although patient confidentiality means that they will not be told the precise diagnosis, only how the infection is spread. It is the nurse's duty to ensure that the appropriate equipment is available, and sometimes special hospital services arranged.

This chapter is concerned with the nurse's role in providing help and advice to those who are either at risk of developing infection, or who already have an established infection. To do this effectively, nurses must draw on their knowledge of:

- counselling,
- teaching,
- health education skills.

All these topics are dealt with separately in a number of excellent texts, and a selection of these can be found in the reading list at the end of the chapter. The material presented here is not intended to be comprehensive or exhaustive; it should be viewed as an attempt to apply some of the existing literature to a group of patients whose needs have often been overlooked in the past. To do this, reference will be made to the framework of stress introduced in Chapter 7.

THE ROLE OF COUNSELLING IN STRESS AND INFECTION

In Chapter 7, the response of the body to infection was introduced by describing the nature of stress, and pointing out that exposure to infection carries all the hallmarks of exposure to a stressful stimulus. Whether or not the body's defence mechanisms succeed in fighting off the infection and avoiding the further stress of established disease will depend on individual circumstances, including the nature of the pathogen, and factors operating within the individual. These may be physical, psychological, or an interaction between the two.

Reactions to stress and the coping mechanisms to deal with it are highly individual. Much depends upon individual perception. This is likely to be influenced by:

- previous experience,
- personality,
- physical and psychological status.

Race, culture, intellect, home circumstances including finance and responsibilities all play a part. The support that can be provided by family, friends or significant others may help to allay the stressful nature of illness and recovery. The quality of reassurance and practical help that can be supplied by health professionals will be of major importance.

Wilson-Barnett (1980), who has conducted extensive research into the stressful nature of hospitalisation, believes that people who are already ill are particularly vulnerable to the effects of both acute and chronic stress. Any illness, whether an infection or not, is stressful. Those who work in hospital become socialised into accepting the discomforts and pain associated with illness, investigations and treatment as everday occurrences, but to the patient his illness is unique. Coping with it may need a lot of courage, even in the absence of complicating nosocomial infections or the sanctions of isolation.

From her numerous research studies, Wilson-Barnett has concluded that people in hospital need a good deal of adaptation to cope with the following stressors:

- unexpected events,
- unpleasant symptoms,
- loss of function,
- loneliness,
- unfamiliar surroundings and relationships,
- altered status and role.

The way in which a patient who requires isolation precautions may experience these can be illustrated by case study 11.1, which concerns Peter, a young man who was found to be a hepatitis B carrier.

Lazarus and Averill (1972) believe that anxiety is generated in patients when they do not understand their situation and cannot anticipate what is going to happen to them. Nurses can help to alleviate these feelings of helplessness by providing explanations in terms that the patient can understand. Wilson-Barnett describes strategies that may enable nurses to reduce the stressful experience of their patients, including:

(1) Preventing, or at least reducing, anxiety by giving information and explanations.
(2) Helping the individual to cope with his problem by providing suggestions for possible coping strategies and a supportive relationship to help reduce the stress of coping alone.

Case study 11.1

A sample of Peter's blood was screened for hepatitis B when he was admitted, and the results of the test became available on the same morning that he was scheduled to undergo laminectomy.

- Unexpected events
  (1) Peter was suddenly told by the nurse that he had an infectious condition carried in his blood, and that for the remainder of his stay in hospital he would be in a single room.
  (2) When Peter was taken to the anaesthetic room the anaesthetist wore disposable gloves to insert the intravenous needle into his vein, and placed a plastic square beneath his arm. Peter had had venepuncture performed on previous occasions, including 2 days before on admission to hospital, and none of these precautions had ever been taken.
- Unpleasant symptoms
  Peter's original infection with hepatitis B had been subclinical. He could remember no symptoms of nausea, upper abdominal pain or mild jaundice that may be associated with the acute infection. Postoperatively he was in pain. He had been told that he could ask for analgesia, but because he was alone in his room the opportunity to ask a nurse came less frequently than if he had been in his old place on the main ward.
- Loss of function
  Postoperatively Peter was nursed lying flat in bed, and the nurses helped him to roll from side to side. When he was allowed to mobilise, he was restricted to his room, and had to use the adjoining WC. Peter felt a keen loss of independence, not just because of his operation, but also because his activities were restricted to a small room and he could not take a bath.
- Loneliness
  When he was admitted to hospital, Peter missed his girlfriend and the company of his flatmates, although they visited each evening. There were other young men on the same ward, however, and before the operation Peter had made friends with them. Postoperatively he missed their companionship, especially in the early days when he was confined to bed. Alone Peter had more time to worry about his problems, especially whether he would be 'infectious forever'.
- Unfamiliar surroundings
  Admission to hospital and the prospect of surgery bring well-documented anxiety. As well as experiencing these, Peter was sent to theatre from his old bed in the main ward, but woke up in a single room that he had never seen before. The nurses wore aprons and disposable plastic gloves when they attended to his wound. The room contained equipment that he had not seen before, and the big disposal box for 'sharps' seemed especially prominent.
- Unfamiliar relationships
  Peter was asked not to allow his visitors to sit on the bed, or to have much close contact with him because he was 'infectious'. These restrictions seemed odd after his formerly close relationship with his girlfriend.
- Altered status and role
  Any formerly well person coming into hospital exchanges his previously healthy condition for the 'sick role' and loses his independence. Peter became more dependent upon the nurses than the average young man in his position, because he could not leave his room until the wound had healed and ceased to drain. All his meals were brought to him, and he had to request the ward telephone to be brought to his room. Items that he might otherwise have purchased from the hospital trolley shop had to be obtained by other people and brought to him. He had to contend with a view of himself as suddenly 'harmful' to others, whereas he had previously been unaware of his carrier status.

The feeling of being alone may be exacerbated for the patient isolated because of infection.

Very little systematic research has taken place into the effects of isolation for infectious conditions. Although there is a growing body of work describing the effects of sensory deprivation, this is probably more applicable to the severely handicapped and those nursed in the artificially constant atmosphere of the intensive care unit. Taylor (1982) points out that many people who might ordinarily prefer the privacy offered by a single room regard it as a prison once isolation is enforced. The use of facilities such as the ward telephone, hospital library and shop may be curtailed. Isolated patients may not see their nurses and doctors as frequently as patients for whom no elaborate gowning procedure is necessary, and nurses may feel less inclined to enter the room unless for a specific purpose. Under these circumstances, the patient's self-esteem may become very fragile.

The approach recommended by Wilson-Barnett implies that sick people may benefit if they are supported by information, and if the nurse responsible for planning their care has some appreciation of the skills acquired during counselling training.

'Patient counselling' and 'patient education' are closely related concepts (Stewart, 1983). Patient counselling is concerned with helping the patient to cope with his condition and treatment, while patient education seeks to help him understand his illness and treatment.

Before patients can either understand or cope with their situation, they must feel involved with the decisions taken by nurses and doctors on their behalf.

Cooperation cannot be expected until this has been achieved. Most nurses can remember incidents where a patient has not complied with them, and this happens quite often when isolation precautions are required. It is not always possible to get to the root of the problem and understand why the patient behaves as he does, but the nurse's relationship with him and his future compliance may be enhanced if they feel able to talk about what has happened. Sometimes there may be a relatively simple explanation. Case study 11.2 illustrates these points.

A few minutes of careful listening can make all the difference to the care that the nurse is able to give, but it is not meant to undervalue the help that professional counsellors provide. Many patients, including a large number who develop infectious illness, require counselling as a major part of their treatment, and the skills of a professional counsel-

---

Case study 11.2

Michael, a diabetic for many years, was 70 years old when he was admitted to hospital with peripheral vascular disease. A decision was taken to amputate his left leg, and after the operation Michael developed a wound infection. The causative organism was *Staphylococcus aureus*, resistant to most of the commonly used antibiotics.

Michael was transferred to a single room to prevent the multiresistant bacteria contaminating the other patients' immediate environment. His dressing was performed after all the others, and his nurse was not responsible for any other dressing. The wound was handled only when the nurse wore disposable plastic gloves, because the dressing was too cumbersome to be handled with forceps. Gloves and aprons were always worn inside Michael's room, to reduce bacterial contamination of the nurse's hands.

Staphylococcus aureus is not a respiratory pathogen, but it commonly inhabits the nasal passages as a commensal, and could be spread by sneezing, leading to infection in other patients' wounds. In the hospital to which Michael had been admitted there had been several cases of infection by staphylococci resistant to the same antibiotics. The infection control team advised masks to be worn in order to limit this avenue of spread.

Michael's nurse explained the need for the mask she wore in his room, and thought that Michael looked rather blank although he made no comment.

He seemed morose when she helped him with his bath, and later when she addressed him he stared out of the window as though he was deliberately ignoring her. The nurse repeated what she had said. Michael had been instructed to do exercises by the physiotherapist, and the nurse had reminded him to do them. Michael still looked away, and his face was expressionless.

When she was reporting Michael's condition to the ward sister, the nurse said that she thought he was reacting poorly to isolation and was becoming uncooperative. The sister was surprised; Michael had been in hospital for some time before his operation, and although he was a solitary man who had few visitors, he had always been friendly and courteous to the nurses. He complied well with the care planned for him, and had said that being in a single room would not worry him, as he would enjoy the peace. Reading was his chief pastime.

During the ward report, the physiotherapist came to see Michael. She had not been told that masks were to be worn, and did not receive this information because she saw that the nurses were busy. She met a very relieved patient indeed, who explained in a trembling voice how glad he was to talk to somebody without a mask – he had always been embarrassed about his impaired hearing, and had compensated by becoming a very competent lip reader.

lor may be valuable. However, the nurse needs to have some insight into the patient's problems if this is to be arranged.

The Royal College of Nursing has recognised counselling as part of the nurse's role. In a paper, published in 1978, the RCN defines counselling as: 'A process through which one person helps another by purposeful conversation in an understanding atmosphere'.

Implicit in this definition is the idea that the discussion must be structured, not aimless, so that when the nurse listens she does so actively. She is not just a passive vessel for the patient's anxieties. Not all communication is verbal; the nurse's posture, gestures and facial expression all convey meaning. This is particularly significant to someone who is deemed an infection risk to others, especially if he is isolated. Unwillingness to enter the room unless for a specific purpose, hurried withdrawal, and a reluctance to come near or touch the patient reinforces the feeling that he is 'unclean'. Communication may be hampered by the wearing of protective clothing, as case studies 11.1 and 11.2 above have shown. Redman (1981) points out that the nurse needs to know how the patient views his illness before she can help him. Key questions to ask the patient, developed from Redman's work, are shown in Table 11.1.

Table 11.1 Key Questions to Ask Before Commencing Patient Education (adapted from Redman, 1981)

(1) What do you think has caused your problem?
(2) Have you any idea why it started at the time it did?
(3) What effects do you think that your problem is having on *you*?
(4) How severe is your problem?
(5) Do you think your problem will be short-term or long-term?
(6) What kind of help do you think you should have?

In case study 11.1 Peter's nurse used Redman's framework to establish his understanding of being a hepatitis B carrier. His answers are shown below:

(1) Peter said that he had been told by the house officer that he had previously had an infectious condition of the blood, probably very mildly, so that he had not noticed many symptoms, but that this had left him a permanent carrier of the virus responsible. He might possibly infect other people, especially if they became contaminated with his blood.
(2) Peter had no idea when he might have been infected with the hepatitis B virus; he had never heard of this type of infection before.
(3) Peter thought that his hospital stay was a great deal more inconvenient because of the infection and he felt much lonelier in a single room.
(4) Peter did not think his problem was severe at the moment, just an inconvenience while he was in hospital, but he enlarged on this in response to the next question.
(5) Peter was concerned, because he had been told by the house officer that he might always carry the virus in his blood, and therefore always be infectious. He was concerned about his flatmates catching the infection from him when he left hospital, and about how his girlfriend would feel; they had been planning to get married the following summer. One of Peter's visiting friends had heard that hepatitis B was associated with drug addiction, and Peter, who had never taken drugs, planned not to tell his parents or workmates that he was a carrier, because he feared the stigma attached to this. He wondered how safely he could conceal his carrier status from other people.
(6) Peter wanted help to find out the extent to which his everyday activities would be affected by being a hepatitis B carrier when he left hospital.

Once Peter's nurse was aware in detail of his worries, she could provide him with information that would go a long way towards giving reassurance and confidence in preparation for his discharge.

In order to provide information and formulate a care plan, the nurse herself needed to know about Peter's condition. It was very important for the nurse responsible for planning Peter's care to appreciate the nature of his infection and its influence on other members of the health care team, as well as on Peter's family. Relevant information about hepatitis B can be found in Chapter 1.

Many episodes of hepatitis B present as subclinical infections, so the patient will be unable to tell when he was first infected. The symptoms are often vague: epigastric pain, nausea, vomiting, tiredness and malaise. If the patient is examined clinically during the acute stages of the illness, there might be signs of mild jaundice, with dark urine and pale stools. Many patients are ill for only a few days, however, and clinical examination never takes place. The chief factor that distinguishes hepatitis B from hepatitis A, which presents in much the same way, is that in about 10% of patients hepatitis B antigens remain in the bloodstream, so the individual becomes a carrier. Over the years, the number of antigens declines, and the patient becomes gradually less infectious. Since the incubation period of hepatitis B is lengthy (up to 160 days) the history taken from the patient is likely to be vague.

Hepatitis B was first recognised as a separate disease entity in the 1960s, when several people became acutely ill after they had received blood transfusions. A viral agent was found responsible, and today the blood of all donors is, of course, screened. In the early 1970s, several outbreaks of acute hepatitis B occurred in hospitals, chiefly in renal dialysis units. Several units were forced to close on a temporary basis, and there were some fatalities.

In recent years hepatitis B has not been implicated in such outbreaks, suggesting that a particularly virulent strain must have been at work in the 1970s. Today, the estimated mortality rate is about 1%, but the hazards attached to hepatitis B have lived on in the minds of nurses and doctors. While the fears of those who witnessed hepatitis B outbreaks in the 1970s are understandable, it is important not to allow these anxieties to become out of proportion. Many people who now work in hospitals have been indoctrinated with irrational fears that have damaged the quality of care they provide for their patients and prevented them establishing meaningful relationships.

When they are dealing with infected patients, nurses may feel that they have little to offer in terms of advice, especially if the infection was a nosocomial one, because under these circumstances the staff concerned may feel that they have 'failed'. Communicable diseases present a different problem. Even in a ward designated to care for infectious patients, diseases like typhoid and meningitis will be encountered sporadically. If the turnover of young, newly qualified staff on the ward is brisk, the number of nurses who have cared for patients with similar problems before may be limited.

Very little research has been conducted regarding the feelings of patients with communicable diseases, although the results of one preliminary study suggest that providing information and telling the patient honestly about the need for isolation seem to be helpful (Genvert, 1979). Bennett (1983), describing the special difficulties experienced by isolated patients, drew attention to the generally unpopular nature of this specialty, which results in poor staff-to-patient ratios. She also considered that a lack of sense of belonging to the life of the ward may cause the isolated patient to feel insecure. There is some evidence that patients nursed together on the same ward may derive support from one another (Wilson-Barnett, 1976). Bennett advocated the provision of written information to isolated patients, to help them understand the purpose behind segregation. She suggested that this should *support* verbal information rather than replace it, and provide a basis for discussion rather than a strict code of rules. Unfortunately, research has indicated that patients require information that is specific (Gould and Wilson-Barnett, 1985). It is difficult to envisage written material that could cover all the needs of patients who have different types of infectious disease, particularly when the mechanism of transmission and the severity of the infection are likely to vary considerably.

Redman's additional questions (Table 11.2) may be useful under these circumstances, to determine the psychosocial and cultural meaning of the illness to the patient. Case study 11.3 shows how these questions provided further information about a patient's feelings towards having shingles.

Table 11.2 Questions Which May Provide Helpful Information About the Patient's View of his Illness (adapted from Redman, 1981)

(1) What do you think your treatment should achieve for you?
(2) What have been your main problems as a result of the illness?
(3) What is your biggest worry in connection with the illness?

Case study 11.3

Jane, 60 years old and single, was treated with the antiviral agent acyclovir (see Chapter 2), and nursed in a single room because of the severe pain in her face associated with the herpetic lesions found in shingles. The exudate that escapes from these lesions contains virus particles, and is the means by which the infection is spread (see Chapter 6). Jane gave the following responses when the nurse asked her the questions shown in Table 11.2.

(1) She had been told by the house officer that the drug she was given should help to prevent the virus multiplying, and reduce the severity of her shingles. The painkillers she had been given had helped her to feel much better, particularly since they enabled her to sleep at night.
(2) Her main problem in connection with the illness had been leaving her elderly, infirm brother to cope on his own at home.
(3) She mentioned three worries in connection with the illness:
- she was upset at the thought of permanent disfigurement from the lesions;
- she was afraid that her frail elderly brother might catch the infection;
- she had heard from a friend that people often develop shingles when they have cancer, and she remembered the doctor asking her about her general health when she was admitted to hospital.

Some of Jane's problems might not have been immediately obvious to her nurse without this close questioning. Pride in one's appearance and the desire to look attractive do not necessarily alter with advancing years, especially when work or social life bring the individual into contact with other people (Webb, 1986). Older people may well suffer a change in body image and decreased self-esteem as a result of illness, and they may dread disfigurement; but they need encouragement to express their feelings, because in western society, preoccupation with appearance is largely seen as the province of the young. Jane had always taken trouble with her appearance, and she enjoyed a busy social life. Working in a shop meant that she was constantly in public view.

Practical help from the social services could be arranged to help Jane's brother, and her nurse was able to reassure her that she would no longer be infectious when she returned home, because the virus is spread only when the lesions are moist.

Previous experience, including interaction with other people influence the ways in which individuals react when they become ill. In Jane's case, remembering an old conversation with a friend had prompted considerable anxieties about her underlying health.

Jane's nurse could not 'solve' all her problems, because unsightly scars may persist for some time after herpes zoster infection, and the disease has often developed in people with some serious underlying health problems, in some cases malignancy. However, given time and encouragement, Jane was helped to explore her feelings, and could be reassured that shingles is by no means inevitably associated with cancer, and that contrary to public opinion cancer is *not* always fatal.

Research by nurses has shown that knowledge is one very important way of helping the individual to cope with the stress of illness and all the threatening events that accompany it. Some of the research studies that have generated these ideas were presented in Chapter 3. It is apparent from communications research that the counselling approach already discussed provides a more effective framework for helping patients than merely giving factual information (Ley, 1977). By providing facts, the nurse treats the patient as a passive object, but the two-way interaction of counselling seeks to involve the patient in his own care.

TYPE OF INFORMATION REQUIRED

The type of information required and the strategies employed to provide it must be geared to the individual needs of the patient and his physical and psychological status. Some people who have developed an infectious condition need explanations and reassurance, while for others new skills must be learnt (for example, the safe disposal of infected material), attitudes may need to be changed, and new behaviour learnt. Much will depend on:

- the severity of the infection,
- its mode of transmission,
- both the short-term and long-term restrictions placed on the individual (if any).

The more severe the infection, and the greater the number of restrictions (especially long-term) placed upon the individual, the greater the challenge presented to his coping mechanisms, and to the nurse helping to ensure that these are adequate.

A review of the literature related to general recovery from illness and patient teaching suggests that there is no general consensus of opinion about the best time to provide information in relation to the acute stage of the illness or recovery (Gould, 1984). This is largely because authors disagree to some extent about when exactly patients in hospital are likely to suffer most anxiety. However, there is evidence that hospital discharge is often unplanned (Turton and Wilson-Barnett, 1981), so that patients likely to experience long-term health problems return to the community with little time to make arrangements. There is a considerable body of evidence to suggest that patients and their families lack support and reassurance once the former have been discharged. This had prompted Webb (1983) to advocate that planning for discharge should begin as soon as possible, preferably on admission to hospital. She argues that the teaching process should parallel the steps of the nursing process, while Stewart (1983) propounds a model of counselling which shares the four stages common to the nursing process. The relationship between these models for teaching, counselling and the nursing process are shown in Table 11.3.

If the individual is faced with major long-term changes in lifestyle, or lasting disability as a consequence of infection, then it is evident that continuing support will be necessary when he goes home. Case study 11.4 illustrates this point.

Table 11.3 Models for Teaching, Counselling and the Nursing Process (after Stewart, 1983)

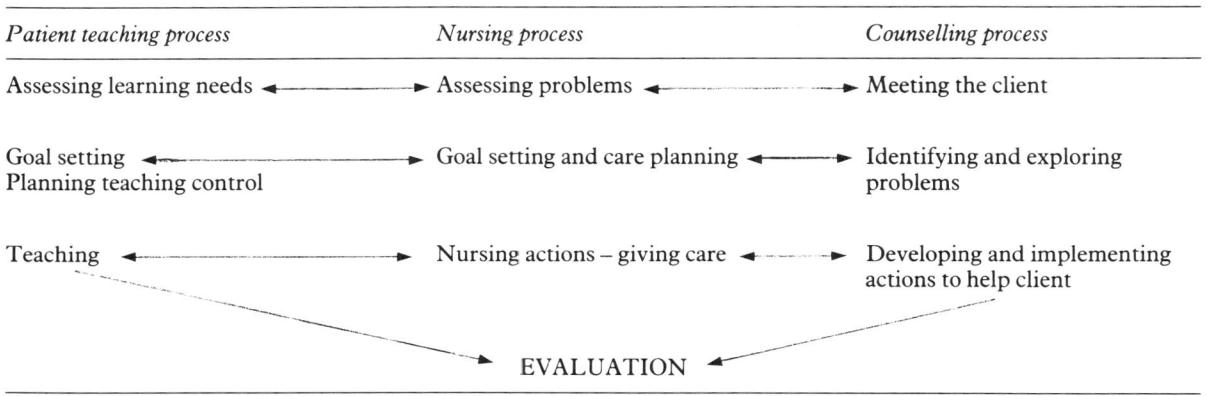

Case study 11.4

Larry was 35 when he came into hospital with a 6 month history of weight loss and poorly defined ill-health. He had suffered a series of chest infections, and was eventually admitted following an acute episode of shortness of breath. He had pneumonia, and the causative organism was found to be *Pneumocystis carinii*. There was evidence of other opportunistic infection, and once on the ward Larry soon developed a sore mouth and perianal lesions due to *Candida*. The type of infections that Larry had developed, his weight loss and lifestyle as a practising homosexual all pointed to a diagnosis of AIDS.

On the ward Larry's infections were successfully treated with a range of antibiotics and antifungal agents, while great care was taken to avoid unnecessary contamination of other patients and the environment with his blood and secretions. At first Larry was expectorating profusely, and required tracheal suction. Under these circumstances, the nurses wore masks, but when Larry's chest infection resolved, the use of masks was discontinued.

Although Larry was very ill when he first came into hospital, attempts were made from the beginning to establish his feelings about his newly diagnosed condition and to prepare for necessary long-term changes in his lifestyle. When the patient's lifestyle does not tie in with the expected norms of society (which may well be the view of the world held by the nurse) she may experience more difficulty, especially if she has to cope with unexpected emotions or feelings in herself.

In recent years, the arrival of patients with AIDS on the wards has drawn particular attention to the problems faced by the sick individual whose way of life is considered at best unconventional, and at worst deviant, and of the difficulties of health professionals who have never before had to examine their own reactions to these people. One of the first publications to help nurses explore their feelings about AIDS, and to provide care for affected patients and the people important to them, was written by members of a Working Party established by the Royal College of Nursing (see Chapter 1). The Working Party drew attention to the severe deficiencies in the ability of some nurses to meet the psychosocial needs of their patients. It was suggested that this is due in large measure to failure of basic nurse education to teach the essential skills required to develop interpersonal relationships. The problem presented by people with AIDS is really only the tip of the iceberg.

Happily in this particular case Larry had a partner of many years' standing, and their home was near the hospital. Larry's family lived in another town and he seldom communicated with them. He wanted his partner, Sean, to be regarded as his next of kin, and it was Sean who was involved in Larry's care and plans for the future.

Some of the many worries and problems about his future that Larry would encounter were discussed with his nurse: his health; his relationship with Sean; the restrictions placed on him by his infection; and his financial situation, since he was too weak to return to work. A few of his concerns have been highlighted below, with suggestions that helped him to face the crisis of developing a serious, long-term infectious condition.

- Larry was very much afraid that Sean might develop AIDS; they were sexual partners who shared the same house. Larry believed that he had acquired the virus the previous summer when he had taken a holiday in California. Sean had not accompanied him, and neither of them had had any other partners except on this occasion.

  It was explained to both men that the possibility of Sean also developing AIDS or lymphadenopathy could not be ruled out, and that in view of the long incubation period it could be months or years before they could be sure. On a more positive note, not everyone who encounters the virus succumbs to it, and Sean could do a lot by adopting a generally healthy lifestyle, and avoiding sex with many partners.

  It was pointed out that transmission of the HIV virus on cooking utensils, bed linen and crockery has never been proven, and that spread in saliva has virtually been ruled out. Sharing the same home, kitchen, and hugging and kissing should not place Sean at risk. If bedclothes became soiled with urine or faeces they should be washed at the highest possible temperature in the domestic washing machine. Sean had expressed a desire to nurse Larry at home if his condition deteriorated, so both men were told about the need to wipe up spilt bodily fluids with hypochlorite solution.

  Larry was still short of breath and unwell, but the nurse was careful to provide both men with information about safe sexual practices in case they should need it. Patients should not be left to seek this kind of help on their own initiative, for many will be too embarrassed to ask. The guidelines provided were those written by the Terrence Higgins Trust, a registered charity with headquarters in London responsible for much of the help and advice that people with AIDS and their friends have received. Many other services are provided and the nurse made sure that Larry and Sean had the address and telephone number of the Trust, and were further informed about the help that could be given to both of them.

- Larry was concerned that his general practitioner would be unwilling to provide treatment, and that home nursing by the district nursing service would be difficult to arrange because of the infectious nature of his condition. A letter had been sent to the general practitioner advising him of his patient's discharge and diagnosis. The district nurse attached to the practice visited the hospital at weekly intervals to be informed about the patients who would soon be discharged into her care. It was arranged for her to meet Larry and Sean, and reassure them that she had a realistic appreciation of the problems involved.

- Larry and Sean had a joint mortgage, and their financial affairs were closely linked. They regarded one another as next of kin, and Larry worried about how Sean would cope financially in the event of his death. This had been troubling both of them for some time, because they had heard of legal wrangles between the natural kin of other homosexuals and their partners in similar circumstances.

  The nurse encouraged both men to discuss this problem as openly as they could. Husbands and wives in the same position know that they must safeguard the spouse who will be left by putting their affairs in order and writing a will, however painful this may be. Larry decided that he would write a will, and soon after he left hospital arranged to see a solicitor who was willing to help.

Nurses using the nursing process, counselling and teaching patients may find their own needs brought to the surface. As the nurse gets to know her patients better it is inevitable that she will become more involved with them. Sometimes this experience can be unsettling, particularly when patients are isolated, as they may be more ready to confide in the nurse when she appears. This is illustrated in case study 11.5.

Nurses are often faced with difficult situations when they look after patients who have become infected. The reluctance of other members of staff to approach a patient in isolation helps to compound the problem. This is shown by case study 11.6.

HEALTH EDUCATION IN THE COMMUNITY

So far in this chapter, attention has been focused on the hospital, on the needs of people who have to cope with the problems of an established infection. But the community also contains large numbers of people who are at some risk of developing infection, and nurses and health visitors who work outside the hospital setting can do much to educate them about the importance of reducing these risks.

Health visitors and community nurses might argue that their teaching is most likely to be effective, because they visit people in the safety of their own homes, when they are not threatened by pain or the anxieties generated by hospital, and because they usually teach individuals or small groups, so that their approach can be tailored as circumstance dictates. Evidence from Chapter 2 suggests, however, that success may be difficult to achieve. A study by Bruce-Quay (1981) showed that when public and professional knowledge about the benefits of infant immunisation was enhanced, the rate of immunisation could be boosted to over 90%. As the experimental scheme was gradually withdrawn, the level declined slowly, suggesting a clear need to keep the levels of awareness in the community high. Redman (1981), in her discussion of patient teaching in hospital, pointed out that although the individual may be motivated to learn new behaviour in hospital, there is no guarantee that compliance will continue in the long term, and that different strategies for promoting this may be necessary.

Redman's suggestion is borne out by a study designed to teach school children about dental hygiene (Addy *et al.*, 1977). This sought to compare the effectiveness of different teaching strategies compared to the knowledge of a control group who received no educational input. On the whole, talks and discussions proved more effective than posters and leaflets, although all levels of knowledge showed decline after 3 months, pointing out the need for reinforcement. The importance of gearing health education according to intellect and social class was evident in this study, for some

---

Case study 11.5

Edward was a newly qualified staff nurse, just starting work on a medical ward when Patrick was admitted. Patrick, a young man the same age as Edward, had been a diabetic for several years, and was admitted into hospital because his blood sugar levels were difficult to control. He was also known to be a hepatitis B carrier. Patrick was self-caring and encouraged to mix with other patients on the ward, but he preferred to spend most of his time reading alone in his room. Edward was pleased that Patrick, who seemed to be such a solitary person, appeared to welcome his company.

One day Patrick mentioned that he had taken drugs in the past, and could still obtain them if he wished. Edward, who had seen the consequences of drug abuse among patients he had nursed, felt deeply shocked that Patrick might be involved in drug pushing and was concerned that Patrick had singled him out as the recipient of this information. He felt himself to be placed in a difficult position, because Patrick's notes made no mention of drug abuse. Edward's immediate impulse was to avoid Patrick, and because the latter tended to stay in his room, this was quite easy to do. However, the ward sister, returning from holiday, noticed that Edward was reluctant to approach Patrick, and asked him about it. At first Edward was reticent, but after the sister drew him out he felt able to mention his conversation with Patrick.

The sister helped Edward to see that Patrick's activities were only part of the problem; the rest was concerned with the way in which Edward had to come to terms with his feelings about Patrick. She pointed out that Edward did not have to approve of Patrick's behaviour in order to accept him, and that despite his own feelings about drug abuse, Edward might still be able to achieve much for Patrick by spending time with him.

Infection: education and counselling

> *Case study 11.6*
>
> Grace had been admitted for surgery from the waiting list. Although the operation belonged to the clean category (see Chapter 9), the incision became inflamed and purulent. Grace had developed a multiresistant staphylococcal infection.
>
> Alison, a student nurse allocated to the ward, had been looking after Grace since she was admitted. While Grace felt unwell with the infection, Alison spent a lot of time talking to her and, with the supervision of the staff nurse, she helped to dress the wound every day and to give Grace her antibiotic injections.
>
> Alison became very upset because she believed that Grace was being neglected. One day she came to work and found that a bedpan had been left in the room all night after it had been used. The doctor had not bothered to dispose of a tray of needles and syringes after performing venepuncture, and Alison noticed during the course of the morning that no domestic staff had entered Grace's room to clean it. The final straw came when a member of the domestic staff pushed the coffee trolley right past Grace's door, refusing to go anywhere near Grace in case she 'caught something'. A furious row broke out. The altercation brought Grace to the door of her room. She announced that she did not want any coffee anyway, she was tired of being bored and shut up by herself, she was tired of Alison, and she was sick of the hospital, which had caused her to feel worse by giving her an infection, rather than clearing up her health problem as had been promised.
>
> When all the fuss had subsided the ward sister called a meeting for everybody who had to work on the ward, nurses, doctors and ancillary staff. She arranged for both the domestic supervisor and the infection control nurse to be present. The outcome of the meeting was positive, because everybody who attended acknowledged that they had been feeling guilty about Grace, first because she had developed the infection, and secondly because they might spread it to other patients. Several people confessed that there were gaps in their knowledge when it came to providing effective care for people like Grace. The sister was able to point out that isolation nursing of the kind required for Grace placed heavy demands on the nurses, and that doctors and domestic staff must cooperate with the plans made for isolation. The expertise of the infection control nurse was welcome, because she was able to update everybody present on the principles necessary to control the spread of infection. She arranged with the domestic supervisor to organise some teaching sessions for her staff.
>
> The sister decided that in future more time should be spent planning the care of patients who had developed nosocomial infections, especially if they had to be isolated. The nursing process was operated on the ward, and every patient was allocated their own nurse, but it had been made apparent that some people, when they are forced to spend much of the day alone, like to see different faces, even though they may appreciate their 'own' nurse. It was important to include the nurses in these plans, especially Alison, who might otherwise have been left to feel that she had been inadequate in the care she had given Grace.

children experienced difficulty understanding the written material provided.

If teaching is to meet the needs expressed by the individual it must accord with his perspectives on health, illness and recovery, because it may otherwise seek to achieve goals that are not realistic for the particular individual concerned. Becker's (1974) health belief model, developed specifically for health education, is based on the premise that the individual's own perceptions are crucial to his motivation to follow advice.

According to Becker's theory, there are five major influences on willingness to take health-related action. The individual must believe that:

- he is susceptible to a disease (or already has it),
- the disease may have serious consequences on some aspect of his life,
- the suggested health action would help to reduce susceptibility to disease,
- the action is feasible.

There must also be some prompt or 'cue to action' that encourages the individual to change behaviour. In summary, Becker's theory envisages the goal of patient/client education to be promotion of an awareness that the possibility of illness exists, together with an appreciation of the options available, including treatment, its consequences and help to carry out a plan geared towards a change in health-related behaviour.

Case study 11.7 shows the way in which a ward sister, then a district nurse, helped Elizabeth (introduced in case study 4.1, pp. 72–73) to change outlook towards health.

Case study 11.7

Elizabeth left hospital 6 days following total abdominal hysterectomy to relieve menorrhagia. Patients undergoing this type of surgery often have a very short hospital stay and Elizabeth had been told about this before the operation. She was surprised, however, to learn that the early discharge would go ahead as planned, because a bloodstained fluid was oozing from the suture line, due to secondary bacterial growth.

Elizabeth had a number of problems that might have contributed to postoperative sepsis. The nurse responsible for her care on the ward identified these as:

- Obesity. The suture line was difficult to keep clean and dry, and dressings were difficult to apply.
- Wound drainage.
- Cigarette smoking (average 20 per day). As well as increasing the risk of postoperative chest infection and coughing, which strains the healing tissues, smoking damages the phagocytic activity of white blood cells. This may be overcome to some extent by a diet rich in vitamin C.

The development of the wound infection caused Elizabeth to lose some faith in the hospital, and she felt anxious about coping when she returned home. Her husband was extremely angry, and thought that the hospital must be 'negligent' to allow an infection to develop, and questioned standards of cleanliness on the ward.

Before Elizabeth left hospital she and her husband were seen by the ward sister, who explained that:

- Unfortunately wound infections are a common event after surgery and have to be considered as one of the risks taken by anybody who has an operation. In Elizabeth's case, the infection did not involve any but the superficial tissues, and should not take long to resolve.
- Elizabeth would not have to cope alone once she left hospital. The district nurse had been requested to dress the wound every day until the infection subsided. If Elizabeth was worried at any time she could telephone the ward.

Elizabeth's husband asked why a course of antibiotics had not been prescribed. It was explained that when infection is of such a superficial nature antibiotics are not normally very helpful in destroying it, but that the district nurse would use a local antiseptic to clean the wound.

When Elizabeth was admitted to hospital the nurse allocated to her care obtained information about her social circumstance. The sister knew that Elizabeth's mother planned to stay for the first 2 weeks that Elizabeth was home and that her teenage daughters would help with housework. The sister gave Elizabeth a leaflet of advice about aftercare following hysterectomy and discussed the main points that it contained. In addition, she provided Elizabeth with more specific information, including her husband in the discussion. The main points were:

- Emphasis was placed on keeping the wound site as clean as possible. A daily bath or shower was recommended, to be taken before the district nurse's visit. The bath should be washed and dried before and after use.
- The value of a diet rich in protein, vitamins and calories to promote healing in tissues damaged by infection was explained. Some women complain that inactivity and boredom during postoperative convalescence contribute to weight gain (there is no hormonal explanation for this) and for Elizabeth, already overweight, this was a positive health risk. Once the wound had healed, a reducing diet might be considered.
- Smoking greatly increases the chances of developing many serious diseases of the heart, lungs and blood vessels. Risk increases rapidly during middle age for women, generally in relation to the time when they experience the menopause. Elizabeth would improve her chances of remaining fit if she could at least reduce the number of cigarettes that she smoked. A selection of pamphlets about the effect of smoking and health was available on the ward and Elizabeth was given some to read at leisure.

The district nurse visited Elizabeth at home next day. Patients tend to behave differently in the security of their own homes compared to hospital, and the district nurse is a guest.

Elizabeth was by herself; her husband had left for work and her mother was shopping. The nurse had already received information from the ward concerning Elizabeth's condition and she now made the following observations:

- Elizabeth's social circumstances were materially good. She lived in a large, detached house, equipped with labour saving devices (washing machine, home freezer) that would remove many of the problems of convalescence.
- The wound was oozing a small quantity of dark, red, offensive fluid; although the edges of the wound did not gape, they looked inflamed.
- Elizabeth herself seemed tense and was clearly

anxious about something, but seemed pleased to see the nurse.

The wound was cleansed with a solution of Savlon and redressed with a non-adherent dressing, ensuring that the tissues were handled gently to avoid further, unnecessary trauma. The nurse knew that the infection had been caused by Gram-negative bacilli, which are generally very resistant to antibiotics, and that it was superficial, having been acquired on the ward. Hygiene would therefore be important in helping to resolve it.

While the wound was being dressed, Elizabeth confessed that she was disappointed in her recovery. She hoped very much that she would not have to delay returning to work, as she became easily bored alone at home. Her daughters seemed to need her less as they grew up and her husband frequently worked overtime.

Over the next few days the wound discharge became serous and scanty, until only a dry dressing was needed to protect Elizabeth's clothes. Performing the dressing provided the nurse with a good opportunity to discuss recovery with Elizabeth and the possible longer-term effects of the operation. It emerged that Elizabeth was concerned about weight gain and very worried indeed about the effects of smoking. Many of her friends who had previously smoked had now given up, but the final trigger had been Elizabeth's own rather indifferent recovery, which the hospital staff had related to her behaviour.

The nurse spent some time encouraging Elizabeth to explore her feelings. She pointed out that much could be done to prevent further problems because their possible existence had already been identified. Elizabeth's problems were clearly divided into long and short term:

- Resolving the infection and healing the wound, to pave the way for recovery from hysterectomy.
- Establishing new patterns of health behaviour, to include:
  (1) weight reduction,
  (2) reduction in the number of cigarettes smoked.

The district nurse was attached to a general practitioner surgery, where several health visitors and practice nurses were employed. She was able to provide Elizabeth with information about the local Weight Watchers group and a support group for people wishing to change their smoking behaviour, run by one of the practice nurses. Elizabeth attended these sessions, and after some time persuaded her husband, also a smoker, to accompany her.

CONCLUSIONS

The point of this chapter has been to discuss the views of infection held by society, and to show how nurses can help their patients by counselling and teaching. Many of the worries that infectious people have do not differ from those of the majority of patients, except that they may be a source of 'danger' to others. Although this risk is often exaggerated, it may nevertheless remain a source of distress, damaging effective communication and impairing return to everyday life. In recent years, nurses, like other members of the public, have been forced to accept that infection is not a thing of the past. The persistence, and in some cases the discovery, of entirely new infectious conditions have provided some of the greatest challenges to nurses. Communication and effective interpersonal relations are central to the care of these people, and placing this chapter at the end of the book instead of at the beginning is intended to emphasise the importance of these skills, rather than suggesting that their role is secondary. Effective communication implies that nurses have information to give, and when caring for people who have infection, or are at risk of developing it, the principles underlying physical care are those of microbiology, and without this the care provided will degenerate into a series of unintelligible rules.

References

Addy, M. et al. (1977). Effectiveness of methods of teaching dental health to 9–10 year olds. *Dental and Oral Epidemiology*, 5: 191–195.

Becker, M. H. (1974). *The Health Belief Model and Sick Role Behaviour. Health Education Monograph*, 2: 409–419.

Bennett, S. M. (1983). The psychological effects of barrier nursing in isolation. *Australian Nurses Journal*, 12 (19): 36–44.

Bruce-Quay, M. (1981). The Calderdale Immunisation Project. *Health Visitor*, 541 (9): 359–362.

Genvert, G. (1979). Isolation information booklet. Stimulates dialogue, allays fears. *Hospitals*, 1–2: 72–75.

Gould, D. J. (1984). Time to explain. *Nursing Mirror*, 158 (8): 20–23.

Gould, D. J. (1985). Isolation procedures in one health district. *Nursing Times Occasional Paper*, **81** (7): 47–50.

Gould, D. J., Wilson-Barnett, J. (1985). A comparison of recovery following hysterectomy and major cardiac surgery. *Journal of Advanced Nursing*, **10**: 315–323.

Lazarus, R. S., Averill, J. R. (1972). Emotion and cognition: with special reference to anxiety. In *Anxiety, Current Trends in Theory and Research*, Speilberger, C. D. (ed.). New York, Academic Press.

Ley, P. (1977). Psychological studies of doctor–patient communication. In *Contributions to Medical Psychology*, Volume 1, Rachman, S. (ed.). Pergamon Press, Oxford.

Redman, B. K. (1981). *The Process of Patient Teaching in Nursing*. C. V. Mosby, St Louis.

Royal College of Nursing (1978). *Counselling in Nursing*. Royal College of London, London.

Stewart, W. (1983). *Counselling in Nursing. A Problem-solving Approach*. Lippincott Nursing Series. Harper and Row, Cambridge.

Taylor, L. (1982). Isolation and barrier nursing. *Nursing*, **2nd series**: 214–215.

Turton, P., Wilson-Barnett, J. (1981). Two aspects of nursing – hospital and community. In *Going Home*, Simpson, J. E. P., Levitt, R. (eds). Churchill Livingstone, London and Edinburgh, pp. 265–280.

Webb, C. (1983). Teaching for recovery from surgery. In *Patient Teaching*, Wilson-Barnett, J. (ed.). Churchill Livingstone, London and Edinburgh, pp. 34–55.

Webb, C. (1986). *Sexuality, Nursing and Health*. H. M. and M. Publishers, Beaconsfield, Bucks.

Wilson-Barnett, J. (1979). *Stress in Hospital*. Churchill Livingstone, Edinburgh and London.

Wilson-Barnett, J. (1980). Prevention and alleviation of stress in patients. *Nursing*, **1st series**: 432–436.

Further Reading

Bille, D. A. (1981). *Practical Approaches to Patient Teaching*. Little, Brown and Co., Boston.

Cohen, S. A. (1981). Patient education: a review of the literature. *Journal of Advanced Nursing*, **6**: 11–18.

Green L. W. (1978). Evaluation and measurement: some dilemmas for health education. *Nursing Digest*, **6**: 69–76.

Narrow, B. W. (1979). *Patient Teaching and Nursing Practice*. Wiley, New York.

Redman, B. K. (1981). *Issues and Concepts in Patient Education*. Appleton-Century-Crofts, New York.

Winslow, E. H. (1976). The role of the nurse in patient education. *Nursing Clinics of North America*, **11**: 213–222.

Wilson-Barnett, J. (ed.) (1983). *Patient Teaching*. Churchill Livingstone, London.

Appendix

A Guide to the Common Bacteria of Medical Significance

Throughout this book emphasis has been placed on the application of basic microbiological principles to nursing care. The properties of bacteria and other microorganisms were outlined in Chapter 1, and throughout this chapter and those that followed, the activities of particular bacteria have been illustrated. Details of the taxonomies and properties of bacteria can be found in any standard medical or microbiology textbook, but this short appendix has been included as a quick reference to readers who are interested in the classification of the most commonly occurring bacteria. This kind of information is helpful to anybody who has to read and interpret reports from the microbiology laboratory. Each group of bacteria will be described under the following headings:

- name
- morphology
- occurrence
- pathogenicity
- method of spread

Streptococcus

- *Morphology* – Gram positive. Oval cocci found in pairs or chains. Often surrounded by capsules.

- *Occurrence* – ubiquitous. Some members of this large group inhabit the human mucous membranes, including mouth, lower intestine and upper respiratory tract. Others live in food, especially dairy products.

- *Pathogenicity* – depends on ability to destroy red blood cells. Haemolytic streptococci grown on solid culture media incorporating blood are surrounded by a clear zone where the red blood cells have been destroyed. Non-haemolytic streptococci do not share this property, and are harmless.

Haemolytic streptococci are categorised according to the antigens on their cell surfaces, which further help to confer virulence upon them. Members of group A are the most virulent, causing tonsillitis, scarlet fever, acute nephritis, acute rheumatic fever, erysipelas, cellulitis and wound infections.

Streptococcus pneumoniae may cause primary pneumonia, peritonitis and meningitis.

Streptococcus viridans can set up subacute bacterial endocarditis.

- *Method of spread* – airborne, contact (hands, fomites), endogenous.

Staphylococcus

- *Morphology* – Gram-positive clusters of cocci.

- *Occurrence* – skin, mucous membranes, air, soil.

- *Pathogenicity* – depends on ability to synthesise the enzyme coagulase. Coagulase negative species like *Staphylococcus epidermidis* and *Staph. citreus* are opportunistic. Coagulase positive *Staphylococcus aureus* can live as a commensal, but is notorious for its ability to set up infections.

- *Method of spread* – air, dust, contact, endogenous.

Corynebacterium

- *Morphology* – Gram-positive rods which show characteristic uneven staining patterns.

- *Occurrence* – skin and mucous membranes, especially the respiratory tract.

- *Pathogenicity* – most members of this group are harmless: *C. hofmannii* and *C. xerosis* are both skin commensals. *C. diphtheriae* causes diphtheria.

- *Method of spread* – human carriers.

Bacillus

- *Morphology* – Gram-positive large rods and spores which form chains.
- *Occurrence* – air, soil, water, dust, wool, hair, animal carcasses.
- *Pathogenicity* – *B. subtilis* is usually harmless. *B. cereus* grows profusely in partly cooked rice and may cause food poisoning. *B. anthracis* is the causative agent of anthrax, usually entering the victim as inhaled or swallowed spores. All members of this group are aerobic, and their spores are unusually resistant to heat and other physical and chemical agents.

Clostridium

- *Morphology* – Gram-positive rods which form spores characteristically wider than the vegetative cells.
- *Occurrence* – soil, especially contaminated with animal faeces.
- *Pathogenicity* – many species are harmless (*Clostridium sporogenes*). All are anaerobic, so that even pathogenic species may not necessarily cause disease unless they are carried deep into the tissues and encounter conditions suitable for toxin production. Pathogenic species include *Cl. tetani*, *Cl. welchii* (*perfringens*), *Cl. botulinum*.
- *Method of spread* – puncture wounds (*Cl. tetani*), food (*Cl. welchii*, *Cl. botulinum*).

Neisseria

- *Morphology* – Gram-negative, kidney-shaped diplococci which often grow inside neutrophils.
- *Occurrence* – mucous membranes, especially conjunctivae, respiratory and genitourinary tracts.
- *Pathogenicity* – several members of the group are harmless commensals, usually inhabiting the respiratory tract (*N. catarrhalis*, *N. pharyngeus*). *N. gonorrhoeae* causes gonorrhoea and neonatal ophthalmic disease. *N. meningitidis* can cause meningococcal meningitis.
- *Method of spread* – *N. gonorrhoeae* – sexual transmission; *N. meningitidis* – entry through mucous membrane of respiratory tract.

Haemophilus

- *Morphology* – very small Gram-negative rods which vary greatly in length.
- *Occurrence* – mucous membranes of man and animals.
- *Pathogenicity* – *H. ducreyi* causes the sexually transmitted disease chancre (soft sore). *H. influenzae* does *not* cause influenza as once thought, but is often found in people who have chronic bronchitis, and can enter the central nervous system to cause meningitis. *Bordetella pertussis* causes whooping cough.
- *Method of spread* – mainly by droplets.

Brucella

- *Morphology* – very small Gram-negative rods.
- *Occurrence* – animals, especially cattle. May enter milk.
- *Pathogenicity* – cause of undulent fever when ingested in unpasteurised milk.
- *Method of spread* – ingestion of unpasteurised milk.

Yersinia

- *Morphology* – small Gram-negative rods.
- *Occurrence* – rat fleas.
- *Pathogenicity* – *Y. pestis* causes plague.
- *Method of spread* – through punctures in skin, via lymphatics to blood. May also be inhaled.

Legionella

- *Morphology* – poorly staining rods, difficult to visualise, does not respond well to Gram's stain.

- *Occurrence* – stagnant water, e.g. water cooling towers and humidifiers, soil.
- *Pathogenicity* – Legionella pneumophila causes a severe, sometimes life-threatening pneumonia, most often, though not invariably, affecting middle-aged men.
- *Method of spread* – in water droplets disseminated through the air.

Intestinal Gram-negative rods:
Escherichia, Klebsiella

- *Pathogenicity* – opportunists. Scourge in hospital. *E. coli* causes urinary tract infections, may be found in wounds, and can give rise to meningitis. Some types are associated with neonatal gastroenteritis. *Klebsiella* can cause urinary, wound and respiratory infections.
- *Method of spread* – contact, autogenous.

Salmonella

- *Morphology* – small, motile Gram-negative rods, distinguishable from *E. coli* only by biochemical and serological tests.
- *Occurrence* – contaminated food and water.
- *Pathogenicity* – *Salmonella typhi* causes typhoid, *S. paratyphi* causes paratyphoid fever. All other species in this group give rise to food poisoning.
- *Method of spread* – human carriers, contaminated food and water.

Shigella

- *Morphology* – Gram-negative rod, distinguishable from *E. coli* and salmonella because it is not motile.
- *Occurrence* – intestinal tract of man and primates.
- *Pathogenicity* – *Sh. dysenteriae* causes bacillary dysentery.
- *Method of spread* – human carriers.

Proteus and Pseudomonas

- *Morphology* – Gram-negative rods.
- *Occurrence* – soil, water excreta of man and animals.
- *Pathogenicity* – infects urine, burns, wounds, respiratory tract, tracheostomies. Scourge in hospitals.

Vibrio

- *Morphology* – motile organism, shaped like a comma. Gram-negative.
- *Pathogenicity* – *V. cholera*, pathogenic only to man, is responsible for cholera. *V. parahaemolyticus* gives rise to food poisoning, usually associated with eating contaminated shellfish. It is especially common in parts of the world like Japan, where much food is eaten raw.

Campylobacter

- *Morphology* – very similar to vibrio.
- *Occurrence* – contaminated food and water.
- *Pathogenicity* – causes food poisoning associated with colic and blood-stained diarrhoea.

Mycobacterium

- *Morphology* – small, slender rods which do not take up microscope stains readily due to their rough, waxy coverings. Described as acid fast because of the technique necessary to visualise them. Grow very slowly on culture media, so that diagnosis can take weeks (average 6–8).
- *Pathogenicity* – *M. tuberculosis* causes tuberculosis of two types: human (pulmonary) TB and bovine TB. *M. lepra* causes leprosy, and is pathogenic only to man.

Spirochaetes:
Leptospira, Treponema

- *Morphology* – very small, delicate rods, best seen under dark ground illumination, when they can be identified by their characteristic corkscrew and flexing movements.

- *Occurrence* – non-pathogenic spirochaetes are found in the mouth, especially the gums, and on the genitalia.
- *Pathogenicity* – species of *Leptospira* are carried by rats and enter via contamination of damaged skin, to cause infectious jaundice, sometimes known as Weil's disease. *Treponema pallidum* causes syphilis and *Treponema pertenue* the less damaging infection yaws, which in tropical countries is spread by direct contact with skin lesions as well as sexually.

Index

abscess formation sites, 113
absorption, 3
acinetobacter, 27
acquired immune deficiency syndrome (AIDS), 14, 20, 24, 35
  counselling, 193
  historically, 45
  patient stress, 107
  transmission of, 30, 46
    via instruments, 71, 89
agammaglobulinaemia, 66
age, as infection factor, 65, 149
airborne infections, 45
amoebic dysentery, 20
amphotericin B, 76
anabolism, 3
anaesthetic equipment, cleaning, 148
angiogenesis, 139, 140
anthrax, 4
  isolation procedures, 95
antibacterial drugs, 44, 45, 71, 74
antibiotic
  resistance, 12, 63, 68
    case history, 14
    in urinary tract infection, 133
  sensitivity, 178
antibiotics, 1, 44, 45, 74, 75
  prophylactic, 147
  side-effects of, 68
antibodies, 117, 118, 121
anticancer drugs, 68
antifungal agents, 19, 71, 74, 76
antigens, 117, 118, 123
antimicrobial drugs, 74, 75
  synthetic, 75
antituberculous drugs, 75, 76
antiviral agents, 71, 74, 76
artificial immunity, 34, 64, 65
ascaris worms, 20
asepsis, principles of, 36, 69
aseptic dressing technique, 49, 155, 159
aspergillus fungus, 18
autoantibodies, 123
autoimmune disease, 123

baby infection risks, 65, 66
  from mechanical ventilation, 70
Bacille Calmette Guérin (BCG) vaccination, 91
bacilli, 5
Bacillus
  anthracis, 4
  cereus, 29
  properties of, 200
bacteraemia, 69, 70
bacteria, 2
  aerobic, 36
  parasitic, 9
  virulent, 8, 9
bacterial
  cell structure, 6
  classification, 4–8
  colony cultures, 177, 178
  contamination, 51, 52
  growth requirements, 8–16
  invasion, 22, 23, 24
    in intravenous therapy, 69
  morphology, 5, 7
  physiology, 5, 6
  reproduction, 11–14
bacteriostatic drugs, 74, 75
B cell lymphocytes, 119, 120, 122, 123
binary fission, 11
bladder irrigation, 129, 130
blood
  and blood product disposal, 89
  specimen collection, 173
bone marrow transplantation, 68
  isolation procedure, 95
Boore's study, 56, 57
botulism, 23
brucella, properties of, 200
bubonic plague, 39
Burkitt's lymphoma, 16

campylobacter bacteria, 5
cancer, and viruses, 16, 17
Candida albicans fungus, 18, 29, 68
cannula insertion, 68, 69
catabolic reaction, 2
catheter
  care guidelines, 132
  case study, 133–135

choice, 130, 131
catheterisation, 68, 78
   indwelling, 125–135
   reasons for, 126
cellular defence mechanisms, 119, 142
cephalosporin drugs, 74
cervical
   carcinoma, 71
   swab specimen collection, 173, 174
Chadwick, E., 40
chemical sterilisation, 88
chemotherapy effects, 67, 68
chest infections, 45, 65
chlamydiae, 4, 20
cholera, 31
   epidemic, 37, 38, 40
   immunisation, 92
   isolation aims, 95
cleaning
   principles, 80–83
   procedures, 83–90
     in isolation unit, 102
Clostridium
   botulinum, 23, 30
   properties of, 200
   tetani, 23
   welchii, 4, 27
cocci, 4, 5
cockroaches, 31
collagen synthesis, 140
communication in nursing, 50, 185–197
community health policies, 63, 91, 92
complement
   fixation tests, 180
   system, the, 116, 117
congenital infection, 24
conjugation of bacteria, 12, 13
contamination risk situation, 80
corynebacterium, properties of, 199, 200
counselling of patients, 186–197
cross-infection, 27
   with food poisoning, 47
Cruse and Foord Study (wounds), 144, 145, 147
cryptococcus fungus, 18

decontamination procedures, 78, 79, 80, 97
dehydrated patient, 67
delirium, 114
DHSS waste disposal coding, 89
diabetes mellitus, 67, 133
diabetic patient risks, 64, 67
dialysis fluid contamination, 71
Dick test (scarlet fever), 180

diffusion, 3, 4
diphtheria, 27, 37, 42, 43
   historically, 41, 42
   vaccination, 91
diplococci, 4, 5
disease
   endemic, 33
   epidemics, 33, 34
disinfectant types, 84–85
disinfection procedures, 83–87
disposal procedures, 78, 79, 88, 89
   of 'sharps', 88, 89
district nurse's role, 196, 197
DNA, 6, 116
   bacterial, 7
dressing technique, aseptic, 49, 155, 159
drug addiction dangers, 64
drug therapy, antibacterial, 44, 45, 68
dysentery (shigella), 23, 31
   amoebic, 20
   isolation aims, 95

education
   in the community, 194
   of patient, 186–197
Ehrlich, P., 44
elderly patient care, 65, 66, 81
   and stress, 107
endemic disease, 33
endocarditis, 74
endogenous infection, 10, 11
endoscopy, 71
endotoxins, 23
entamoeba histolytica, 20
enteral feeding, 70
enteric isolation categories, 95
environmental
   cleaning in hospitals, 81
   health policies, 64
enzyme secretion, by bacteria, 22, 23
epidemics, 33, 34
   historically, 38–41
epidemiological
   curves, 33, 34
   research studies, 50, 51, 59–61
epidemiology, 33, 38
epithelial migration, 140
Epstein–Barr (EB) virus, 16, 17
Escherichia coli, 2, 5, 70
   bacterial properties of, 201
evaluative research, 58, 59
excreta, infected, 101
excretion, 4

exogenous infection, 10, 11
exotoxins, 23
eye infection defences, 26

feeding
  enteral, 70
  intravenous, 69
fever (pyrexia), 66
fimbriae, 7, 8
flatworms, 20, 21
flora, of skin, 26, 27, 69
Florey, H., 44
fluid balance monitoring, 66, 67
food
  hygiene, 29, 30, 31, 45, 63, 70
  poisoning, 5, 23, 27, 29, 47
    case studies, 28, 47
    epidemics, 34, 65
    from enteral feeding, 70
    patient care, 98, 99
fungal disease (mycosis), 18
fungi, 9, 10
  structure of, 17, 18

gas gangrene bacillus, 4
gastrointestinal system defences, 25
genetic
  engineering, and interferons, 116
  factors, and infection, 66
  information, in cells, 6
genitourinary system defences, 26
Giardia lamblia infection, 19, 20
glandular fever, 95
gonorrhoea, 4, 23, 24, 31
  treatment of, 74
Gram-negative
  bacilli, 7, 10, 27
    contamination, 71
  infections, 70, 74
Gram-positive bacilli, 7, 10, 27
Gram's stain, 7
griseofulvin antifungal agent, 76

Haemophilus
  influenzae, 22
    properties of, 200
hand-washing techniques, 63, 79
  with isolated patient, 99
hay fever, 123
healing process (wounds), 138–144
  illustrated, 143
health
  education in community, 194, 195

visitor's role, 64, 65, 194
heat
  disinfection, 86, 87
  sterilisation, 88
helminths (worms), 4, 20, 21
hemiplegic patient, 27
hepatitis B virus, 24, 46
  case history, 108, 187
  patient care plan, 97
  and stress, 107, 108
  theatre precautions with, 90
  transmission, 30, 64
Herpes simplex virus, 16
homeostasis, 2, 72
  and stress, 105
hospital
  cleaning, 80–90
  infection control policies, 64, 78, 79
    key factors, 80
hospital-acquired infection, 10
  patient risk factors, 63
human immunodeficiency virus (HIV), 14, 45
  patient stress, 107
  waste disposal from, 89
humidifier disinfection, 70
humoral defence mechanisms, 119, 142
hygiene
  education, 64
  in hospitals, 80–90
hysterectomy case study, 72, 73

immigrant family risks, 65
immobility dangers, 67
immune system, 123
  maturity, 65
immunisation
  artificial, 34, 41, 65
  community health programme, 91, 92
  historically, 41–44
  physiological basis of, 120–123
immunity, 34, 38
  artificial, 64, 65
  influencing factors, 64–68
  innate, 65
  natural, 64, 65
  to smallpox, 41
immunofluorescence techniques, 181
immunoglobulins, 119
incineration of waste, 89, 90
  infected, 100
incubation
  of culture media, 176, 177
  of infections, 34

infected linen precautions, 101
infection
    congenital, 24
    control team, 13, 70, 161, 163–165
    development, 4–21
    historically, 35–45
    hospital-acquired, 10, 63
    nosocomial, 1, 4, 68
    prevention, 63, 96–103
    response, physiological, 109–124
    spread, 28–31, 33, 34
    wound, 24, 49, 144–151
infectious patient nursing, 93–103
    after death, 102
    isolation categories, 95
inflammation, 68, 109–113
    from cannula insertion, 69, 73
inflammation response (wounds), 138, 147
influenza vaccination, 65, 91
injection, intravenous, 68
innate
    immune deficiency diseases, 66
    immunity, 65
inoculation, 24
insect bites, 31
instrument sterilisation, 71, 87, 88
interferons, 116
interview data (research), 53, 54
intravenous therapy, 68, 69, 70, 74
isolated patient stress, 107
isolation
    categories, 95
    clothing, 99, 100
    facilities, 93–99
    techniques, 2, 55, 99–103

Kaposi's sarcoma, 46
Keddi, F., 35
Klebs and Loeffler research, 37
klebsiella, 5
    bacterial properties of, 201
Koch's postulates, 37

Lassa fever, 31
    isolation precautions, 95
legionella, properties of, 201
leprosy, 35
leptospira, 5
leukaemia, 68
    isolation aims, 95
linen, infected, 101
living organisms, 2–4
'lockjaw', 23

lymph node structure, 121
lymphocytes, 119, 121, 123

macrolides antibiotics, 75
macrophages, wandering, 111
malaria, 19, 20, 24, 31
malnutrition, 66, 67
Marburg fever, 95
measles immunisation, 34, 44, 91
mechanical ventilation, 70
Medical Officer of Environmental Health (MOEH), 167
Medical Research Council, 167
meningitis, 1
    meningococcal, 22
    treatment of, 74
    viral, isolation of, 95
mesangial cells, 26
metabolism, 2
microbiology
    diagnostic, 44
    request forms, 175
    test result interpretation, 181, 182
        case study, 183
microorganisms, and infection, 4–31
monocytes, 110
morphology, of bacteria, 4, 5
mouth care, 67
    postoperative, 73
    with mechanical ventilation, 70
mycobacterium, bacterial properties of, 201
mycoplasmas, 4, 20
mycoses (fungal disease), 18

nasogastric tubes, 70
National Childhood Encephalopathy Study, 43, 60, 61
National Prevalence Study, The, 60, 145
natural immunity, 64, 65
needle
    disposal, 88, 89
    injection risks, 64
Neisseria
    meningitidis, 22, 23
    properties of, 200
nerve cells, 5
Nightingale, F., 39, 40
non-specific urethritis (NSU), 20
normal flora, of body, 26, 27, 69
nose swab specimen collection, 173
nosocomial infection, 1, 4, 68
    isolation, 93–103
    spread, 71
notifiable diseases, listed, 167
nursing research processes, 49, 50

nutrition, of patient, 66, 67, 70
    and tissue infection, 149, 150
nutritional supplements, 70
nystatin antifungal agent, 76

obesity, 67
    postoperative effects of, 72
Occupational Health Department, 65
ophthalmia neonatorum, 24
osmosis, 3, 4

pandemic, 33
Pasteur, L., 35–37
pathogens, 9
patient care
    counselling, 186–197
    individual, 63, 64, 81
    research, 50–61
penicillin(s), 44, 45, 74
    resistance, 30
peptides, 75
peripheral vascular disease, 67
pertussis (whooping cough), 43, 44
pH values, and bacteria, 9
phage typing, 181
phagocytosis, 22
Pharaoh's ants, 31
physiotherapy preventative care, 66
Pneumocystis carinii infection, 20
polio
    vaccination, 91
    virus, 23
polymorphs, 109, 110, 112
pressure sore, 67
    treatment, 48
primary closure, of wounds, 142, 143
    delayed, 142
prokaryotic cells, 6
prophylactic antibiotics, 147
protective
    clothing, for isolation nursing, 99, 100
    isolation, 103
        categories, 95
protein
    deficiency, 66, 67
    synthesis, 7
proteus, 5
    bacterial properties of, 201
    infections, 74
protozoa, 19
pseudomonas, 5
    infections, 74
psittacosis, 20

Public Health Laboratory Service (PHLS), 166
pyrexia (fever), 66, 113–115

questionnaire construction (research), 52, 53

rabies, 40
    immunisation, 92
    isolation procedures, 95
radiation sterilisation, 88
radiotherapy effects, 67, 68
research
    clinical, 35–45
    nursing, 49, 50–61
respiration, 4
respiratory
    infections, from antibiotic therapy, 68
    isolation categories, 95
    system defences, 25, 26
rheumatoid arthritis, 123
rickettsiae, 4, 20
RNA, 14, 116
roundworms, 20
rubella vaccination, 91

'safe' environment, 63–92
salmonella, 5, 7, 23, 27, 30, 47, 71
    bacterial properties of, 102
    isolation aims, 95, 97
    patient care, 98
Schick test (diphtheria), 42, 180
secondary intention healing, 143
sepsis
    from sutures, 147, 148
    risks, 69, 71
    treatment in bones and joints, 75
serology, 179, 180
sexually transmitted infection, 30, 31, 45
    isolation aims, 95
'sharps' disposal procedures, 88, 89
shaving, and wound infection, 146
sheepskin contamination, 51, 81
shigella (dysentery), 23, 31
    bacterial properties of, 201
    isolation aims, 95
shingles patient care, 97
skin
    flora, 26, 27, 69
    infection defences, 24
smallpox, 41
Snow, Dr. J., 37, 38, 40
specimen
    collection, by type, 172–174
    handling, 174

laboratory procedures, 175–184
spirochaetes bacteria, 5, 201, 202
sputum specimen collection, 172
staphylococci, 4, 5
Staphylococcus
   aureus, 10, 23, 27
     bacterial properties of, 199
     on contaminated sheepskin, 51
   epidermidis, 10, 23, 27
     infection of cerebrospinal fluid shunts, 71
sterilisation
   of instruments, 71
   procedures, 87–88
steroid drugs, 68
stool specimen collection, 172
streptococcal infection, 5
Streptococcus
   bacterial properties of, 199
   pneumoniae, 22
stress
   and infection, 104–108
   effects, 63, 68, 71
   from hospitalisation, 186, 187
     case study, 188
strict isolation categories, 95
study compilation (research), 55–59
sulphonamides, 44, 75
surgical
   incision risks, 68, 147
   intervention (wounds), 142
syphilis, 5, 24, 31, 202
   congenital, 24, 31
   treatment of, 74
syringe disposal, 88, 89

tapeworms, 20, 21
T cell lymphocytes, 119, 120, 122, 123
temperature regulation, 114
   case study, 115
testing, of new products (research), 49, 56
tetanus vaccination, 91
tetracycline antibiotics, 74, 75
theatre precautions
   with hepatitis B carrier, 90
   with wounds, 145
therapy
   antibiotic, 147
   drug, 44, 45, 68
   intravenous, 68, 69, 70
   x-ray, deep, 68
thermometer storage, 81
third world infection risks, 66
threadworms, 20

throat swab specimen collection, 173
thrombophlebitis, 74
ticks, 20
tissue repair, 138–141, 147
toxaemia, 23
toxin production, 23
Toxoplasma gondi, 20
Treponema pallidum, 5, 24
Trichomonas vaginalis, 19, 24
Trexler isolator, 94
tuberculosis, pulmonary, 22
   patient care plan, 96
tumour formation, 16, 17
typhus, 31
   immunisation, 92

upper respiratory tract infection, 45
urinary
   catheterisation, 68, 78
     indwelling, 125–135
     reasons for, 126
   stasis, 67
   tract infection, 5, 27, 75, 127, 129, 183
     hospital-acquired, 127
     in dehydrated patient, 67
     occurrence research, 59, 60
     patient care, 99, 127–135
     prevention, 131
urine
   monitoring (microbiological), 131
   specimen collection, 172
   tests, 182, 183

vaccination, 1, 43, 44
Vaccine Damaged Children, Assoc. of Parents for, 43
vaginal
   swab specimen collection, 173
   thrush, 18
van Leeuwenhoek, A., 37
varicose ulcers, 67
vascular insufficiency, 67
vasodilatation, 111
vector transmission of infection, 31
ventilation, mechanical, 70
vibrio, bacterial properties of, 5, 201
viral immunity, 34
virulence, in bacteria, 8, 22
virus, 4
   activity, 16
   and cancer, 16, 17
   multiplication, 15
   structure, 14

waste disposal procedures, 88, 89, 90
   DHSS colour coding for, 89
   infected, 100
water-borne infections, 31, 40, 45
Weil's disease, 5, 202
white blood cell(s)
   and inflammation, 109
   count depression, 68, 75
   defences, 26
whooping cough (pertussis)
   immunisation, 43, 44
   isolation aims, 95
World Health Organisation, 45
   vaccination recommendations, 92

worms, parasitic, 4, 20, 21
wound
   classification, 141, 144
   drainage, 148
   dressing, 151–159
      preparations, 156, 157, 158
   healing, 138–141, 151–154
      historically, 137–138
   infection, 24, 49, 144–151
   research survey, 60
   swab specimen collection, 172

x-ray therapy, deep, 68

GOT YOUR FACTS RIGHT...?

Here are two books from Heinemann Nursing which give you all the basic clinical information you need. And show you how to apply your facts and give good nursing care.

ORTHOPAEDIC NURSING
Cynthia Smith
Course Teacher at the Portsmouth District School of Nursing.
With over 150 clinical line illustrations, this textbook is clear, comprehensive and a pleasure to use.
Using a problem-solving approach, it describes the nursing care of the orthopaedic and trauma patient. It covers the full range of conditions which you will see, particularly as a specialist in orthopaedic areas.
It also outlines management plans which give sound advice on how to deal with the more complex aspects of patient care — psychological well-being, comfort, education and rehabilitation.
246 x 189mm, limp, 336 pages, illus   433 30490 1

SURGICAL NURSING
Joan Bickerton, Director of Nurse Education, Winchester and Basingstoke School of Nursing.
"an excellent basis for detailed study and a useful reference"   Nursing Times

This is a highly illustrated book which can be used as a core text by student nurses and includes sufficient detail to be useful to qualified nurses too. Section I examines general aspects of surgery and surgical nursing: pain, infection, preoperative and postoperative care, haemodynamics, nutrition and others. Section II follows the structures of the body — from the gastrointestinal tract to the structures of the head — and describes operations and procedures and related nursing care.
246 x 189mm, limp, 352 pages, illus   433 02832 7

NEW NURSING CATALOGUE
For details of these books and our full range of titles please send for our complete catalogue:

Heinemann Nursing
FREEPOST EM17, 22 Bedford Square, LONDON, WC1B 3BR